T0327745

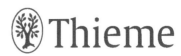

Sagittal Balance of the Spine

From Normal to Pathology: A Key for Treatment Strategy

Pierre Roussouly, MD
Senior Surgeon
Spinal Surgery Unit
Croix Rouge Française-CMCR des Massues
Lyon, France

João Luiz Pinheiro-Franco, MD, AFS
Neurosurgeon and Spine Surgeon
Samaritano Hospital of São Paulo
São Paulo, Brazil

Hubert Labelle, MD
Professor of Surgery
Division of Orthopedic Surgery
University of Montreal
Montréal, Québec, Canada

Martin Gehrchen, MD, PhD
Associate Professor and Head of Spine Surgery
Spine Unit
Department of Orthopaedic Surgery
Rigshospitalet and University of Copenhagen
Copenhagen, Denmark

259 illustrations

Thieme
New York • Stuttgart • Delhi • Rio de Janeiro

Executive Editor: Timothy J. Hiscock
Managing Editor: Sarah Landis
Director, Editorial Services: Mary Jo Casey
Production Editors: Naamah Schwartz and Torsten Scheihagen
International Production Director: Andreas Schabert
Editorial Director: Sue Hodgson
International Marketing Director: Fiona Henderson
International Sales Director: Louisa Turrell
Director of Institutional Sales: Adam Bernacki
Senior Vice President and Chief Operating Officer: Sarah Vanderbilt
President: Brian D. Scanlan

Library of Congress Cataloging-in-Publication Data

Names: Roussouly, Pierre, editor. | Pinheiro-Franco, João Luiz, editor. | Labelle, Hubert, editor. | Gehrchen, Martin, editor.
Title: Sagittal balance of the spine : from normal to pathology : a key for treatment strategy / [edited by] Pierre Roussouly, João Luiz Pinheiro-Franco, Hubert Labelle, Martin Gehrchen.
Description: New York : Thieme, [2019] | Includes bibliographical references.
Identifiers: LCCN 2019010292| ISBN 9781626237322 (hardback) | ISBN 9781626237339 (e-book)
Subjects: | MESH: Spinal Curvatures–physiopathology | Spinal Curvatures–surgery | Spine–surgery | Spine–physiology | Postural Balance–physiology | Spondylolisthesis
Classification: LCC RD768 | NLM WE 735 | DDC 617.4/71–dc23 LC record available at https://lccn.loc.gov/2019010292

© 2019 by Thieme Medical Publishers, Inc.

Thieme Publishers New York
333 Seventh Avenue, New York, NY 10001 USA
+1 800 782 3488, customerservice@thieme.com

Thieme Publishers Stuttgart
Rüdigerstrasse 14, 70469 Stuttgart, Germany
+49 [0]711 8931 421, customerservice@thieme.de

Thieme Publishers Delhi
A-12, Second Floor, Sector-2, Noida-201301
Uttar Pradesh, India
+91 120 45 566 00, customerservice@thieme.in

Thieme Publishers Rio de Janeiro, Thieme Publicações Ltda.
Edifício Rodolpho de Paoli, 25º andar
Av. Nilo Peçanha, 50 – Sala 2508
Rio de Janeiro 20020-906 Brasil
+55 21 3172-2297 / +55 21 3172-1896
www.thiemerevinter.com.br

Cover design: Thieme Publishing Group
Typesetting by DiTech Process Solutions

Printed in Germany by CPI books, Leck

5 4 3 2 1

ISBN 978-1-62623-732-2

Also available as an e-book:
eISBN 978-1-62623-733-9

Important note: Medicine is an ever-changing science undergoing continual development. Research and clinical experience are continually expanding our knowledge, in particular our knowledge of proper treatment and drug therapy. Insofar as this book mentions any dosage or application, readers may rest assured that the authors, editors, and publishers have made every effort to ensure that such references are in accordance with **the state of knowledge at the time of production of the book.**

Nevertheless, this does not involve, imply, or express any guarantee or responsibility on the part of the publishers in respect to any dosage instructions and forms of applications stated in the book. **Every user is requested to examine carefully** the manufacturers' leaflets accompanying each drug and to check, if necessary in consultation with a physician or specialist, whether the dosage schedules mentioned therein or the contraindications stated by the manufacturers differ from the statements made in the present book. Such examination is particularly important with drugs that are either rarely used or have been newly released on the market. Every dosage schedule or every form of application used is entirely at the user's own risk and responsibility. The authors and publishers request every user to report to the publishers any discrepancies or inaccuracies noticed. If errors in this work are found after publication, errata will be posted at www.thieme.com on the product description page.

Some of the product names, patents, and registered designs referred to in this book are in fact registered trademarks or proprietary names even though specific reference to this fact is not always made in the text. Therefore, the appearance of a name without designation as proprietary is not to be construed as a representation by the publisher that it is in the public domain.

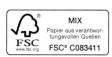

Contents

Foreword

What is balance?

This question may first appear to all of us evident: how could we stand, sit, or walk properly without balance? Artists must have an intimate sense or feeling of balance in order to master the main law of beauty: harmony. For us spine surgeons, a few years ago, our only means to evaluate post-operative balance was to observe a match between good functional result and good-looking, harmonious profile restoration. This intuitive feeling, even if efficient in some hands, was difficult to explain and transmit.

It is only with the routine use of long-standing lateral X-rays that we became able to describe sagittal balance parameters. Hundreds of discussions, sometimes heated, allowed for a better scientific approach. This book is a cornerstone of what we have progressively understood in the last few years with our successes and failures.

If the principle of harmony is unique to the individual, everyone also has his own answer to find balance according to his own characteristics: shape, muscle strength, age. Gravity imposes inescapable forces of control on the human body. A good profile is the one which minimizes muscle action and negative compensations. What we call harmony is the best sagittal shape allowing an ideal muscle action. Gravity, spinal shape, and muscles are the three main components working together to achieve good balance. However, even if simplified, it is impossible to standardize the human body balance and any attempt to do so is bound to fail.

Despite important progress, we must keep in mind that this book is mainly based on static studies. Dynamic analyses are currently missing but should not be forgotten.

We hope that even if the aesthetic point of view remains important, a better scientific approach will help spine surgeons provide more appropriate treatment of spinal deformities.

Daniel Chopin, MD
(retired)
Spinal Unit
Neuro-Orthopedic Department
University of Lille, France
Spine Center
Institut Calot Berck sur Mer, France

Preface

In 1998, when Duval-Beaupère published a new pelvic parameter, the pelvic incidence, and demonstrated its influence on the spinal shape, sagittal balance was not a very hot topic as only five publications had addressed this specific subject in the international literature. By comparison, in the past two years more than two hundred publications have approached the subject. This underlines the importance of sagittal balance evaluation in the daily practice of a spinal specialist today.

Even if pelvic and spinal parameters and their combination organizing sagittal body alignment are well defined, the use of this knowledge in understanding spinal pathology and developing treatment strategies remains uncertain, and practitioners continue to face unexpected treatment failures.

In this book, we have tried to develop a global concept: "from normal to pathology." Of course, it is impossible to define "normal" because of the wide range of a normal status; for humans, normality is the fantastic property of permanent verticality acquired with evolution. The human body is the only one able to sustain the standing position with a balanced and economical status. Anatomical evolution of the pelvic shape is the mechanical key of verticality, changing from flat and high in the first tree-dwelling primates to large and retroverted in humans. This heredity explains the large range of pelvic shapes characterized by the pelvic incidence angle (PI). The strong relation between spinal shape and the sacral plateau allowed for the development of a classification of normal spinopelvic alignment related to PI values. These different spinal shapes deriving from PI variation demonstrate their own mechanical behavior.

In young adults, every type of sagittal alignment is able to provide an economical system, but with increasing age and stress, degeneration can occur and progressively changes alignment orientation and balance features. To maintain verticality, the human body has to develop compensatory mechanisms, and loses the initial economic status.

Balancing between flexion and extension stresses, each type develops its own degenerative evolution resulting in specific degenerative shapes following PI and compensation ability.

Various parameter combinations have been described to characterize a balanced or unbalanced status, but they are focused on L1-S1 lumbar lordosis and pelvic parameters. This is insufficient to determine a treatment strategy, since it ignores PI specificities and spinal curvature reciprocity. Even if it is well known that an unbalanced result induces a bad functional result, it is still not well understood what a balanced system is and how to reach it.

In order to settle the concept "from normal to pathology," we need to reverse the approach and address "from pathology to normal." In a pathology, we have evidence of the previous "normal" status using PI that may offer guidance for how to restore an appropriate shape. Following PI values, we may anticipate the better "normal" shape fitting with the pelvis specificity. It is not just a matter of angle restitution, since curve repartition has to be respected to avoid mechanical failures such as PJK.

The reader will observe that this book is not based on technical descriptions. Our aim was to emphasize the treatment strategy following spinopelvic shape identification. It was a difficult challenge: some assertions are still hypothetical and will have to be demonstrated in future studies. As a global concept, we have tried to define each step of sagittal balance evolution during life and following each shape specificity. Probably as the basis of treatment strategy, it would have been too ambitious to use this shortcut as a title: "How to return to normal from normal." We hope that this book will help you in understanding the fascinating story of sagittal balance.

Pierre Roussouly, MD
João Luiz Pinheiro-Franco, MD, AFS
Hubert Labelle, MD
Martin Gehrchen, MD, PhD

Contributors

Mohanad Alazzeh, BS
Department of Neurosurgery
University of California at San Francisco
San Francisco, California, USA

Abdulmajeed Alzakri, MD, MS, DESC Ortho
Clinical Spine Surgery Fellow at the University
of Montréal
Department of Orthopaedics
College of Medicine, King Saud University
Riyadh, Saudi Arabia

Christopher P. Ames, MD
Professor
Department of Neurological Surgery
University of California, San Francisco
San Francisco, California, USA

Hideyuki Arima, MD, PhD
Research Fellow
Department of Orthopaedic Surgery
Norton Leatherman Spine Center
Louisville, Kentucky, USA
Clinical Instructor
Department of Orthopaedic Surgery
Hamamatsu University School of Medicine
Hamamatsu, Shizuoka, Japan

Carl-Eric Aubin, PhD, ScD (hc), PEng
Professor
Department of Mechanical Engineering
Polytechnique Montreal
Researcher
Sainte-Justine University Hospital Center
Montréal, Québec, Canada

Cédric Y. Barrey, MD, PhD
Chairman
Department of Spine and Spinal Cord Surgery
Hôpital Pierre Wertheimer
Hospices Civils de Lyon
Université Claude Bernard Lyon 1
Lyon, France

Théo Broussolle
Surgical Specialty Intern
Department of Neurosurgery C
Neurological Hospital
Lyon, France

Leah Y. Carreon, MD, MSc
Clinical Research Director
Norton Leatherman Spine Center
Louisville, Kentucky, USA

Jean-Etienne Castelain, MD
Fellowship
Department of Orthopaedics and Traumatology
Spine Unit 1
University Hospital of Bordeaux,
Bordeaux, Aquitaine, France

Derek T. Cawley, MMedSc, MCh, FRCS
Consultant Spine Surgeon
Tallaght University Hospital
Dublin, Republic of Ireland

Daniel Chopin, MD
(retired)
Spinal Unit
Neuro-Orthopedic Department
University of Lille, France
Spine Center
Institut Calot Berck sur Mer, France

Thibault Cloché, MD
Orthospine Department
Bordeaux Nord Aquitaine Hospital
Bordeaux University
Bordeaux, Nouvelle Aquitaine, France

Anthony M. DiGiorgio, DO, MHA
Resident
Department of Neurosurgery
Louisiana State University Health Sciences Center
New Orleans, Louisiana, USA

Amir El Rahal, MD
Department of Neurosurgery
University Hospital of Geneva, HUG
Geneva, Switzerland

Martin Gehrchen, MD, PhD
Associate Professor and Head of Spine Surgery
Spine Unit
Department of Orthopaedic Surgery
Rigshospitalet and University of Copenhagen
Copenhagen, Denmark

Steven D. Glassman, MD
Professor
Department of Orthopedic Surgery
University of Louisville
Louisville, Kentucky, USA

Martin Haeusler, PhD
Head Evolutionary Morphology and Adaptation Group
Institute of Evolutionary Medicine
University of Zurich
Zurich, Switzerland

Shahnawaz Haleem, MSc(Tr&Orth), MRCSEd, MRCSI, FRCS(Tr&Orth)
Complex Spine Fellow
Honorary Associate Clinical Lecturer
St. George's University Hospital
Oxford University Hospitals
London, United Kingdom

Hyoungmin Kim, MD, PhD
Clinical Associate Professor
Department of Orthopedic Surgery
Seoul National University Hospital
Seoul, South Korea

Hubert Labelle, MD
Professor of Surgery
Division of Orthopedic Surgery
University of Montreal
Montréal, Québec, Canada

Fethi Laouissat, MD
Consultant Orthopaedic Surgeon
Spine Surgery Unit
Hôpital Privé de l'Est Lyonnais
Saint-Priest, Rhône, France

Darryl Lau, MD
Chief Resident
Department of Neurological Surgery
University of California, San Francisco
San Francisco, California, USA

Amélie Leglise, MD
Orthopédie Department
Bordeaux Pellegrin Hospital
Bordeaux University
Bordeaux, Nouvelle Aquitaine, France

Jean-Charles Le Huec, MD, PhD
Professor
Department of Orthospine
Bordeaux Nord Aquitaine Hospital
Bordeaux University
Bordeaux, Nouvelle Aquitaine, France

Praveen V. Mummaneni, MD
Joan O'Reilly Endowed Professor in Spinal Surgery
Vice Chairman
Deptartment of Neurosurgery
University of California, San Francisco
San Francisco, California, USA

Nishant Nishant, MD
Orthopedic and Spine Surgeon
Rameshwaram Orthopedic
Spine & Ent Clinic
Patna, Bihar, India

Colin Nnadi, MBBS, FRCS(Orth)
Spine Unit
Oxford University Hospitals NHS Foundation Trust
Oxford, Oxfordshire, United Kingdom

Ibrahim Obeid, MD, MSc
Consultant
Spine Department
Bordeaux University
Bordeaux, France

Stefan Parent, MD, PhD
Full Professor of Surgery
Chair, Academic Chair in Pediatric Spinal Deformities of CHU Ste-Justine
Chief, Division of Pediatric Orthopedic Surgery
CHU Sainte-Justine
Department of Surgery
Université de Montréal
Montréal, Québec, Canada

Charles Peltier, MD
Department of Spine Surgery
Hôpital P.-Wertheimer, Hospices Civils de Lyon
Lyon, France

Marion Petit, MD
Orthopédie Department
Bordeaux Pellegrin Hospital, Bordeaux University
Bordeaux, Nouvelle Aquitaine, France

João Luiz Pinheiro-Franco, MD, AFS
Neurosurgeon and Spine Surgeon
Samaritano Hospital of São Paulo
São Paulo, Brazil

Pierre Roussouly, MD
Senior Surgeon
Spinal Surgery Unit
Croix Rouge Française-CMCR des Massues
Lyon, France

Amer Sebaaly, MD, BS
Department of Orthopedic Surgery
Hotel Dieu de France Hospital
Saint Joseph University
Beirut, Lebanon

Jacques Sénégas, MD
Spine Surgeon
Professor
Département of Anatomy
University Bordeaux II
Bordeaux, France

Christine Tardieu, PhD
Director of Research CNRS
Research Unit "Adaptativ Mecanisms and Evolution"
Department "Adaptation du Vivant"
National Museum of Natural History
Paris, France

Jean-Marc Mac-Thiong, MD, PhD
Associate Professor
Department of Surgery
Université de Montréal
Montréal, Québec, Canada

Wendy Thompson, MD
Orthospine Department
Bordeaux Nord Aquitaine Hospital, Bordeaux University
Bordeaux, Nouvelle Aquitaine, France

Jean Marc Vital, MD, PhD
Spinal Unit
Universitary Hospital Pellegrin
Bordeaux, France

Xiaoyu Wang, PhD
Research Fellow
Department of Mechanical Engineering
Polytechnique Montreal
Montréal, Québec, Canada

Part I

Introduction to Sagittal Balance

1 Historical Background of Spinal Sagittal Balance

Pierre Roussouly and Nishant Nishant

Abstract

The concept of normal sagittal spinal curvatures was first described by Hippocrates in ~ 400 BC. Galen confirmed the succession of curves limited by areas where vertebrae were characterized by the same anatomy. He was the first to use the Greek names lordosis and kyphosis. This anatomical segmentation in cervical lordosis, thoracic kyphosis, lumbar lordosis, and sacral kyphosis remained the reference, and Leonardo da Vinci was the first to design the sagittal anatomy of the full human spine. Although many biomechanical studies were achieved regarding spinal resistance and the role and positioning of gravity on the spine between the 17th and 19th centuries, it is only during the second part of the 20th century that a new way of analyzing the spinal curvatures was initiated. Delmas introduced the important relation between sacral orientation and the spinal shape. He described variations in human spinal curvature related to the sacral plateau inclination from very curved (static) to very flat (dynamic). Later, During and Duval-Beaupère demonstrated the direct correlation between a pelvic shape angle and pelvis positioning. Duval-Beaupère gave the name "pelvic incidence" to this fundamental angle and by a simple pelvimetry demonstrated the geometrical relation: pelvic incidence equals pelvis tilt plus sacral slope. Berthonnaud and Dimnet proposed a new spinal curvature segmentation based on the inflection point where lordosis transitions into kyphosis. This geometry introduced a new vision of spinal curvatures no longer limited by anatomical area but possibly longer or shorter than the thoracolumbar limit (T12-L1). Since the beginning of the 21st century, many other studies have shown the importance of respecting the sagittal balance in functional results after spine surgery, and sagittal balance became one of the most important topics in clinical research on spinal pathologies.

Keywords: During J, Duval-Beaupère G, Hippocrates, pelvic incidence, spinal curvatures

1.1 Introduction

Sagittal balance of the spine is a recent concept developed by pioneers in the latter part of the 20th century and which has become well established currently in beginning of the 21st century. Before the modern age, many concepts on spinal curvatures were described by Hippocrates in ancient Greece,[1] and are still used in the majority of anatomical publications. Lordosis and kyphosis have Greek etymologies, and it was probably Galen[2] who first used the terminology "ithioscoliosis," to describe the natural curves of the spine in the sagittal plane.

During the 16th century, human dissection brought to light precise descriptions of vertebrae anatomy, although it was centered on local description rather than Hippocrates curve segmentation. Pelvic positioning as a compensatory method secondary to certain spinal pathologies was first analyzed by some authors in the 19th century as a way of balance compensation. Global changes in the aging population became well known during this era. But it was not until the 20th century,

with the advent of X-ray images of the spine, that it began to come into focus. During the golden era of the 1970s and 1980s, a plethora of information on spinal biomechanics was published, however only with a segmental focus.[3]

Few authors expressed interest in global assessment of the spine either with relevance to anatomy or pathology. In 1953, Delmas,[4] a French anatomist, described the changes in spinal curvatures in asymptomatic individuals. His point of view had very few applications in the traditional treatment of spinal pathologies at that time. Spinal curvature concepts were exclusively relegated to manual therapy proposed by some investigators as a global rehabilitation technique, albeit as an empirical approach based on clinical assessment.

During et al[5] revolutionized spinal biomechanics by proposing a new pelvimetry that integrated both the spine and pelvis with respect to their shapes and positioning. Although this landmark paper was published in *Spine* in 1985, it failed to receive wide acceptance in the scientific community. Not until 2008, with Duval-Beaupère's scientific paper that detailed the sagittal layout of the spine and pelvis, was sagittal parameter catapulted to the forefront of spinal research and accepted as one of the most fundamental criteria for understanding spinal pathologies and their treatment.[6]

In this chapter, the authors pursue the historical background of spinal theory from the earliest Indus Valley civilization of ancient India to the Greeks and, finally, to the beginning of modern concepts to enlighten our readers on how ideas on spinal balance progressively evolved to become an undeniable element in understanding the spine.

1.2 Ancient India

The oldest reference available is written in the ancient Hindu mythological epics *Srimad Bhagvat Mahapuranam*[7] (3500 BC and 1800 BC), where it is mentioned how Lord Krishna corrected the hunchback of one of his devotees, Kubj, by pressing down on his feet and pulling up on his chin.[8,9] A detailed description of the human body, including spinal anatomy, was known to the religious Aryans between 2500–2000 BC up to 750–500 BC.[10] In the Vedic period, which began in 1800 BC mainly after the age of the *Brahmanas*, the term "scoliosis" was never used, rather it was described in Sanskrit.

1.3 Ancient Greece

For the Greek philosopher Plato (427–347 BC),[11] nature was a perfect divine creation and motion was a unique attribute of animals. He emphasized the flexibility of the spine, which was created to allow for body movements. Spinal flexibility was seen as being in harmony with a perfect body. Aristotle (490–430 BC)[12] considered spinal flexibility an absolute necessity for bipedal motion. Among the animal kingdom, by comparing birds and human bipedalism, Aristotle demonstrated that human bipedal capability was the source of human superiority. However, these considerations were more philosophical than practical.

Hippocrates (460–370 BC), the father of medicine,[13,14,15] was born on the Greek island of Kos (▶ Fig. 1.1). He was responsible for changing medicine from what was previously religious and supernatural phenomena into a scientific and observational discipline. As human dissections were forbidden at that time, his observations were extracted from animal dissections, bodies in motion at gymnasiums, and cadavers on the battlefield. In his famous opus, *On Articulations*, he described the spinal curvatures following their sagittal orientation:

Regarding the rachis, it is inflected along its whole length: from the sacral extremity to the great vertebra (fifth lumbar), with which the lower limbs are connected, spine is convex backward. From there to the diaphragm insertion, the spine is convex forward for the whole length. This area is covered anteriorly by muscles: the psoas. From there to the great vertebra above the shoulders (seventh cervical), rachis is on the whole length, convex backward; but due to the length of the spinous processes, longer in the middle of the back, it appears more bent than in reality. Regarding the cervical area itself, it is convex forward....
(French translation by Émile Littré 1844)

Hippocrates identified spinal deformities with the term "scoliosis." He showed that the forward bending of the spine changes with age and work culture. More than a century before Percivall Pott, Hippocrates related progressive severe kyphosis with the presence of tubercles in the lungs. He described many systems of treatment for deformities using a combination of traction and pressure. His description of the spinal curvatures remains in use to this day and will continue to be the basic mainstay of global spinal anatomy forever.

Archimedes (287–212 BC) was a well-known mathematician, physicist, inventor, and astronomer of his age. He had the most profound influence on the future of spinal biomechanics through his work on the equilibrium of planes.

1.4 Roman Empire

Galen of Pergamon (130–210 AD)[16] was initially a physician of gladiators, which afforded him vast expertise in trauma. He was Greek but worked in Rome, serving Emperor Marc Aurèle and his son, Commode. He wrote several medical books where he reviewed Hippocrates. His anatomic doctrines became the basis for medical education for more than 1200 years.

It was assumed that Galen was the first to use the terms lordosis and scoliosis, dividing spinal deformities into lordosis, where the spine bends backward, kyphosis, where it bends forward, and scoliosis for lateral deformities. Because of variable translations and interpretations, it remains questionable whether Galen used the words lordosis and kyphosis in their modern significations. Lordosis (Greek λόρδωση), which can be translated into curvature, was used initially for any kind of normal curvature, bent forward or backward. Kyphosis (Greek κύφωση), translated as "hump," had a pathological signification: abnormal forward curvature. This sagittal subdivision of the normal spine, initiated by Hippocrates, with its modern translation sacral kyphosis, lumbar lordosis (LL), thoracic kyphosis, and cervical lordosis, came to us without any change and still remains the gold standard in anatomical descriptions of the spine. As an official surgeon of gladiators in amphitheaters, he was accepted as "the father of sports medicine." Galen also improved some devices described by Hippocrates for spinal trauma (▶ Fig. 1.2).

Oribasius (325–400 AD),[17] another Roman physician, added a bar to the Hippocratic reduction device and used it to treat both spinal trauma and spinal deformity.

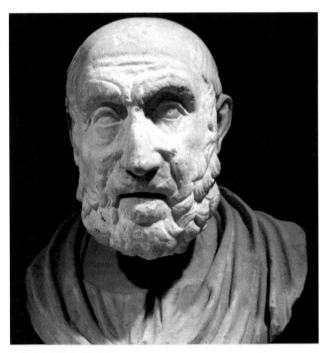

Fig. 1.1 Hippocrates.

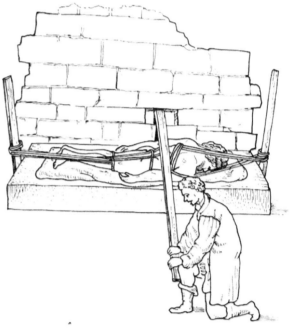

Fig. 1.2 Device of spinal deformity reduction first described by Hippocrates then improved by Galen.

Paul of Aegina (625–690 AD)[18] performed the first known laminectomy using a red-hot iron. He also collected the medical work of 1000 years in a seven-volume encyclopedia.

1.5 Middle Ages (330–1453 AD)

After a period of great activity during antiquity in medicine, contributions during the Middle Ages was paltry in comparison, especially in Europe. Translations of documents salvaged from ancient Greek were relegated to copyists in monasteries. Because of the proximity of Byzantium where most Greek archives were stored, Persian and Arabian physicians were able to translate Greek into Arabic and use and comment on the teachings of Hippocrates and Galen. The most famous, Avicenna (980–1037 AD), was a physician from what is presently Uzbekistan. Among his writings is the book, *The Canon of Medicine*, which became the reference book for students of medieval medicine. In the first volume, he analyzes the anatomy of the spine and precisely describes intervertebral motions in flexion, extension, and lateral flexion; spinal pathologies were treated in the third and fourth volume.[19] Following Hippocrates, he considered that kyphosis may have external (trauma) or internal causes and that good health was dependent upon a regular flux of humors (i.e., one of the four fluids entering into the constitution of the body). He considered degeneration and subsequent articular rigidity as a decrease of flux. He may have recognized spinal diseases such as Pott's disease as an ankylosing spondylitis.[20]

Abulcasis (936–1013 AD),[21] a famous Arabian surgeon of the 11th century, wrote a treatise on surgery, *At-Tasnif*, in which he describes surgical disorders, including low back pain, sciatica, scoliosis, and spinal trauma, and advocates the use of chemical or thermal cauterization for several spinal disorders. He also developed a device to reduce the dislocated spine.

Şerefeddin Sabuncuoğlu (1385–1468 AD),[22] a Turkish physician, wrote an illustrated atlas of surgery, describing scoliosis, sciatica, low back pain, and spinal dislocations. He devised a technique for the reduction of spinal dislocations using a frame similar to that designed by Abulcasis.

1.6 15th to 17th Centuries

The Renaissance was a fertile period where humanists rediscovered Ancient Greek and Arabian works and spurred development of a new way of thinking in all arts and sciences. Until Andreas Vesalius (1514–1564),[23] medicine and anatomy described by Greek authors were considered an absolute truth. He was the first to criticize Galen in his book, *De Humani Corporis Fabrica*, where he made accurate revisions of spine anatomy using direct and precise observations on human cadavers, a technique not allowed in Ancient Greece and limited to animal dissections, especially monkeys. Andreas Vesalius' work, however, was limited to vertebrae description; nothing was written on the global assessment of the spine. Even the rich iconography of his work on human dissection was done in an artistic manner where spinal shape was not identifiable (▶ Fig. 1.3).

In only one drawing did Leonardo da Vinci (1452–1519)[24] give a perfect lateral view of the whole spine, respecting Hippocrates' orientation and segmentation of the spinal curvatures with the right number of vertebrae (▶ Fig. 1.4).

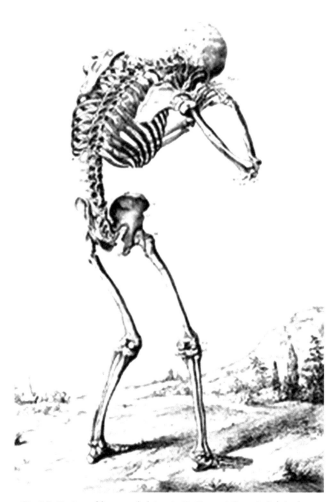

Fig. 1.3 Design of human skeleton in *De Humani Corporis Fabrica* by Vesalius.

He sensed the mechanical interaction of bone and muscles and, for him, the power of motion in animals was necessarily the result of mechanical means.

Although lesser known, Giovanni Alfonso Borelli (1608–1679)[25,26] is considered the "father of biomechanics." In his book, *De Motu Animalium*, he begins the introduction with these words: "Bodies and movements are the subject of mathematics. Such scientific approach is exactness of geometry...." His main observation was that muscles act on bony articulations in a manner akin to short lever arms. By extrapolation on the spine, he was able to calculate the forces acting on each intervertebral disk under a charge on the neck (▶ Fig. 1.5). He detailed the contact force on the fifth lumbar vertebra as the addition of weight-bearing and muscle forces. He was the first to experimentally define the position of the body's center of gravity.

1.7 18th to 19th Centuries

The 18th century is marked by the advent of a scientific approach that was focused apart from the mirage that the human body as a godly creation. Even Vesalius, when describing perfectly the anatomy of vertebrae after human dissection, was describing in effect a perfect work of God.

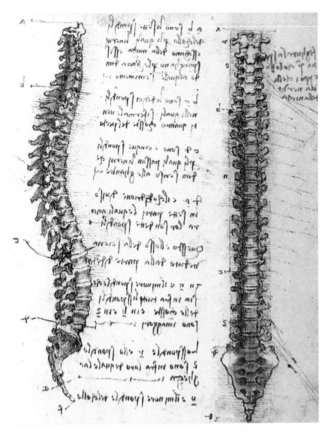

Fig. 1.4 The first lateral view of human spine designed by Leonardo da Vinci.

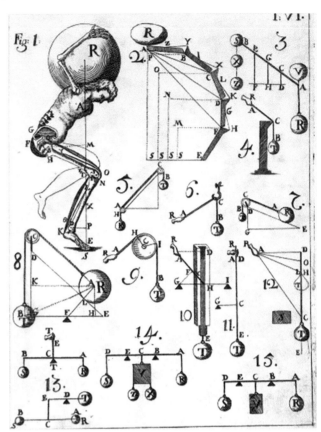

Fig. 1.5 Physical calculation of mechanical forces acting on the human body in weight-bearing action.

This philosophical change of this period was formulated by Immanuel Kant (1724–1804) in his book *Critique of Pure Reason*. He showed that in a scientific approach, instead of placing the subject (actor of research) under the object rules (presupposition), it is the subject who applies his own rules onto the object under observation. In other words, when a scientific analysis presents a contradiction with previous observations, it is necessary to criticize objectively and, over time, change former ideas and understanding.

During the 18th century, few studies were undertaken with regard to the anatomy and biomechanics of the spine. Leonhard Euler (1707–1783)[27,28] was a Swiss mathematician who, while studying the curvature of the spine, effectively demonstrated that a curved structure had a superiority in terms of resistance to a straight structure. Later, Jean Cruveilhier, in his *Treatise of Descriptive Anatomy* published in 1833, uses this relation to explain the spinal resistance: $R = N^2 + 1$, where N is the number of curvatures of the structure, and gave a ratio of 1:16 for the normal spine resistance.

Two fundamental clinical descriptions of spinal disease were written. Bernard Connor in 1697 described the spontaneous fusion of the sacrum and vertebrae in *Ankylosing Spondylitis*. Percivall Pott (1714–1788)[29] was the first to describe the arthritic tuberculosis of the spine and its severe kyphotic evolution.

Because of an explosion of engineering and biomechanical advancements in the 19th century, many of these methods were introduced into the science of the spine. Center of gravity positioning in the human body was the most pursued challenge of the time. It must be taken into account that radiology had not yet

been invented. Ernst and Wilhelm Weber,[30] in 1836, published a description on the movement of center of gravity during gait in their landmark publication *Die Mechanik der Menschlichen Gehwerkzeuge* (Mechanics of the Human Gait),[31] which laid the foundation of the modern concept of locomotion. In 1891, Wilhelm Braune and Otto Fischer,[32] in their book *Der Gang des Menschen* showed the positions of the center of gravity for each segment of the body in a tridimensional study. Using frozen cadavers and a special balance plate, they determined the body mass center for each body segment measured. A hundred years later, Duval-Beaupère[33] performed the same measurements by way of a barycentremeter using X-ray measurements. Hermann von Meyer, a German anatomist, and Karl Culmann[34] used a crane model to explain the mechanical effect of muscles on bony structures. In 1892, Julius Wolff[35] published, *The Law of Bone Remodelling*, stating that, "...Structure is nothing else than the physical expression of function under pathological conditions. The structure and form of the parts change according to the abnormal conditions of force transmission."

1.8 20th Century

It is at the very end of the 19th century that Wilhelm Conrad Röntgen in 1895 performed the first radiograph of his wife Anna's hand. Because of the high risk of irradiation and the negative effects resulting from prolonged and large exposure, the use of long-standing X-rays arrived late and were mainly used for spinal deformities such as scoliosis. Lateral long X-rays

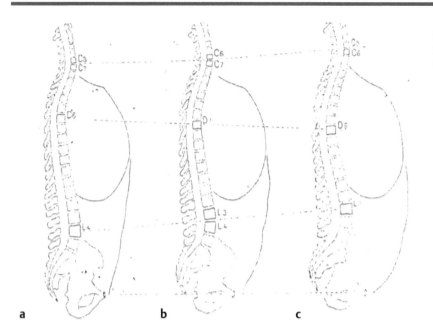

Fig. 1.6 Delmas classification of spinal shapes: (a) dynamic straight back, (b) average normal shape, and (c) static curved back.

were performed exceptionally for severe kyphosis and almost never in idiopathic scoliosis check-ups. It would not be until the very end of the 20th century when lateral long-standing X-rays would be used routinely for spinal diseases, thanks to the decreased irradiation of numerical X-rays, and more recently with the use of the EOS technique. In the first half of the 20th century, even as the number of publications on biomechanics increased, very few were published papers on the spinal profile. However, interest was triggered in spine biomechanics. Jules Amar (1879–1935) published his work, *The Human Motor*, on analysis of the physical and physiologic components of gait and task performance in thousands of disabled veterans in France.[36,37]

In the 1950s, André Delmas (1910–1999),[38] a French professor and anatomist at Paris University, dedicated part of his research to anthropology. His interest was human bipedalism and he went on to analyze variations in spinal curvatures. He focused on 6000 specimens in the Delmas-Orfila-Rouvière collection, now within the Medical School at the University of Montpellier. In 1951, Delmas described an index of spinal curvature: (spinal height × 100)/spinal length. Both measurements were done from the atlas to the lower plate of L5. For a straight spine, the index would be 100; the more the spine is curved, the greater the index decreases. Through this technique, he classified three kinds of spine: straight spine (index > 96), normal spine (94 < index < 96), and curved spine (index < 94). He called the first spine type "dynamic" and the third one "static" (▶ Fig. 1.6). He was, however, probably mistaken when he considered the "dynamic" straight spine as a feature of strong men, Nordics, and Black Africans. In another publication in 1960, he proposed the hypothesis of L3 as a constant position of the LL apex. Even though it is known today through long-standing X-rays that there is a variability of apex positioning, Delmas had published a figure that perfectly represented the sacrum shapes relative to the value that was to be later identified as the "pelvic incidence" (▶ Fig. 1.7).

In 1982, Pierre Stagnara[39] was the first to publish the analysis of long-standing lateral X-rays in 100 young adult volunteers, using a very standardized standing position to capture lateral

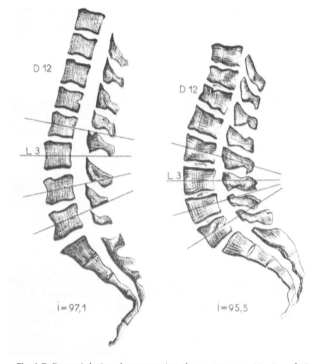

Fig. 1.7 Dumas' design demonstrating the constant positioning of L3 as lordosis apex. Without knowing the pelvic incidence (PI) angle, the sacral shape was well identified corresponding to flat lordosis on the left (low PI) and curved lordosis on the right (high PI).

X-rays. To the best of our knowledge, this was one of the first studies using the treatment of each X-ray on a digitalizing table, identifying vertebral bodies using four points. Statistical analyses of these results were performed using a computer. Kyphosis and lordosis were bounded by an intermediate vertebral body where both curves were transitioning (▶ Fig. 1.8). Lordosis inferior limit was the sacral plateau. Despite this modern segmentation, the authors were unable to identify morphological groups and to give a classification of normal

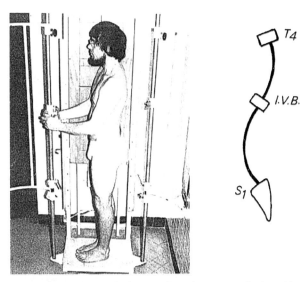

Fig. 1.8 Stagnara: Standardization of standing position for lateral long-standing X-rays. Both curves kyphosis and lordosis were separated by the intermediate vertebral body (IVB).

sagittal alignment. They concluded that "the morphologic types appear much more varied than those described by Delmas." Nonetheless, they confirmed a good correlation between the lordosis and sacral slope (SS). Stagnara used the legend of Procrustes from Greek mythology to argue that there is no "ideal" sagittal shape.

During the 1980s, several authors published various studies on sagittal spinal alignment in asymptomatic elderly patients with lower back pain with the same conclusions.

In 1985, During et al[5] suggested that "aberrations of posture" might cause low back pain as a result of patterns of stress concentrations. Their concept was quite advanced for the time and, as can be noticed, the term "sagittal balance" was not mentioned. The authors studied lateral radiographs in a standing position in 52 asymptomatic individuals and 77 patients with diverse lumbar spine pathologies. Insights from mechanical engineering led During, an engineer, and his colleagues to consider lumbar spine as a multisegmental crankshaft fixed to its base, the pelvis, with a modifiable position. The authors affirmed that "to generate a homogeneous stress distribution, the instantaneous shape of the crankshaft, its position in relation to the direction of the force, and the position of the base are of paramount importance." This position was the cradle of sagittal balance knowledge.

Furthermore, During et al proposed a skeletal outline of the spinopelvic complex and defined the angles (▶ Fig. 1.9). The α angle corresponded to the presently well-known SS angle. They defined the center of the hips as the midpoint between the centers of the femoral heads. Furthermore, they described the pelvisacral angle "β," which is the complement of pelvic incidence (PI) described later by Duval-Beaupère (PI = 90° − β) and the pelvic tilt (PT) (α + β), which is the complement of the pelvis tilt also described by Duval-Beaupère. The instantaneous shape of rotation of the lordotic curve R was approximated to a circle, including the upper anterior vertices of L4, L5, and S1. The size of the circle could be easily measured using a jig, with "M" being the center and "R" the radius.

During et al also observed that the morphology of lordosis was dependent on the inclination of the sacral endplate. They

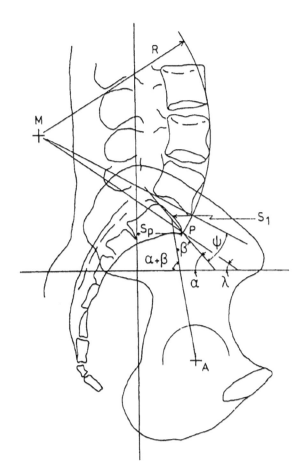

Fig. 1.9 During's sagittal parameters.

concluded that the equilibrium is linked by a chain of spinopelvic parameters in which the positioning of the pelvis (angle α + β) determines the SS (α) with a close relation between α + β and the pelvisacral angle β. Their first results in a "normal" population were: β = 39.2° (corresponding PI = 50.8°), α = 40°, α + β = 79.2° (corresponding PT = 10.8°) (▶ Fig. 1.10). It was very close to the well-known measurements done in more recent publications. In pathology, another relevant result was the average β value in spondylolisthesis of 26.5° (corresponding PI = 63.5°). Labelle et al also found the same average value for PI in spondylolisthesis.

During is undisputedly the pioneer of sagittal balance assessment. He was the first to describe the pelvis parameters regarding the hip joints as a paramount factor in the LL adaptation to manage the spinopelvic sagittal balance. Unfortunately, this paper was held back for being highly confidential and never found any place in the literature. Probably inspired by During et al, Itoi[40] published a study of 100 osteoporotic kyphotic patients and analyzed the respective correlations of spinal curvatures (he used the functional segmentation), pelvic parameters, and lower limbs positioning. Itoi defined a chain of compensation beginning with lordosis increasing the pelvic retroversion. He demonstrated the role of the hips in motion and the necessity of knee flexion and subsequent femoral shaft inclination when hip extension was overpassed (▶ Fig. 1.11). He integrated the possibility of sacroiliac

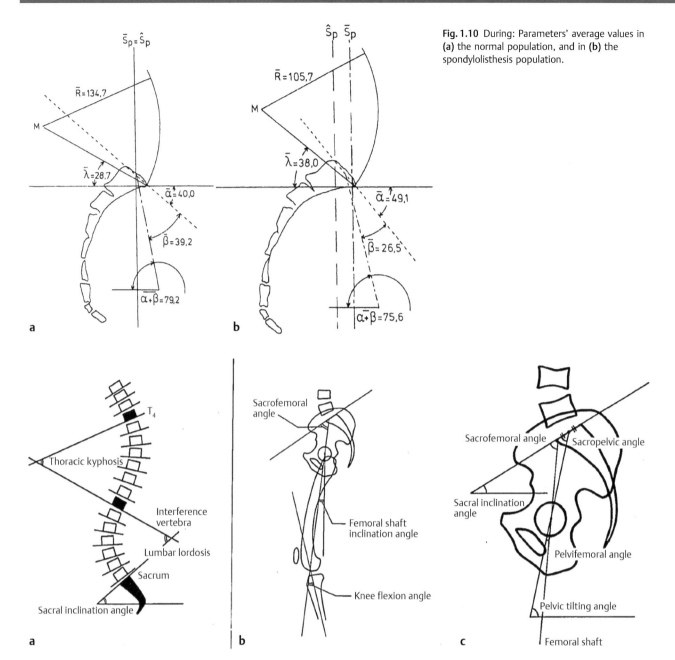

Fig. 1.10 During: Parameters' average values in (**a**) the normal population, and in (**b**) the spondylolisthesis population.

Fig. 1.11 (a-c) Itoi: Spinal segmentation and lower limbs mechanism of compensation.

joint mobility in the mechanism of adaptation but he did not invest any interest in shape variation of the pelvis designed by the sacropelvic angle (SPA = PI + 90°). At the same time, Takemitsu et al[41] classified LL evolution in a population of aging people (▶ Fig. 1.12).

Subsequently, 10 years after During et al, Legaye and Duval-Beaupère[6] published a paper describing the fundamental pelvic parameter: pelvis incidence (▶ Fig. 1.13). They used the same angles described by During et al before but, as a complement, the newly presented angles took on a better visibility and allowed a better understanding of their interrelations. They emphasized the relation PI = PT + SS, previously described by During. Legaye et al and Duval-Beaupère et al concluded there was a direct relation between PI and LL, through the strong correlation between PI and SS, then between SS and LL (small PI,

flat LL, high PI, curved LL). They also proposed an equation to determine ideal LL, which was never well used.

As this momentum grew, Jackson and Hales[42] published several articles on LL structure, and its relation to sacral plateau orientation. Legaye et al[6] established a new pelvimetry, introducing a relation between femoral heads and the sacral plateau. Instead of the sacral plateau midpoint as a reference landmark, they proposed using the posterior edge of the sacral plateau. Jackson and Hales described the pelvis radius as the line between the femoral heads and the posterior edge of the sacral plateau. The angle between the pelvis radius and the sacral plateau (PRS1) had the same significance as the PI of Duval-Beaupère (▶ Fig. 1.14). In the end, between both propositions, it was the PI relative to pelvic radius that has remained the more cited pelvic parameter in current publications.

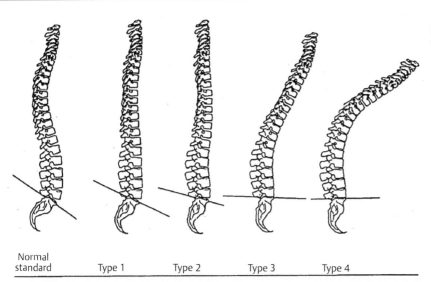

Fig. 1.12 Takemitsu: Classification of variation of degenerative lumbar lordosis.

Normal standard   Type 1   Type 2   Type 3   Type 4

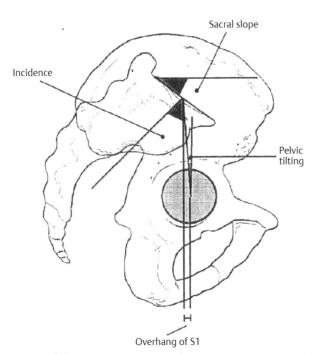

Fig. 1.13 Legaye and Duval-Beaupère: First design of pelvic incidence, pelvis tilting, and sacral slope.

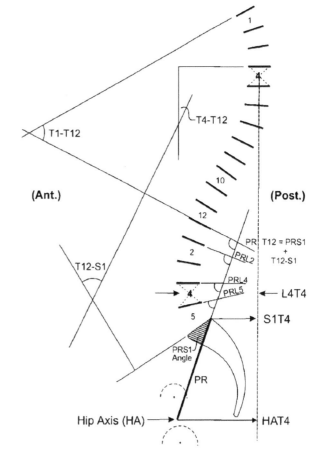

Fig. 1.14 Jackson's parameters using the posterior edge of the sacral plateau.

Several studies[43,44,45,46,47] were conducted on the role of gravity on sagittal balance, based on the theory that the cone of oscillation is centered on the projection on the ground of the global axis of gravity described by Dubousset. Duval-Beaupère et al, using the barycentremeter measurement[33] were able to give the proper barycenter for each part of the body. Other authors[48,49,50,51] used a force plate to take standing radiographs and were able to show the position of the axis of gravity regarding anatomical landmarks. Proximity of this axis with the femoral heads was demonstrated in asymptomatic populations. Superposition of these studies with C7 plumb line alignment was done in normal and aging populations. Lafage et al used this analysis to describe the evolution of sagittal balance in aging people. The lack of pertinent information (gravity line falls always between the feet) did not permit useful clinical applications of the gravity assessment.

In recent papers, some authors seemed to have discovered the role of the lower limbs in sagittal balance. Mangione et al[52] described the angle between the vertical line and the femoral shaft when the knees are in flexion. Yoshimoto et al,[53]

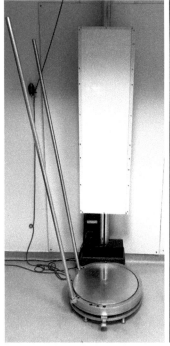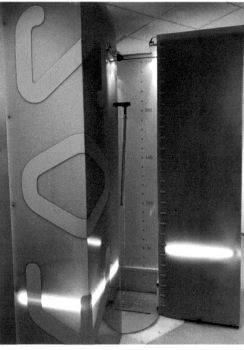

Fig. 1.15 Turning force plate allowing simultaneous X-ray and gravity line positioning used in Lyon. On the right is an EOS cabin.

describing the hip-spine syndrome, demonstrated the relation of spinal curvatures, pelvic retroversion, and the acetabulum orientation. Lazennec et al[54,55] demonstrated the hip prosthesis behavior in degenerative spinal kyphosis. Trojani et al[56] described the hip extension reserve that is consumed when the pelvis is retroverted, inducing femoral tilt and knees flexion if this reserve is overpassed. Le Huec et al[57] described the full balance index that introduced the angle of femoral tilt in a reduction strategy.

To improve the accuracy and repeatability of measurements, software has been developed to assess the spinal shape either in 2D or 3D. Stagnara was the first to use computerized measurements with a digitized table. At the close of the 1980s, Graf, Dubousset, Berthonnaud, and Dimnet[58,59,60,61] developed different systems for 3D reconstruction of the spine based on crossing frontal and lateral long-standing X-rays. Research at that time was mainly dedicated to scoliosis. Even though the use of the Harrington rods was a significant improvement in scoliosis surgical treatment, the pure 2D distraction used in this technique neglected profile reduction inducing a flattening of the back, a major complication known as "failed back." Introduction of 3D conceptualization using the Cotrel–Dubousset technique was revolutionary in the 1980s.[62] The simultaneous reduction of both frontal and lateral deformities had begun to become mandatory.[63]

Several studies on populations of asymptomatic volunteers or patients with specific spinal disease have been done using computerized analyses.[64,65,66,67,68,69,70] These studies convert average values of various parameters and also allow for extracting valuable guidelines for obtaining good balance. Lafage, combining balance parameters with a quality of life questionnaire, was able to predict ideal or pathological limits for key parameters such as LL and PT.

From graphic software, the Templier group,[71] working at the ENSAM in Paris with Lavaste and Skalli, designed software for sagittal analysis that is derived from the well-known, yet still active Surgimap, which was improved upon by Lafage. In Lyon, France, Dimnet and Berthonnaud developed Optispine, which was used on all spondylolisthesis studies of the Spinal Deformity Study Group. Currently, based on Optispine studies, SMAIO developed the KEOPS software. All recent reconstruction software are able to simulate a surgical reduction and may also be useful in correction strategies. Most recently, the EOS standing X-ray capture technique allows full body analysis, introducing the lower limbs position. This technique is based on Charpak theory, which allows for irradiation reduction while avoiding image distortion by vertical displacement of the sources. Reconstruction of radiological images have become easier with greatly enhanced accuracy (▶ Fig. 1.15).

1.9 Conclusion

The author emphasizes, in the subsequent chapters of this book, that different schools of thought have divergent but complementary hypotheses. A grounded understanding of sagittal balance is mandatory to attain biomechanical stability of the spine. Furthermore, spinal assessment has gone beyond the critical point of no return; there is now no possibility of reverting back to the old concepts in modern assessment of spinal evaluation and treatment.

References

[1] Breasted JH. The Edwin Smith Surgical Papyrus [published in facsimile and hieroglyphic transliteration with translation and commentary in two volumes]. Chicago, IL: University of Chicago Press; 1930

[2] Galen. On the Affected Parts [translated from the Greek by Siegel RE]. Basel, Switzerland: S. Karger; 1976:113

[3] White AA, Panjabi MM. Clinical Biomechanics of the Spine. Philadelphia, PA: Lippincott Williams & Wilkins; 1990

[4] Saban R. André Delmas (1910–1999). Hist Sci Med. 2000; 34(2):187–188

[5] During J, Goudfrooij H, Keessen W, Beeker TW, Crowe A. Toward standards for posture. Postural characteristics of the lower back system in normal and pathologic conditions. Spine. 1985; 10(1):83–87

[6] Legaye J, Duval-Beaupère G, Hecquet J, Marty C. Pelvic incidence: a fundamental pelvic parameter for three-dimensional regulation of spinal sagittal curves. Eur Spine J. 1998; 7(2):99–103

[7] Subramaniam K. Srimand Bhagavatam. Mumbai, India: Bharatiya Vidya Bhavan; 1979

[8] Kumar K. Spinal deformity and axial traction. Spine. 1996; 21(5):653–655

[9] Kumar K. Did the modern concept of axial traction to correct scoliosis exist in prehistoric times? J Neurol Orthop Med Surg. 1987; 8:309–310

[10] Satapatha Brahmana. Part XII.2,4,12,14

[11] Martin RB. The origin of biomechanics. http://www.asbweb .org/about-bio-mechanics. Accessed October 19, 2015

[12] Braun GL. Kinesiology: from Aristotle to the twentieth century. Res Q. 1941; 12(2):164–173

[13] Hippocrates. On joints. In: Capps E, Page TE, Ruse WH, eds. Hippocrates: The Loeb Classical Library. Vol. 3. London, UK: W. Heinemann; 1927:200–397

[14] Naderi S, Andalkar N, Benzel EC. History of spine biomechanics: part I—the pre-Greco-Roman, Greco-Roman, and medieval roots of spine biomechanics. Neurosurgery. 2007; 60(2):382–390, discussion 390–391

[15] Dugas R. A History of Mechanics. New York, NY: Dover; 1988

[16] Goodrich JT. History of spine surgery in the ancient and medieval worlds. Neurosurg Focus. 2004; 16(1):E2

[17] Vasiliadis ES, Grivas TB, Kaspiris A. Historical overview of spinal deformities in ancient Greece. Scoliosis. 2009; 4:6

[18] Gurunluoglu R, Gurunluoglu A. Paul of Aegina: landmark in surgical progress. World J Surg. 2003; 27(1):18–25

[19] Naderi S, Acar F, Mertol T, Arda MN. Functional anatomy of the spine by Avicenna in his eleventh century treatise Al-Qanun fi al-Tibb (The canons of medicine). Neurosurgery. 2003; 52(6):1449–1453, discussion 1453–1454

[20] Aciduman A, Belen D, Simsek S. Management of spinal disorders and trauma in Avicenna's canon of medicine. Neurosurgery. 2006; 59(2):397–403, discussion 397–403

[21] Spink MS, Lewis GL. Albucasis, on Surgery and Instruments: A Definitive Edition of the Arabic Text with English Translation and Commentary. London, UK: The Wellcome Institute of the History of Medicine; 1973

[22] Naderi S, Acar F, Arda MN. History of spinal disorders and cerrahiyetülhaniye: a review of a Turkish treatise written by Şerefeddin Sabuncuoğlu in 15th century. J Neurosurg. 2002; 96:352–356

[23] Benini A, Bonar SK. Andreas Vesalius 1514-1564. Spine. 1996; 21(11):1388–1393, 1514–1564

[24] Novell JR. From da Vinci to Harvey: the development of mechanical analogy in medicine from 1500 to 1650. J R Soc Med. 1990; 83(6):396–398

[25] Maquet P. Iatrophysics to biomechanics. from Borelli (1608–1679) to Pauwels (1885–1980). J Bone Joint Surg Br. 1992; 74(3):335–339

[26] Middleton WEK. A little-known portrait of Giovanni Alfonso Borelli. Med Hist. 1974; 18(1):94–95

[27] Gribbin J. Science: A History. London, UK: Penguin; 2003:1453–2001

[28] Richardson JA. History of biomechanics and kinesiology. http://biomechanics. vtheatre.net/doc/history.html. Accessed October 19, 2015

[29] Gruber P, Boeni T. History of spinal disorders. In: Boos N, Aebi M, eds. Spinal Disorders: Fundamentals of Diagnosis and Treatment. Berlin, Germany: Springer; 2008:1–35

[30] Weber W, Weber E. Die Mechanics of the Human Walking Apparatus (Mechanics of the Human Walking Apparatus) (in German). Böttingen, Germany: Dietrich; 1836

[31] Weber EH. Anatomical and physiological tests on some systems of human spine mechanism (in German). Arch Anat Physiol. 1827; 1:240–271

[32] Braune W, Fischer O. Der gang des menschen (Human gait) (in German). Saech Gesellsch Wissensch. 1895; 21:153–322

[33] Duval-Beaupère G, Schmidt C, Cosson P. A barycentremetric study of the sagittal shape of spine and pelvis: the conditions required for an economic standing position. Ann Biomed Eng. 1992; 20(4):451–462

[34] Skedros JG, Brand RA. Biographical sketch: Georg Hermann von Meyer (1815–1892). Clin Orthop Relat Res. 2011; 469(11):3072–3076

[35] Wolff J. The Law of Bone Remodelling (in German) Berlin, Germany: Verlag von August Hirschwald; 1892:419–426

[36] Amar J. The Human Motor, or the Scientific Foundation of Labour and Industry. New York, NY: Routledge; 1920

[37] Drewlinger DM. Biomechanics: Emergence of an Academic Discipline in the United States. Denton, TX: Texas Woman's University; 1996

[38] Delmas A, Depreux R. Spinal curves and intervertebral foramina. Rev Rhum Mal Osteoartic. 1953; 20(1):25–29

[39] Stagnara P, De Mauroy JC, Dran G, et al. Reciprocal angulation of vertebral bodies in a sagittal plane: approach to references for the evaluation of kyphosis and lordosis. Spine. 1982; 7(4):335–342

[40] Itoi E. Roentgenographic analysis of posture in spinal osteoporotics. Spine. 1991; 16(7):750–756

[41] Takemitsu Y, Harada Y, Iwahara T, Miyamoto M, Miyatake Y. Lumbar degenerative kyphosis. Clinical, radiological and epidemiological studies. Spine. 1988; 13(11):1317–1326

[42] Jackson RP, Hales C. Congruent spinopelvic alignment on standing lateral radiographs of adult volunteers. Spine. 2000; 25(21):2808–2815

[43] Preston CB, Evans WG, Rumbak A. An evaluation of two methods used to determine the centre of gravity of a cadaver head in the sagittal plane. J Dent Assoc S Afr. 1996; 51(12):787–793

[44] Shirazi-Adl A, Parnianpour M. Role of posture in mechanics of the lumbar spine in compression. J Spinal Disord. 1996; 9(4):277–286

[45] Vernazza S, Alexandrov A, Massion J. Is the center of gravity controlled during upper trunk movements? Neurosci Lett. 1996; 206(2–3):77–80

[46] Vital JM, Senegas J. Anatomical bases of the study of the constraints to which the cervical spine is subject in the sagittal plane. A study of the center of gravity of the head. Surg Radiol Anat. 1986; 8(3):169–173

[47] Richards BS, Birch JG, Herring JA, Johnston CE, Roach JW. Frontal plane and sagittal plane balance following Cotrel-Dubousset instrumentation for idiopathic scoliosis. Spine. 1989; 14(7):733–737

[48] El Fegoun AB, Schwab F, Gamez L, Champain N, Skalli W, Farcy JP. Center of gravity and radiographic posture analysis: a preliminary review of adult volunteers and adult patients affected by scoliosis. Spine. 2005; 30(13):1535–1540

[49] Schwab F, Lafage V, Boyce R, Skalli W, Farcy JP. Gravity line analysis in adult volunteers: age-related correlation with spinal parameters, pelvic parameters, and foot position. Spine. 2006; 31(25):E959–E967

[50] Lafage V, Schwab F, Skalli W, et al. Standing balance and sagittal plane spinal deformity: analysis of spinopelvic and gravity line parameters. Spine. 2008; 33(14):1572–1578

[51] Vaz G, Roussouly P, Berthonnaud E, Dimnet J. Sagittal morphology and equilibrium of pelvis and spine. Eur Spine J. 2002; 11(1):80–87

[52] Mangione P, Sénégas J. Sagittal balance of the spine. Rev Chir Orthop Repar Appar Mot. 1997; 83(1):22–32

[53] Yoshimoto H, Sato S, Masuda T, et al. Spinopelvic alignment in patients with osteoarthrosis of the hip: a radiographic comparison to patients with low back pain. Spine. 2005; 30(14):1650–1657

[54] Lazennec JY, Brusson A, Rousseau MA. Hip-spine relations and sagittal balance clinical consequences. Eur Spine J. 2011; 20 Suppl 5:686–698

[55] Lazennec JY, Riwan A, Gravez F, et al. Hip spine relationships: application to total hip arthroplasty. Hip Int. 2007; 17 Suppl 5:S91–S104

[56] Trojani C, Chaumet-Lagrange VA, Hovorka E, Carles M, Boileau P. Simultaneous bilateral total hip arthroplasty: literature review and preliminary results [in French]. Rev Chir Orthop Repar Appar Mot. 2006; 92(8):760–767

[57] Le Huec JC, Cogniet A, Demezon H, Rigal J, Saddiki R, Aunoble S. Insufficient restoration of lumbar lordosis and FBI index following pedicle subtraction osteotomy is an indicator of likely mechanical complication. Eur Spine J. 2015; 24 Suppl 1:S112–S120

[58] Graf H, Hecquet J, Dubousset J. 3-dimensional approach to spinal deformities. Application to the study of the prognosis of pediatric scoliosis. Rev Chir Orthop Repar Appar Mot. 1983; 69(5):407–416

[59] Lafage V, Dubousset J, Lavaste F, Skalli W. 3D finite element simulation of Cotrel–Dubousset correction. Comput Aided Surg. 2004; 9(1–2):17–25

[60] Courvoisier A, Drevelle X, Vialle R, Dubousset J, Skalli W. 3D analysis of brace treatment in idiopathic scoliosis. Eur Spine J. 2013; 22(11):2449–2455

[61] Berthonnaud E, Labelle H, Roussouly P, Grimard G, Vaz G, Dimnet J. A variability study of computerized sagittal spinopelvic radiologic measurements of trunk balance. J Spinal Disord Tech. 2005; 18(1):66–71

[62] Cotrel Y, Dubousset J. A new technic for segmental spinal osteosynthesis using the posterior approach. Rev Chir Orthop Repar Appar Mot. 1984; 70 (6):489–494

[63] Farcy JP, Roye DP, Weidenbaum M. Cotrel-Dubousset instrumentation technique for revision of failed lumbosacral fusion. Bull Hosp Jt Dis Orthop Inst. 1987; 47(1):1–12

[64] Illés T, Somoskeöy S. Comparison of scoliosis measurements based on three-dimensional vertebra vectors and conventional two-dimensional measurements: advantages in evaluation of prognosis and surgical results. Eur Spine J. 2013; 22(6):1255–1263

[65] Berthonnaud E, Papin P, Deceuninck J, Hilmi R, Bernard JC, Dimnet J. The use of a photogrammetric method for the three-dimensional evaluation of spinal correction in scoliosis. Int Orthop. 2016; 40(6):1187–1196

[66] Pinel-Giroux FM, Mac-Thiong JM, de Guise JA, Berthonnaud E, Labelle H. Computerized assessment of sagittal curvatures of the spine: comparison between Cobb and tangent circles techniques. J Spinal Disord Tech. 2006; 19 (7):507–512

[67] Vialle R, Ilharreborde B, Dauzac C, Guigui P. Intra and inter-observer reliability of determining degree of pelvic incidence in high-grade spondylolisthesis using a computer assisted method. Eur Spine J. 2006; 15(10): 1449–1453

[68] Rajnics P, Templier A, Skalli W, Lavaste F, Illés T. The association of sagittal spinal and pelvic parameters in asymptomatic persons and patients with isthmic spondylolisthesis. J Spinal Disord Tech. 2002; 15(1):24–30

[69] Dumas R, Steib JP, Mitton D, Lavaste F, Skalli W. Three-dimensional quantitative segmental analysis of scoliosis corrected by the in situ contouring technique. Spine. 2003; 28(11):1158–1162

[70] Labelle H, Roussouly P, Berthonnaud E, et al. Spondylolisthesis, pelvic incidence, and spinopelvic balance: a correlation study. Spine. 2004; 29 (18):2049–2054

[71] Rajnics P, Pomero V, Templier A, Lavaste F, Illes T. Computer-assisted assessment of spinal sagittal plane radiographs. J Spinal Disord. 2001; 14(2):135–142

2 The Acquisition of Human Verticality

Christine Tardieu and Martin Haeusler

Abstract

The shift from facultative to permanent bipedalism was a pivotal step in human evolution. Skeletal adaptations to efficient sagittal balance of the trunk are therefore key to identify fossils as our ancestors, the hominids. Morphological modifications of the pelvis and spine had a major role in this process. Here, we review these evolutionary adaptations that resulted in the formation of the spinopelvic functional unit. We suggest that the double S-shape of the vertebral column evolved secondary to the functionally linked pelvic modifications. Together with the lumbar lordosis, the approximation of the sacroiliac and hip joints brought the center of body mass closer to the hip joints, thus minimizing muscular work to maintain equilibrium. A prerequisite for the adoption of lumbar lordosis in early hominids was a long and mobile lumbar spine. As great apes have a rigid spine with three to four lumbar vertebrae, different scenarios have been proposed for the evolution of the human spinal segmentation. We argue that the common ancestor of chimpanzees and humans already possessed five lumbar vertebrae, and a pelvic incidence of ~ 30° that increased during evolution as the sacro-acetabular distance decreased. The strong correlation in humans between pelvic incidence and lumbar lordosis points toward an elaborated functional link that was shaped by natural selection. A review of the hominid fossil record, including *Sahelanthropus, Orrorin, Ardipithecus ramidus, Australopithecus afarensis, Australopithecus africanus, Australopithecus sediba, Homo erectus*, and Neanderthals, suggests that this link between pelvis and spine was probably only established with *H. erectus* 1.5 million years ago.

Keywords: bipedalism, hominid evolution, lumbar lordosis, pelvis, sagittal balance, spine

2.1 Introduction

The adaptation to bipedalism represents the primary change during human evolution that permits to diagnose fossils as our ancestors, the hominids. This group includes all forms in the lineage leading to modern humans after the split from the chimpanzee lineage some 5 to 8 million years ago. Adaptation to bipedalism therefore occurred long before the production of stone tools, the loss of dense body hair, and the increase in brain size.

Nonhuman primates live mostly in trees and show a diverse locomotor repertoire. This polyvalence with versatile locomotor abilities is therefore also expected in our earliest hominid ancestors. Their varied arboreal locomotor repertoire included quadrupedalism, vertical climbing, suspension, and occasional bipedalism. It was the percentage of terrestrial bipedalism that increased in our first ancestors in relation to the environment, together with its advantages and its constraints. Only later during human evolution, our ancestors became permanent bipeds, which represents a strong specialization.

Sagittal balance of the trunk over the hip joints is essential for efficient bipedal locomotion. Consequently, its acquisition during the evolution of hominids was crucial in the shift from a facultative to a permanent form of bipedalism. The modification of the sagittal morphology of the pelvis and spine played a major role in the process of this evolutionary adaptation, which resulted in the formation of a spinopelvic functional unit.[1] We suggest that the double S-shape of the vertebral column, often considered as one of the most important evolutionary adaptations to bipedal locomotion, evolved secondary to the functionally linked modifications of the pelvis.

2.2 Compared Anatomy: The Axial Skeleton in Quadrupeds, Apes, and Hominids

To understand and interpret the evolution of the human morphology, we must use the tool of comparative anatomy. Here, we focus on a comparison of quadrupeds, great apes, and humans with australopithecines. This group of fossil hominids lived in South and East Africa 2 to 4 million years ago and is considered to represent the first true bipeds. Their growth period was short and they became mature at an age of around 12 years, similar to chimpanzees.

In the sagittal view, the skeletons of a quadrupedal monkey, a great ape, and a human reveal very different body proportions (▶ Fig. 2.1a). The prehensile foot of macaques and gorillas contrasts with the human foot that is strongly adapted to provide support and propulsion during bipedal locomotion. The cranial capacity is around 400 to 600 cm³ in great apes, while the mean is 1400 cm³ in modern humans (▶ Fig. 2.1b). Facial prognathism is strong in great apes and the canines are very salient. The occipital foramen is positioned posteriorly in the cranial base, and the nuchal musculature is powerful. This cranial morphology results in a distinctive balance of the head on the cervical spine. Australopithecines have a cranial capacity of around 400 cm³, which implies an increased brain size relative to their small body size compared to great apes. The prognathism is reduced, the position of the occipital foramen is more anterior and the nuchal musculature is modified. The small canines are aligned with the other teeth.

2.2.1 Pelvis and Rib Cage in Frontal View

Pelvis

In frontal view, the marked reduction of the distance between the hip joint and the sacroiliac joint is clearly visible in humans. This played a key role in the evolution of bipedalism and was present in australopithecine pelves (▶ Fig. 2.1c). The approximation between the sacroiliac and hip joints reduces the rotational moments of the iliac segment transmitting trunk weight to the lower limbs, thus reducing muscular work to maintain the equilibrium.[2]

Another important difference is the loss of the tail in hominoids (i.e., great apes and humans). Monkeys such as macaques

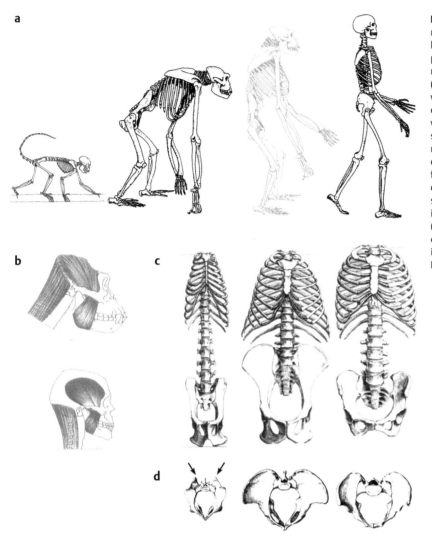

Fig. 2.1 Skeletal differences among quadrupedal monkeys, great apes, and humans. **(a)** macaque, knuckle-walking gorilla, fictive gorilla in bipedal posture with bent hips and bent knees, and modern human (adapted from Ref. 52). **(b)** Differences in head posture: head of a gorilla with projecting face, powerful jaws, strong chewing muscles, and strong neck muscles, whereas modern humans show a reduced facial skeleton with relatively weak chewing and neck muscles. **(c)** Trunk skeleton: narrow thorax and elongated lumbar spine in a macaque; broad, funnel-shaped thorax, short lumbar spine and elongated ilium in a chimpanzee, and barrel-shaped thorax with long lumbar spine and short ilium in modern humans (adapted from Ref. 5). **(d)** Cranial view of the pelvis of a macaque, chimpanzee, and modern human; arrows, strong iliac tuberosities in macaque (adapted from Ref. 5).

possess a long tail with strong caudal muscles that originate on the sacrum. Their erector spinae muscles are inserted on the very developed iliac tuberosities (► Fig. 2.1d). In hominoids that have lost their tail, the erector spinae is inserted on the iliac crest and the sacrum. Humans differ from great apes by a broad sacrum with an extended insertion area of the erector spinae. The entire iliac blade of great apes and humans is considerably broader than that of monkeys. In the brachiating great apes, this provides an extensive area of origin for the latissimus dorsi and the quadratus lumborum, important muscles that support the trunk and pelvis during arm suspension (► Fig. 2.1d). In humans, the latissimus dorsi has a smaller area of origin, and the iliac crest can be divided in three sections that provide origin for the muscles balancing the trunk. From the lateral section of the iliac blade originate the oblique and transverse abdominal muscles, in the intermediate section latissimus dorsi and quadratus lumborum, and in the medial section the trunk erectors and gluteus maximus (► Fig. 2.2). While in great apes the origin of the gluteus maximus does not reach higher than the base of the sacrum, it has in humans a very high origin on the pelvis at the level of the iliac crest. The capacity of this muscle for trunk erection is thus far greater in humans than in great apes (► Fig. 2.2).

Humans also have an anteriorly curved lateral section of the iliac blades that modified the position of the lesser gluteal muscles. They thus became abductors on an extended hip while they were medial rotators on a flexed hip in great apes. This implies a different mechanism of lateral pelvic balance during bipedalism[3] (► Fig. 2.1).

The pelvis of australopithecines has laterally flaring and frontally oriented iliac blades similar to great apes with an extensive area of origin of the latissimus dorsi.[4] This implies a different hip abductor mechanism and thus a different mode of bipedalism than in modern humans.[3] On the other hand, they resemble the human condition in having a broad sacrum, and the gluteus maximus muscle originated from the posterior ilium.[4]

Rib Cage

The rib cage is funnel-shaped in great apes and barrel-shaped in modern humans[5] (► Fig. 2.1c). This conforms to the wide and frontally oriented iliac blades in great apes and an anteriorly curved iliac crest in modern humans. The long and robust last rib of great apes provides an ideal attachment for the quadratus lumborum. Together with the reduced gap between the thorax and the iliac crest, this provides the necessary rigidity for the

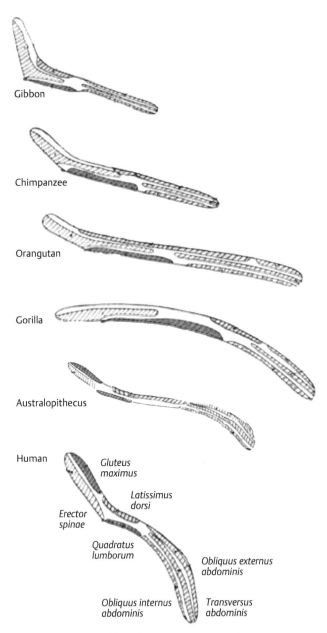

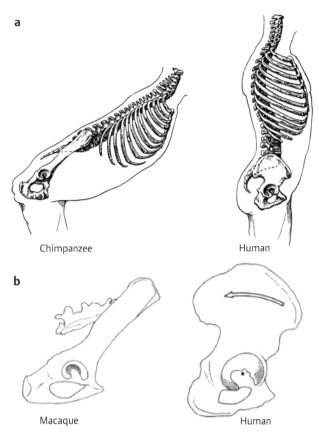

Fig. 2.2 Iliac crest with muscle origins. Great apes show an extensive area of origin of latissimus dorsi and quadratus lumborum that are important during forelimb dominated locomotion, while in hominids gluteus maximus also originates on the ilium (adapted from Ref. 53).

Fig. 2.3 Spinal curvature and pelvis. (a) Nonhuman primates possess a single thoracolumbar curve, while humans additionally have a marked lumbar lordosis that contributes to bring the center of body weight close to the hip joint (adapted from Ref. 55). (b) In humans, the sacrum, ischium, and pubis are oriented similar to quadrupeds, whereas the ilium is curved lordotically, leading to the development of the greater sciatic notch (adapted from Ref. 2).

trunk in the forelimb-dominated locomotion of great apes.[6] Humans have a relatively wide upper thoracic aperture. This allows a greater respiratory efficiency and heavy breathing used for running while it reduces shoulder mobility. On the other hand, the lower thorax is narrower compared to great apes, and together with the longer lumbar spine this leads to a slim waistline. This plays an important role for our ability to run as it allows to exploit the greater flexibility of the lumbar spine.[6]

Australopithecines such as the 3.2 million years old Lucy (*Australopithecus afarensis*, Ethiopia), also show a funnel-shaped thorax. Together with their cranially oriented shoulder girdle, this reflects their adaptation for climbing that they retained from

the common ancestor with chimpanzees.[6,7] However, these characters make them unable to run long distances.[6,7]

2.2.2 Sagittal View of Spine and Pelvis

Spine

Spinal Curvature

Modern humans have a double S-shaped vertebral column with four curvatures (i.e., a cervical lordosis, a thoracic kyphosis, a lumbar lordosis, and a sacral kyphosis). Great apes, in contrast, possess a weak kyphotic thoracolumbar curvature and a relatively short and stiff neck, which mainly results from a highly positioned shoulder girdle and massive pectoral muscles[6] (▶ Fig. 2.1, ▶ Fig. 2.3). In association with a narrow sacrum and a short lumbar column there is an "entrapment" of the lumbar vertebrae between the iliac blades in great apes and thus a reduced lumbar mobility.

Number of Vertebrae

The length of the spinal regions and particularly of the lumbar region plays an important role for its mobility and capacity for lordosis. A long lumbar region is thought to be fundamental for having facilitated the adoption of bipedal locomotion in early hominids. The evolution of a human-like segmentation of the vertebral column is therefore of particular interest. In primates, the total number of precaudal vertebrae is surprisingly stable at 29. Quadrupedal monkeys have 12 to 13 thoracic vertebrae coupled with a long and flexible lumbar spine of six to seven elements and a short sacrum of three segments (▶ Fig. 2.1).[5] This allows them extensive flexion–extension movements needed for quadrupedal climbing, running, and springing. In contrast, apes show a stiffer and more rigid trunk adapted to forelimb-dominated locomotion. By integrating the last one or two lumbar vertebrae into the sacrum, their lumbar spine is accordingly reduced to five segments in gibbons and to four in orangutans, chimpanzees, and gorillas, while the sacrum became compensatorily elongated to four in gibbons and five elements in great apes on average.[5] A large percentage of chimpanzees and gorillas even possesses only three lumbar vertebrae and a correspondingly elongated sacrum. Such vertebral border shifts are associated with alterations in the expression of Hox genes that control the regional identity of vertebrae.

Another border shift occurred at the thoracolumbar junction in the ancestors of modern humans, leading to 12 thoracic and 5 lumbar segments on average, which makes the lumbar spine longer and more flexible than in great apes. This flexibility is a prerequisite for our lumbar lordosis, which cannot be achieved with the short and stiff lumbar spine of chimpanzees and gorillas. Different scenarios have been proposed for the evolution of this characteristic of modern humans: the short-backed scenario[8] suggests that the short lumbar column of chimpanzees and gorillas is primitive. The long-backed scenario proposes that a six-segment-long lumbar spine was retained in the ancestors of apes and humans.[9] This hypothesis was rejected by the discovery of new vertebral fossils that demonstrate the presence of five lumbar vertebrae in early hominids and not six as claimed before.[10,11,12] We therefore argue for an intermediate scenario with five lumbar vertebrae as the primitive condition in great apes and humans. Such a scenario is further supported by *Oreopithecus*, a great ape that lived 8 million years ago in Italy and also had five lumbar vertebrae.[13] The scenario has the advantage that the last common ancestor of chimpanzees and humans already had five lumbar vertebrae, which facilitated the adoption of lumbar lordosis and thus of bipedal locomotion.

Orientation of Facet Joints at the Thoracolumbar Junction

Early hominids seem to have differed from humans in the orientation of the facet joints at the thoracolumbar junction. In modern humans, the transition from thoracic to lumbar-like orientation is usually at T12, but in up to 40% of the population at T11. In contrast, all early hominid fossils show the transition at T11,[11,12,14,15] and it is likely that in the future hominid fossils will be discovered with the transitional vertebra at T10. Lumbar-like facet joints allow flexion–extension but restrict spinal rotation, while thoracic-like facet joints do not restrict mobility. The functional implication of a more cranially located transitional vertebra in early hominids might be related to a greater rotational stability of the trunk.[16] This might represent a climbing adaptation in early hominids, while a greater rotational capacity was needed in later *Homo* for running.

Pelvis

Quadrupedal-Like Orientation of the Human Sacrum, Ischium, and Pubis (▶ Fig. 2.3)

Very early it was noticed that the longitudinal axis of the sacrum is only slightly inclined with respect to the horizontal plane in upright standing humans, thus closely corresponding to the spatial orientation in quadrupeds (▶ Fig. 2.3a).[17] Also, the longitudinal axis of the pubis and ischium has retained the same angulation with the femur as in quadrupeds; only the ilium axis is bent backward (▶ Fig. 2.3b). It has, therefore, been asserted that the acquisition of upright posture in hominids occurred only above the pelvis with the lumbar lordosis, and that the hominid lower pelvis is essentially that of quadrupeds. Because of the relatively stiff lumbar spine of great apes, they have to rotate their trunk in the hip joints when they want to stand up on their hind legs (▶ Fig. 2.1a). This brings the ischium into a vertical orientation, which would offset the lever arm of the hamstrings if the femur is fully extended, and forces great apes to stand upright with bent hips and bent knees.[2] The quadrupedal-like posteroinferior angulation of the ischium in modern humans is therefore important for preserving an optimal lever arm for the hamstrings as extensors of the hip joint, and the backward rotated ilium together with the S-shaped curvature of the spine is crucial to shift the whole trunk backward, thus bringing the body's center of gravity close to the hip joints.[2]

The Angle of Pelvic Incidence in Human and Nonhuman Primates

The interpretation of the sagittal aspect of the pelvis was greatly aided by the description of the angle of pelvic incidence by the research team of G. Duval-Beaupère in Paris. This new pelvic parameter was initially called "angle of sacral incidence."[18,19,20] It is defined by the line from the midpoint between the two femoral heads to the center of the upper surface of the sacrum and perpendicular to the upper surface of the sacrum (▶ Fig. 2.4a). The incidence angle is an anatomical variable that is specific to each individual. It represents the sum of the two positional parameters, sacral slope (α) and pelvic tilt (β), and determines the amount of lordosis that provides the most economical upright posture for each individual at a given pelvic tilt in terms of muscle fatigue and vertebral strain.

The first paper that introduced the pelvic incidence in (palaeo) anthropology was published in 2006 by Tardieu et al.[21] It described the variability of the angle of incidence and its correlation with other pelvic parameters in an osteological sample of 51 macerated adult modern human pelves (of 26 men and 25 women) (▶ Fig. 2.4b). This study showed that a low angle of incidence is correlated with a weak sacral slope, a less curved sacrum, and a higher sacral position in relation to the iliac crests. A high angle of incidence is correlated with a strong sacral slope, a curved sacrum, and a low position of the sacrum in relation to the iliac crests. These observations were confirmed by the negative correlation obtained between incidence and sacroacetabular distance (pelvic thickness) (-0.52, p < 0.0001). A tendency to a backward displacement of the sacrum in relation to the acetabulum is observed with a high pelvic incidence.

Tardieu et al.[22] compared intact pelves of newborns and adults. The mean angle of incidence was 27° in the newborns

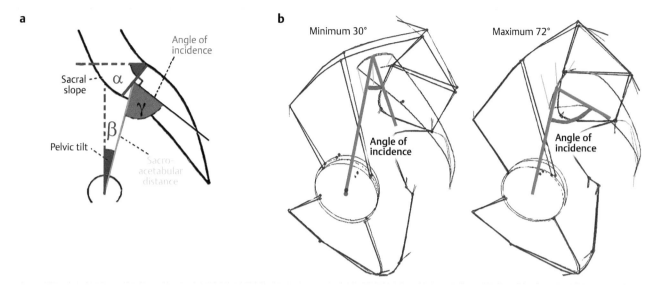

Fig. 2.4 Angle of pelvic incidence. **(a)** Description of the pelvic incidence. **(b)** Relationship of the angle of incidence, sacral slope, and sacro-acetabular distance (see text for details; for methods, see Refs. 21 and 22; figures adapted from Ref. 1).

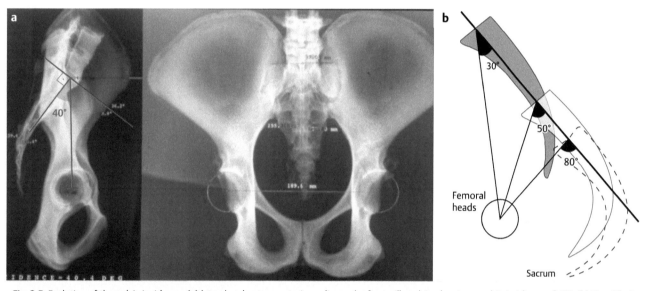

Fig. 2.5 Evolution of the pelvic incidence. **(a)** lateral and anteroposterior radiograph of a gorilla pelvis, showing a pelvic incidence of 40°. **(b)** Simplified model of pelvic evolution. The sacral slope is kept constant to emphasize the inverse relationship of the sacro-acetabular distance with increasing incidence (adapted from Ref. 1).

compared to 54° in the adults. The newborn pelves showed a correspondingly low sacral slope and the sacrum was straight and anchored high upon the ilia. In lateral view, the plane through the centers of the superior sacral surface and the hip joints was almost parallel to the plane of Lewinnek and thus aligned vertically. As this configuration does not favor the balance of the trunk, the sacrum moves backward from gait acquisition until the end of the growth period. At the same time, the sacrum rotates anteriorly, so that it becomes more horizontally in its cranial part and more curved caudally.

Radiographic measurements of the angle of incidence of nonhuman primates were presented by Tardieu et al.[21,22] In nonhuman primates, the pelvic incidence is small and always inferior to 40° as expected from the long distance between the sacroiliac and hip joints (▶ Fig. 2.5a; see also Table 4 in Ref. [1]).

It is important to specify that this angle does not offer any correlation with the spinal curvature in nonhuman primates.

Sagittal Model of the Evolution of the Pelvis

We proposed a simplified model of the evolution of the pelvis in lateral view (▶ Fig. 2.5b).[1] Because the mean angle of incidence of great apes seems to be identical to that of quadrupedal monkeys such as baboons, it can be hypothesized that the last common ancestor of chimpanzees and hominids also possessed a pelvic incidence between 30° and 40°. Corresponding to the inverse relationship between the angle of incidence and the sacro-acetabular distance observed both during the growth of the human pelvis and within adults, we proposed a similar inverse relationship in hominid evolution. While the angle of incidence progressively increased, the sacro-acetabular distance decreased at the same time by a more and more backward positioned superior sacral surface in relation to the hip joints. We also suggested that the increase in incidence would have been under positive selection at the same time as the distance between the sacroiliac and hip joints was reduced, as it provided a clear advantage to improve sagittal balance of the trunk during bipedal walking in early hominids. For the interpretation of hominid fossils, it is very important to recall the fundamental positive correlation that links the angles of incidence and lumbar lordosis in extant humans[1] ($R = 0.55$, $p < 0.0001$). This correlation establishes a functional link between the spine and the pelvis, which distinguishes the spinal balance of humans from extant nonhuman primates during occasional bipedalism. The association between two very different elements, the mobile vertebral column and the rigid pelvis, is a critical process of functional integration. Moreover, it is very delicate to decipher this process as it becomes only manifest during postnatal growth in tight association with gait acquisition and takes place very progressively. Are we able to recognize some traces of the establishment of this crucial link in the history of fossil hominids?

2.3 Interpretation of Hominid Fossils

In this chapter, we present hominid fossils that preserve an associated pelvis and spine or give other indications for sagittal balance. The earliest claimed hominid fossils still had a very polyvalent locomotor repertoire and their taxinomic interpretation is controversial. This includes *Sahelanthropus*, which is known from a 7-million-year-old crushed skull from Chad. Based on an anteriorly placed foramen magnum, it was inferred that *Sahelanthropus* walked bipedally upright.[23] However, the skull needed extensive reconstruction and the neck musculature seems to have been unusually powerful for a biped, which raised doubts regarding its hominid status.[24]

The second oldest early hominid fossil is *Orrorin tugenensis*, which was found in 6-million-year-old sediments in Kenya. *Orrorin* is mainly known from skull and teeth fragments as well as isolated femora. They have been described to show evidence for upright bipedalism, including an elongated femoral neck and an asymmetric distribution of cortex in the femoral neck.[25]

A more complete, though severely crushed skeleton is known for the 4.4-million-year-old *Ardipithecus ramidus* from Ethiopia. With limb proportions similar to monkeys, it was a palmigrade tree climber, and showed no adaptations for suspensory or knuckle-walking behavior characteristic of living great apes. Although lumbar vertebrae are not preserved, the relatively short ilium associated with a wide sacrum does suggest that *Ardipithecus* did not have a rigid lumbar spine. The morphology of this hominid would thus imply that a long ilium that entraps the last lumbar vertebrae, a narrow sacrum, and a reduced number of lumbar vertebrae are derived rather than primitive characteristics in great apes (i.e., they were acquired during the course of evolution of gorillas and chimpanzees rather than present in the last common ancestor of chimpanzees and hominids).[26] It is, however, also conceivable that *Ardipithecus ramidus* belonged to an extinct ape genus not closely related to the human lineage.[27]

The earliest fossils that are undisputedly hominids belong to australopithecines. Their pelvis demonstrates a human-like reduction of the sacro-acetabular distance and a pelvic incidence close to the mean of modern humans. The reconstructions of Häusler and Schmid[28] indicates an incidence of approximately 52° in the 3.2-million-year-old Lucy skeleton AL 288–1 (*A. afarensis*), 45°–54° in the 2.4 million-year-old Sts 14 (*Australopithecus africanus*), and 50° in the 2.0-million-year-old MH2 *Australopithecus sediba*[29] (▶ Fig. 2.6).

The Lucy skeleton preserves six thoracic and a midlumbar vertebra. Other partial skeletons with vertebral columns are Sts 14 and Stw 431 (*A. africanus*)[10] as well as the *A. sediba* skeletons

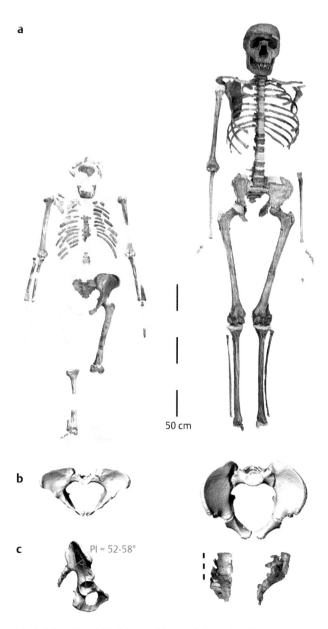

Fig. 2.6 Fossil hominid skeletons. **(a)** Lucy skeleton (AL 288–1, *Australopithecus afarensis*) and KNM-WT 15000 (*Homo erectus*). **(b)** Superior view of the pelvis of Lucy and a modern human. **(c)** Lateral view of Lucy and frontal and sagittal view of the sacrum and lower lumbar vertebrae of MH2 (*Australopithecus sediba*) (adapted from Ref. 14).

MH1 and MH2.[14] Their vertebral wedging suggests a well-developed lumbar lordosis that was made up of five lumbar vertebrae as in modern humans[11,12] (► Fig. 2.7). Both Lucy and Sts 14 show changes suggestive of Scheuermann's disease[30] and several isolated australopithecine vertebrae show similar

alterations.[31] This high prevalence of Scheuermann's disease might indicate a greater loading of the vertebral column during juvenile growth period than in modern humans, which is perhaps related to the relatively small cross-sectional area of the early hominid vertebrae[31] (► Fig. 2.8).

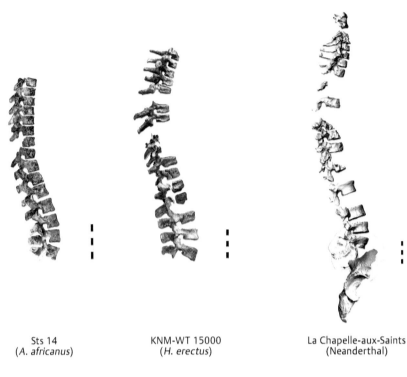

Sts 14
(*A. africanus*)

KNM-WT 15000
(*H. erectus*)

La Chapelle-aux-Saints
(Neanderthal)

Fig. 2.7 Fossil hominid vertebral columns: Sts 14 (*Australopithecus africanus*), KNM-WT 15000 (*Homo erectus*), and the Neanderthal from La Chapelle-aux-Saints showing well-developed spinal curvatures (adapted from Ref. 54).

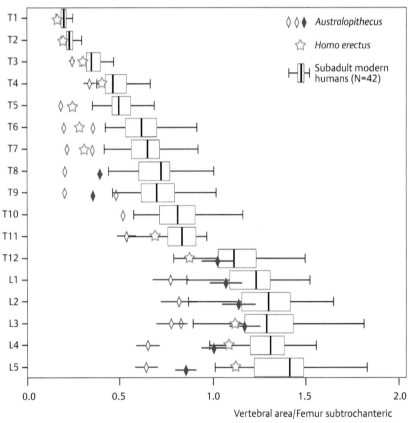

Fig. 2.8 Superior endplate area of the vertebrae relative to proximal femur size as a measure for body size for *Australopithecus* (open diamonds, AL 288–1; light blue diamonds, Sts 14; dark blue diamonds, Stw 431), *Homo erectus* (stars, KNM-WT 15000), and subadult modern humans (box plots).

The human-like pelvic incidence in australopithecines, on the other hand, does not necessarily imply that they possessed an identical spinopelvic balance as modern humans. Thus, the large, funnel-shaped thorax and the prominent face suggest a more ventrally located center of body weight, and their frontally oriented ilium implies a different mechanism of lateral pelvic stabilization. With its short lower limbs, *Australopithecus* was not as adapted to long distance walking and running (e.g., *Homo erectus*). *Australopithecus* was therefore called a "compromise biped" who still possessed a surprisingly versatile locomotor repertoir.[32] The modern human-like functional link between the pelvis and the vertebral curvatures therefore seems to have been a long process of trial and error. The strong correlation between lordosis and incidence in extant humans is tightly linked with our exclusive bipedalism and stereotypical gait pattern, expressed by periodicity of the movement.[33,34] Before the acquisition of a regular and stereotypical gait, the correlation was likely absent or only weak. A progressively stronger correlation was only established when bipedalism became a major element within the locomotor repertoire so that early hominids became "committed" bipeds and developed a similarly specialized postcranial morphology.[32]

H. erectus is known by the almost complete skeleton KNM-WT 15000, which is dated to 1.5 million years ago. Its skeletal age is roughly similar to a 15-year-old modern human boy, and it demonstrates that the growth period in *H. erectus* was longer than in *Australopithecus*.[35] It only misses the first six cervical and two midthoracic vertebrae and displays fully human-like body proportions and thoracic shape.[36] This is confirmed by a reanalysis of KNM-WT 15000 that refutes earlier claims for disproportions because of congenital skeletal dysplasia but indicates that this individual suffered from juvenile disk herniation.[11,12,37,38,39,40] *H. erectus* demonstrates an almost modern bauplan of the axial skeleton. Its long lower limbs emphasize its capacity for running. *H. erectus*, therefore, can be considered an obligate biped with a posture and mode of locomotion close to modern humans. Although there are some uncertainties in Walker and Ruff's[41] reconstruction of the KNM-WT 15000 sacroiliac joint, its pelvic incidence of about 49°–52° is close to the mean of the modern human range of variation.[22] A recent new reconstruction of its pelvis will provide more precise insight into the mode of walking and running of this individual.[42] A second *H. erectus* pelvis, an adult female from Gona, Ethiopia, has a very similar incidence angle of 48°–50°.[22] Interestingly, however, the wedging angles of lumbar vertebrae L3-L5 of KNM-WT 15000 are in the upper range of modern humans, while the degree of anterior wedging at L1 also clearly exceeds the mean of modern humans.[39] This might imply a more marked lumbar lordosis in this specimen than on average today, and thus a stronger curve than expected from the pelvic incidence.

Neanderthals are the successors of *H. erectus* and lived in Europe and large parts of Asia between about 400,000 and 40,000 years ago. Several different skeletons have been discovered. One of the earliest fossils of the Neanderthal lineage from Spain shows an isthmic spondylolisthesis at L5,[43] a typical pathology that is exclusively associated with bipedalism.[44] Moreover, the lumbar vertebrae of this individual are anteriorly wedged and elongated, which is suggestive of the lumbar form of Scheuermann's disease.

All Neanderthals have been described to possess a much weaker cervical lordosis, thoracic kyphosis, and lumbar lordosis than modern humans and their pelvic incidence is said to be in the range of great apes.[45,46] However, the small sample size, pathological changes, and deformations by earth pressure call for further study of incidence and spinal curvature in Neanderthals. Thus, a new reconstruction of the La Chapelle-aux-Saints Neanderthal demonstrates that this individual possessed a pelvic incidence of 56° and a human-like degree of lumbar lordosis.[1,47,48]

From this review of the fossils, it appears that the pelvis and the vertebral column might have become a functional unit in human evolution during the transition from occasional to permanent bipedalism. This functional link was probably established at the stage of *H. erectus*. Developmental data suggest that this process of integration possesses a solid genetic basis, for which selection acted both on the pelvis and the vertebral column.[1] The genetic modifications of the pelvis included the reduction of the distance between sacroiliac and hip joints, which entailed an increase in the angle of incidence and the widening of the sacrum with respect to the last common ancestor with African great apes. Concomitantly, the preservation of a five-segment-long lumbar spine permitted the development of the vertebral curvatures. The superior part of the vertebral column was of course also involved in this process of integration as the target of selection was the efficiency of the bipedal balance of the whole body. The correlation between the thoracic kyphosis and the lumbar lordosis ($R = 0.50$)[1] illustrates this association as the geometries of the lumbar and thoracic curvatures are tightly interrelated.[49] The balance of the head on the cervical spine, which was very important in this context, also involved an adaptation of the morphology of the head.[50] We therefore can speak of a complex process of integration, which we are only beginning to understand.

2.4 Conclusion

In an evolutionary point of view, the establishment of the relationship between the angle of incidence, a fixed anatomical pelvic parameter specific to each individual, and variable positional parameters pertaining to the pelvis and vertebral curvatures were crucial steps in the acquisition of hominid sagittal balance. We interpret this relationship as the foundation of an optimal compromise between stability and mobility that is necessary for balancing the trunk above the lower extremity.[51] Mobility is necessary for the vertebrae to modulate the degree of spinal curvature, while stability in the pelvis is necessary to allow the exploitation of these curvatures, and it guarantees the dampening effect of the four compensatory spinal curvatures.

The strong correlation between the angle of incidence and the degree of lumbar curvature in extant humans points toward an elaborated functional response of the postcranial skeleton that was shaped by natural selection. It corresponds to a very derived process of integration between sagittal pelvic morphology and the lumbar spine, which was probably progressive and of long duration. It reveals an advanced stage of specialization to permanent bipedalism and to an economical sagittal balance in extant humans. This specialization was not present among australopithecines. It might only have been reached among *H. erectus* populations, and thus we may expect that an effective step of integration had begun at this stage of evolution.

References

[1] Tardieu C, Hasegawa K, Haeusler M. How the pelvis and vertebral column became a functional unit during the transition from occasional to permanent bipedalism? Anat Rec. 2017; 300(5):912–931

[2] Kummer BKF. Functional adaptation to posture in the pelvis of man and other primates. In: Tuttle RH, ed. Primate Functional Morphology and Evolution. The Hague, Netherlands: Mouton; 1975:281–290

[3] Stern JT, Jr, Susman RL. The locomotor anatomy of Australopithecus afarensis. Am J Phys Anthropol. 1983; 60(3):279–317

[4] Haeusler M. New insights into the locomotion of Australopithecus africanus based on the pelvis. Evol Anthropol. 2002; 11(S1):53–57

[5] Schultz AH. The Life of Primates. Hampshire, United Kingdom: Weidenfeld and Nicolson; 1969.

[6] Schmid P. The trunk of the australopithecines. In: Coppens Y, Senut B, eds. Origine(s) de la Bipédie chez les Hominidés. Paris, France: CNRS; 1991: 225–234

[7] Schmid P, Churchill SE, Nalla S, et al. Mosaic morphology in the thorax of Australopithecus sediba. Science. 2013; 340(6129):1234598

[8] Williams SA, Middleton ER, Villamil CI, Shattuck MR. Vertebral numbers and human evolution. Am J Phys Anthropol. 2016; 159 Suppl 61:S19–S36

[9] McCollum MA, Rosenman BA, Suwa G, Meindl RS, Lovejoy CO. The vertebral formula of the last common ancestor of African apes and humans. J Exp Zoolog B Mol Dev Evol. 2010; 314(2):123–134

[10] Haeusler M, Martelli SA, Boeni T. Vertebrae numbers of the early hominid lumbar spine. J Hum Evol. 2002; 43(5):621–643

[11] Haeusler M, Schiess R, Boeni T. New vertebral and rib material point to modern bauplan of the Nariokotome Homo erectus skeleton. J Hum Evol. 2011; 61 (5):575–582

[12] Haeusler M, Schiess R, Boeni T. Modern or distinct axial bauplan in early hominins? A reply to Williams (2012). J Hum Evol. 2012; 63:557–559

[13] Harrison T, Rook L. Enigmatic anthropoid or misunderstood ape? The phylogenetic status of Oreopithecus bambolii reconsidered. In: Begun DR, Ward CV, Rose MD, eds. Function, Phylogeny, and Fossils: Miocene Hominoid Evolution and Adaptations. New York, NY: Plenum; 1997:327–362

[14] Williams SA, Ostrofsky KR, Frater N, Churchill SE, Schmid P, Berger LR. The vertebral column of Australopithecus sediba. Science. 2013; 340 (6129):1232996

[15] Ward CV, Nalley TK, Spoor F, Tafforeau P, Alemseged Z. Thoracic vertebral count and thoracolumbar transition in Australopithecus afarensis. Proc Natl Acad Sci U S A. 2017; 114(23):6000–6004

[16] Haeusler M, Frater N, Bonneau N. The transition from thoracic to lumbar facet joint orientation at T11: functional implications of a more cranially positioned transitional vertebra in early hominids. Am J Phys Anthropol Suppl. 2014; 58:133

[17] Schultz AH. The skeleton of the trunk and limbs of higher primates. Hum Biol. 1930; 2(3):303–438

[18] Duval-Beaupère G, Schmidt C, Cosson P. A barycentremetric study of the sagittal shape of spine and pelvis: the conditions required for an economic standing position. Ann Biomed Eng. 1992; 20(4):451–462

[19] Legaye J, Duval-Beaupère G, Hecquet J, Marty C. Pelvic incidence: a fundamental pelvic parameter for three-dimensional regulation of spinal sagittal curves. Eur Spine J. 1998; 7(2):99–103

[20] Duval-Beaupère G, Legaye J. Composante sagittale de la statique rachidienne. Rev Rhum. 2004; 71(2):105–119

[21] Tardieu C, Hecquet J, Barrau A, et al. Le bassin, interface articulaire entre rachis et membres inférieurs: analyse par le logiciel DE-VISU. Comptes Rendus Palevol. 2006; 5(3–4):583–595

[22] Tardieu C, Bonneau N, Hecquet J, et al. How is sagittal balance acquired during bipedal gait acquisition? Comparison of neonatal and adult pelves in three dimensions. Evolutionary implications. J Hum Evol. 2013; 65(2):209–222

[23] Zollikofer CPE, Ponce de León MS, Lieberman DE, et al. Virtual cranial reconstruction of Sahelanthropus tchadensis. Nature. 2005; 434(7034):755–759

[24] Wolpoff MH, Hawks J, Senut B, Pickford M, Ahern J. An ape or the ape: is the Toumaï cranium TM 266 a hominid? Paleoanthropology. 2006:36–50

[25] Pickford M, Senut B, Gommery D, Treil J. Bipedalism in Orrorin tugenensis revealed by its femora. C R Palevol. 2002; 1:191–203

[26] Lovejoy CO, Suwa G, Simpson SW, Matternes JH, White TD. The great divides: Ardipithecus ramidus reveals the postcrania of our last common ancestors with African apes. Science. 2009; 326(5949):100–106

[27] Sarmiento EE. Comment on the paleobiology and classification of Ardipithecus ramidus. Science. 2010; 328(5982):1105–, author reply 1105

[28] Häusler M, Schmid P. Comparison of the pelves of Sts 14 and AL 288–1: implications for birth and sexual dimorphism in australopithecines. J Hum Evol. 1995; 29:363–383

[29] Haeusler M, Frémondière P, Fornai C, et al. Virtual reconstruction of the MH2 pelvis (Australopithecus sediba) and obstetrical implications. Am J Phys Anthropol Suppl. 2016; 62:165

[30] Cook DC, Buikstra JE, DeRousseau CJ, Johanson DC. Vertebral pathology in the afar australopithecines. Am J Phys Anthropol. 1983; 60(1):83–101

[31] Haeusler M, Frater N, Mathews S, et al. Are musculoskeletal disorders evolutionary trade-offs of bipedalism? Proc Europ Soc Hum Evol. 2015; 4:107

[32] Rose MD. The process of bipedalization in hominids. In: Coppens Y, Senut B, eds. Origine(s) de la Bipédie chez les Hominidés. Paris, France: CNRS; 1991:37–48

[33] Tardieu C. Étude comparative des déplacements du centre de gravité du corps pendant la marche par une nouvelle méthode d'analyse tridemensionelle. In: Coppens Y, Senut B, eds. Origine(s) de la Bipédie chez les Hominidés. Paris, France: CNRS; 1991:49–58

[34] Tardieu C, Aurengo A, Tardieu B. New method of three-dimensional analysis of bipedal locomotion for the study of displacements of the body and body-parts centers of mass in man and non-human primates: evolutionary framework. Am J Phys Anthropol. 1993; 90(4):455–476

[35] Tardieu C. Short adolescence in early hominids: infantile and adolescent growth of the human femur. Am J Phys Anthropol. 1998; 107(2):163–178

[36] Walker A, Leakey R, eds. The Nariokotome Homo erectus Skeleton. Berlin, Germany: Springer; 1993

[37] Haeusler M, Schiess R, Boeni T. Evidence for juvenile disc herniation in a Homo erectus boy skeleton. Spine. 2013; 38(3):E123–E128

[38] Schiess R, Haeusler M. No skeletal dysplasia in the Nariokotome boy KNM-WT 15000 (Homo erectus)—a reassessment of congenital pathologies of the vertebral column. Am J Phys Anthropol. 2013; 150(3):365–374

[39] Schiess R, Boeni T, Rühli F, Haeusler M. Revisiting scoliosis in the KNM-WT 15000 Homo erectus skeleton. J Hum Evol. 2014; 67:48–59

[40] Meyer MR, Haeusler M. Spinal cord evolution in early Homo. J Hum Evol. 2015; 88:43–53

[41] Walker A, Ruff C. The reconstruction of the pelvis. In: Walker A, Leakey R, eds. The Nariokotome Homo erectus Skeleton. Berlin, Germany: Springer; 1993:221–233

[42] Fornai C, Haeusler M. Virtual reconstruction of the pelvic remains of KNM-WT 15000 Homo erectus from Nariokotome, Kenya. Am J Phys Anthropol. 2017; 162 Suppl 64:183

[43] Bonmatí A, Gómez-Olivencia A, Arsuaga JL, et al. Middle Pleistocene lower back and pelvis from an aged human individual from the Sima de los Huesos site, Spain. Proc Natl Acad Sci U S A. 2010; 107(43):18386–18391

[44] Mays S. Spondylolysis, spondylolisthesis, and lumbo-sacral morphology in a medieval English skeletal population. Am J Phys Anthropol. 2006; 131 (3):352–362

[45] Been E, Peleg S, Marom A, Barash A. Morphology and function of the lumbar spine of the Kebara 2 Neandertal. Am J Phys Anthropol. 2010; 142(4):549–557

[46] Been E, Gómez-Olivencia A, Shefi S, Soudack M, Bastir M, Barash A. Evolution of spinopelvic alignment in hominins. Anat Rec (Hoboken). 2017; 300 (5):900–911

[47] Haeusler M, Fornai C, Frater N, Been E, Bonneau N. Neanderthal vertebral curvature and spinal motion—the evidence of spinal osteoarthritis in the La Chapelle-aux-Saints skeleton. Proc Europ Soc Hum Evol. 2016; 5:115

[48] Haeusler M, Fornai C, Frater N, Bonneau N. The vertebral column of La Chapelle-aux-Saints: the evidence of spinal osteoarthritis for Neanderthal spinal curvature. Am J Phys Anthropol. 2017; 162 Suppl 64:206

[49] Roussouly P, Pinheiro-Franco JL. Biomechanical analysis of the spino-pelvic organization and adaptation in pathology. Eur Spine J. 2011; 20 Suppl 5: 609–618

[50] Been E, Shefi S, Raviv Zilka L, Soudack M. Foramen magnum orientation and Its association with cervical lordosis: a model for reconstructing cervical curvature in archeological and extinct hominin specimens. Adv Anthropol. 2014; 4(3):133–140

[51] Putz RLV, Müller-Gerbl M. The vertebral column—a phylogenetic failure? A theory explaining the function and vulnerability of the human spine. Clin Anat. 1996; 9(3):205–212

[52] Napier JR. The antiquity of human walking. Sci Am. 1967; 216(4):56–6

[53] Waterman HC. Studies on the evolution of the pelvis of man and other primates. Bull Am Mus Nat Hist. 1929; 58:585–642

[54] Haeusler M, Trinkaus E, Fornai C, et al. Morphology, pathology and the vertebral posture of the La Chapelle-aux-Saints Neandertal. Proc Natl Acad Sci USA. 2019; 116:4923–4927

[55] Schultz AH. 1957. Past and present views on man's specializations. Irish J Med Sci:341–56

Part II

Biomechanics of Sagittal Balance

3 From the Head to the Feet: Anatomy of the Upright Position

Jean Marc Vital, Jacques Sénégas, and Jean-Etienne Castelain

Abstract

The sagittal anatomy of the vertebral column cannot, at present, be studied in an isolated fashion. The surgeon should include it together with the skeleton, from the head to the feet in the standing position. This is characteristic of the biped *Homo sapiens*. Studies must comprise balance during movement, primarily walking. This chapter (1) summarizes animal phylogenesis to review the various mechanisms of implementation of this fragile upright posture, which is difficult to maintain comfortably because of the aging of the vertebral column; and (2) describes the various ways to evaluate this henceforward classic sagittal balance, in particular with the EOS system without forgetting to consider the behavior of the spine during ambulation. The authors describe the systems of compensation in pathological situations.

Keywords: aging process, compensation, pelvic ring, upright position, sagittal balance, walking

3.1 Phylogenesis

3.1.1 The Skull

From an embryological and descriptive point of view, the skull is very different from vertebrae. However, Jean Dubousset coined the terms "cranial vertebra" to include the skull—situated above the cervical spine—together with the vertebral column. It is demonstrated in this chapter the phylogenetic evolution that animals developed so that the gaze of quadrupeds and, later, that of bipeds would be horizontal.

Numerous angles have been described by anthropologists to study the course of the shape of the skull according to animal species and in the evolution of hominids. These angles are employed to clarify the orientation of the great occipital foramen (or foramen magnum) and of the eye sockets. The occipital angle of Broca (▶ Fig. 3.1) is measured between the line joining the nasion (point situated at the nasal root) and the opisthion (posterior edge of the great occipital foramen) and a line joining the same opisthion to the basion (the anterior edge of the foramen magnum). This angle decreases from a skull of a quadruped (45°) to a human skull (10°). The decrease in the occipital angle of Broca corresponds to a horizontalization of the foramen magnum, which could be designated "intracranial horizontalization." This horizontalization is very marked when comparing the skeleton of primates, which presents a whole spine kyphosis (cervical, thoracic, and lumbar kyphosis) and a human skeleton, which presents lumbar and cervical lordosis (▶ Fig. 3.2). The second angle described by anthropologists is the orbito-occipital angle drawn between the axis of the eye and the line joining the basion and the opisthion. This angle, with 63° to 90° in quadrupeds, have lower values of 30° to 69° in monkeys and reaches 20° in modern humans. Beauvieux, an anatomist from Bordeaux, clearly demonstrated that the nasion–opisthion line is parallel to the external semicircular canal of the internal ear (▶ Fig. 3.3). In agreement with that, one may consider that the nasion–opisthion line is the reference line of the horizontal plane. The axis of the eye (and consequently that of the gaze) is directed 30° downward and forward. This gaze directed 30° anteriorly and downward corresponds to the reference position of the head as proposed by many ergonomists (▶ Fig. 3.4).

From the posterior to the anterior in the skull base, the foramen magnum locates more posteriorly in chimpanzees, with intermediary position in Australopithecus, and to Pithecanthropus and being located more anterior (or less posterior) in *Homo sapiens*. This morphology is in line with the direction of greater leverage of the trapezius muscle to augment its action of stabilization of the head[1] (▶ Fig. 3.5).

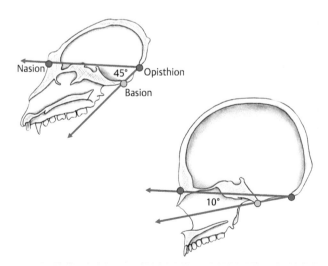

Fig. 3.1 Occipital angle of Broca; "intracranial horizontalization" of foramen magnum.

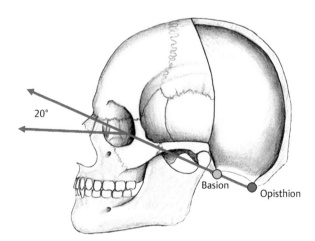

Fig. 3.2 Orbito-occipital angle in man (20°).

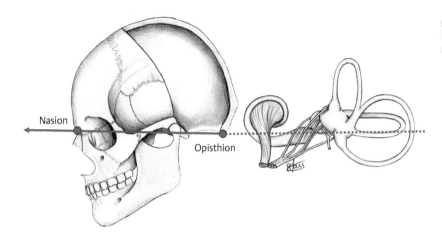

Fig. 3.3 According to Beauvieux, the lateral (or horizontal) semicircular canal is parallel to the nasion–opisthion line.

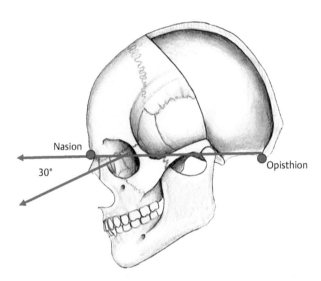

Fig. 3.4 Reference position of the cranium; nasion–opisthion line is horizontal and orbit axis forms a 30° angle with this line.

3.1.2 The Pelvic Ring

The phylogenetic evolution of the shape and orientation of the various constituents of the pelvic ring (sacrum, iliac wings, ischium, and pubis) has been extensively described notably in the other chapters of this book. Nevertheless, it is necessary to review the main concepts.

Tardieu et al[2] studied the 3D anatomy of the pelvic ring of 19 infant and 50 adult hominid fossils. These authors investigated the evolution of the shape of the hips and sacrum during acquisition of biped walking and during growth. They used two angles, pelvic incidence (PI)[3] and an original angle they called "bow angle" (designated here as the iliopubic angle) limited by the line joining the middle of the sacral endplate and the middle of the acetabulum or the femoral heads (FHs) and the line from the middle of the FHs and the pubis in front (▶ Fig. 3.6). This angle, which increases with the width of the pelvis in front, increased during the evolution of primates toward bipedalism in the same way as PI, which increases with the width of the pelvis.

According to Tardieu et al[2] and Morvan et al,[4] the iliac wings widen and become more sagittal (▶ Fig. 3.7) during the evolution of bipedalism. Thus, the pelvis enlarges in its anteroposterior (AP) dimensions (accounting for the increase in PI) (▶ Fig. 3.8), grows anteriorly (accounting for the increase in iliopubic angle), and opens upward to better support internal organs and the trunk.

Tardieu et al[2] studied the pelvic ring of the *Australopithecus afarensis* named Lucy, that lived 3 million years ago. The authors observed that the pelvis was retroverted, with a small PI and a shape and orientation of the iliac wings intermediate between chimpanzees and *H. sapiens* (▶ Fig. 3.9).

Recently, Schlösser et al[5] introduced a new angle, the ilioischial angle (▶ Fig. 3.10), between the line connecting the middle of the sacral endplate to the center of the acetabulum and a line along the middle of the ischium. This angle decreases with the acquisition of bipedalism and also with growth. It decreases with the increase of the width of the posterior part of the pelvis to supplement the "bow angle" of Tardieu et al,[2] which increases with the increase of the width of the pelvis in the front and the PI angle, which increases with the increase of width of the pelvis in the middle. The decrease in the ilioischial angle tends to increase the leverage of hamstrings, indispensable to maintain the femurs extended while standing.

The sacrum—the base of the ship's mast that is the spine (▶ Fig. 3.11)—represents one-seventh of the spine's height. It has widened and gained in height during evolution of hominids until *H. sapiens*. The sacrum also evolved by curving anteriorly (▶ Fig. 3.12). Abitbol[6] used the angle of the sacral curve between the line following the anterior wall of the S1 vertebral body and the line following the anterior wall of L5. The sacrococcygeal angle (▶ Fig. 3.12) described by Marty et al[7] is drawn between a line perpendicular to the upper endplate of S1 and a line perpendicular to the endplate of S5. According to Tardieu et al,[2] this angle increases with the acquisition of bipedalism (▶ Fig. 3.12, ▶ Fig. 3.13).

During the acquisition of bipedalism, anatomical modifications such as the widening and sagittal orientation of the iliac wings, the anterior curving of the sacrum, along with the increase in lumbar lordosis are explained, according to Tardieu et al,[2] by the action of the extensor muscles (lumbosacral muscles, glutei, and hamstrings) but also, notably for the sacrum, by the tension of the strong sacrospinal ligaments (▶ Fig. 3.13, ▶ Fig. 3.14, ▶ Fig. 3.15).

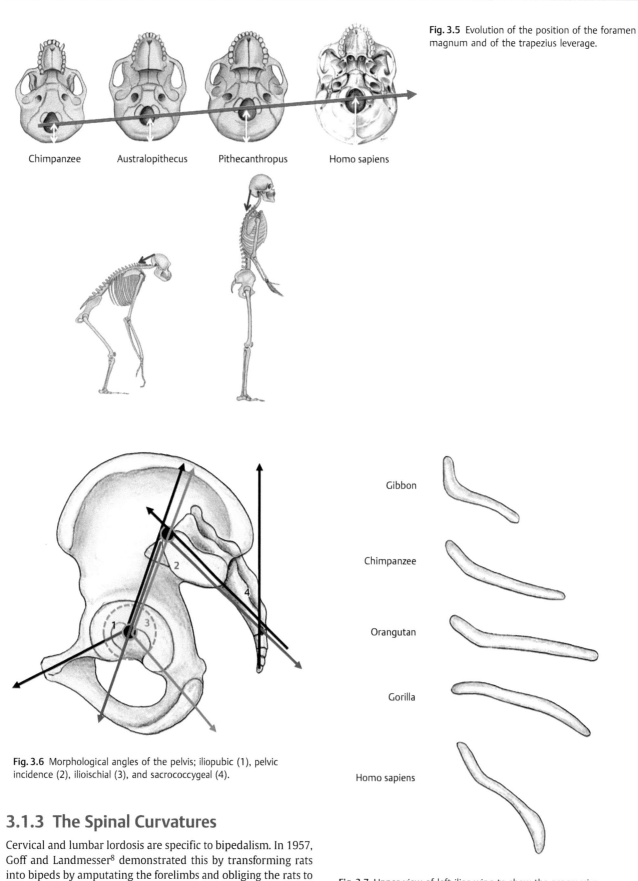

Fig. 3.5 Evolution of the position of the foramen magnum and of the trapezius leverage.

Chimpanzee   Australopithecus   Pithecanthropus   Homo sapiens

Gibbon

Chimpanzee

Orangutan

Gorilla

Homo sapiens

Fig. 3.6 Morphological angles of the pelvis; iliopubic (1), pelvic incidence (2), ilioischial (3), and sacrococcygeal (4).

Fig. 3.7 Upper view of left iliac wing to show the progressive sagittalization with evolution.

3.1.3 The Spinal Curvatures

Cervical and lumbar lordosis are specific to bipedalism. In 1957, Goff and Landmesser[8] demonstrated this by transforming rats into bipeds by amputating the forelimbs and obliging the rats to feed on their hindlimbs to survive by placing their feeders high. Long-term spine X-rays of these rats rendered bipedal showed

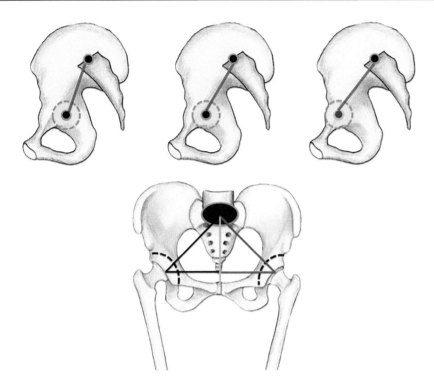

Fig. 3.8 Anteroposterior enlargement of the pelvis during evolution with increase of the pelvic incidence.

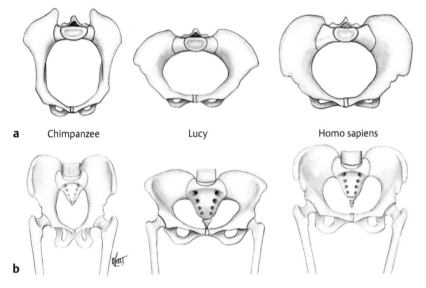

Fig. 3.9 Upper (**a**), and anteroposterior (**b**) views of the pelvis.

a   Chimpanzee   Lucy   Homo sapiens

b

an increase in the cervical lordosis and a flattening of the lumbar kyphosis (▶ Fig. 3.16).

Hominids such as gorillas or orangutans have the ability to remain upright. However, because of the lack of lumbar lordosis combined with a very flat pelvis inducing a PI inferior to 10°, they are forced to maintain an almost seated position with marked retroversion of the pelvis and flexion of the knees. These two compensatory phenomena are observed in human pathology when there is substantial loss of lumbar lordosis and severe anterior imbalance. The four-legged gait most often used by nonhuman hominids is facilitated by the length of their forelimbs (or upper limbs) with a much higher intermember index than in humans. Lumbar lordosis and pelvic anteversion

are intimately linked and maintained thanks to the action of the paravertebral muscles and the gluteus maximus, making the contour of the buttocks characteristic of the real biped *H. sapiens* ("only humans have buttocks" said Buffon). The lumbar lordosis is lacking in other hominids, which have flat buttocks.

3.2 The Aging Process of the Spine

The aging process is inexorable and may be accelerated by genetic and especially mechanical influences (i.e., repetition of professional or sporting activity constraints of the spine). The intervertebral disk begins to dehydrate very early, at the age of 18 years old. There may occur a reduction of the physiological lordosis (▶ Fig. 3.17) estimated at 25° in L5-S1, 15° in L4-L5, and 10° to 12° in the upper lumbar spine. Indeed, the aging of the lumbar spine is "propagated" from bottom to top in the whole spine, as a result of the hinged position of the lower segments L5-S1 (and even L4-L5) relative to the pelvis (▶ Fig. 3.18). This results in a very significant loss of lordosis between L4 and S1, where two-thirds of the lumbar lordosis is located. The same phenomenon exists in the cervical spine with loss of disk height initially occurring in the lower cervical disks (C7-T1, C6-C7, and C5-C6) because of a tightening effect and extended preservation of the height of the upper disks, which often remain hypermobile notably in extension to maintain a horizontal gaze.

In parallel with the loss of intervertebral disk height, which contributes to lumbar or cervical kyphosis, there is an enlargement of the facet joints that creates posterior bulk, limiting the straightening (or extension) of the patient in the same way as the increase in height of lumbar spinous processes (▶ Fig. 3.19), as demonstrated by Aylott et al,[9] using a longitudinal computed tomography (CT) study.

The aging of paravertebral muscles is characterized by a loss in the number of both type 1 and type 2 muscle fibers. Atrophy of muscle fibers is also observed and especially affects type 2, fast twitch fibers. Degenerative change or fatty involution is a natural aging phenomenon of muscles. It was quantified in the lumbosacral muscles by Hadar et al[10] who described three stages of fatty degenerative changes in posterior muscles:
- Stage 1: less than half of the cross sectional area of the affected muscles.
- Stage 2: 50% fatty transformation.
- Stage 3: more than 50% fatty tissue (▶ Fig. 3.20).

The fatty involution progresses from the deepest zone toward the surface, the multifidus being the first muscle affected, and also from below upward (i.e., from the lumbosacral junction toward the thoracolumbar junction). Cruz et al[11] demonstrated a direct correlation between aging, loss of lumbar lordosis, and degree of fatty involution of the paravertebral muscles.

Fortin et al[12] conducted a longitudinal magnetic resonance imaging study of multifidus over 15 years and observed an atrophy more marked in L5-S1 than in L1-L2 with fatty replacement independent of physical activity (work or sport) but dependent on the body mass index. In patients with degenerative (or arthrogenic) kyphosis, signs even more marked; we found almost complete disappearance of type 2 fibers, with severe fibrous and fatty involution involving both lumbar and thoracolumbar muscles, and an abnormal number of moth-eaten, core or targetoid, and ragged red fibers. All these histopathologic signs are observed in myopathies[13] (▶ Fig. 3.21).

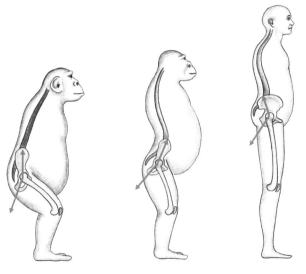

Fig. 3.10 Evolution of the ilioischial angle.

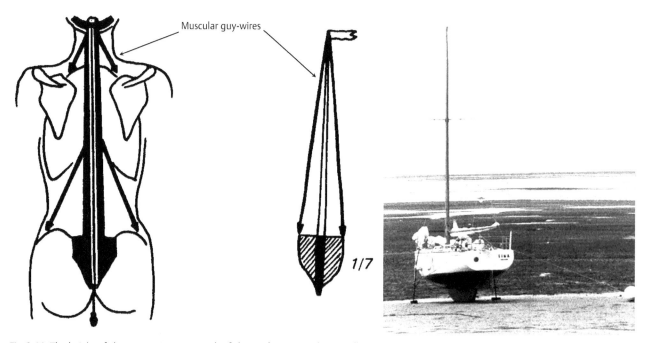

Fig. 3.11 The height of the sacrum is one-seventh of the total spine, similar to sailboats.

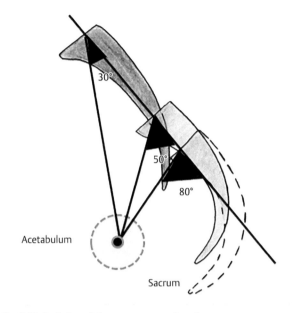

Fig. 3.12 Evolution of the sacrococcygeal angle.

The aging processes affecting disks, facet joints, ligaments, and muscles lead to a progressive loss of lumbar lordosis. It may cause limitation of bipedalism with obligation for aging subjects to use mechanisms of compensation. The first is pelvic retroversion, then flexion of the knees and, when these two means are insufficient, canes may be necessary. Senile osteoporosis, leading to kyphosis-induced vertebral compression fractures, which often occur one after the other like dominoes, only exacerbates this anterior imbalance.

The mechanisms of compensation[14] for the control of the balance in the sagittal plan include the following:

- Cervical hyperlordosis.
- Displacement of the cranial center of gravity.
- Extension of the vertebral column.
- Retroversion of the pelvis.
- Extension of hips.
- Flexion of the knees.
- Flexion/extension of the ankles.
- Inversion/eversion of the feet.

Compensations involving the lower limbs are very often overlooked by the clinical examination and imaging studies.

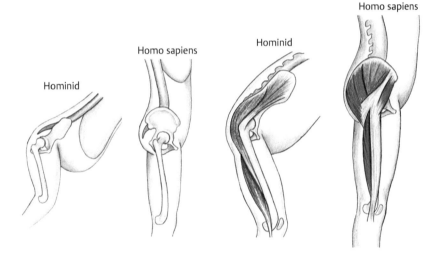

Fig. 3.13 Evolution of the pelvis and the surrounding muscles.

Fig. 3.14 Action of the muscles and ligaments for trunk straightening during phylogenesis.

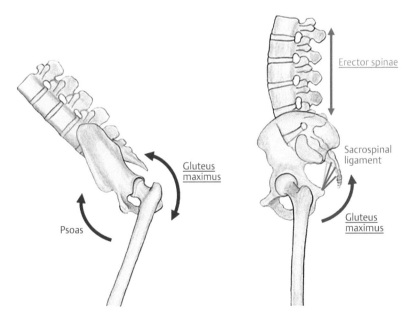

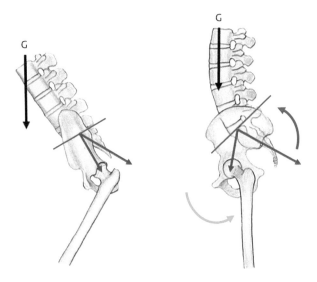

Fig. 3.15 Evolution of the shape and position of the pelvis during phylogenesis.

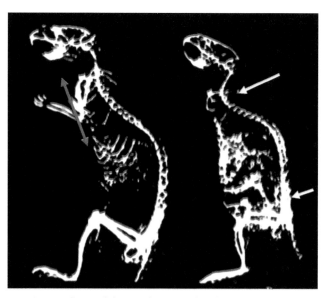

Fig. 3.16 Evolution of the spinal curves in biped rats with increase of cervical and lumbar lordosis.

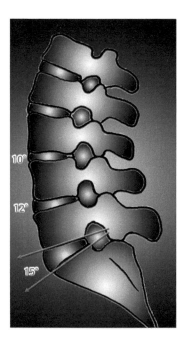

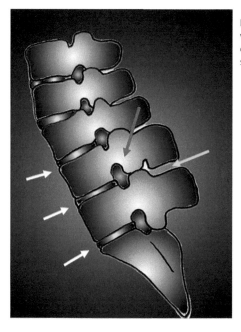

Fig. 3.17 Natural decrease in lumbar lordosis with aging as a result of flattening of the lower disks and hypertrophy of the articular and spinous processes.

Two strategies of compensation are most typically adopted by the patient, depending on the level and type of thoracic kyphosis, whether there exists a reserve of lumbar extension (in some cases at a single level), and, above all, the residual capacity of the gluteal and hamstring muscles. In some patients with proximal thoracic kyphosis, with preservation of lumbar lordosis (or with a single abnormally mobile lumbar segment), and when the muscles are still somewhat effective, the compensation strategy adopted by the patient consists in straightening the spine as much as possible while maintaining hips and knees extended and flexing the ankles (▶ Fig. 3.22, ▶ Fig. 3.23, ▶ Fig. 3.24a). The trade-off is the head/neck segment in a position of R1 retraction, but fatigue can also lead to loss of

a horizontal gaze. Only a certain degree of hip and knee flexion may then restore it.

The most usual strategy employed—when there is no possibility of lumbar extension—consists in compensating for the thoracolumbar kyphosis and for the posterior pelvic tilt by using maximum femoral extension (while on imaging studies, one might conclude in a flexion of the hips). Knees and ankles are stabilized in flexion. This posture lowers the center of mass very effectively. A horizontal gaze is consequently possible (▶ Fig. 3.22, ▶ Fig. 3.23b). However, if the patient extends the knees, this results in anterior imbalance (▶ Fig. 3.23b).

When the vertebral curvatures become worse and the cervical and thoracolumbar extensor muscles become weaker,

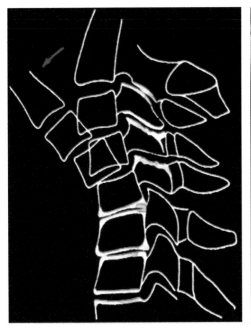

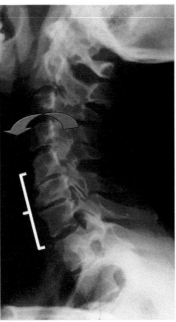

Fig. 3.18 Natural aging evolution of the cervical spine with hypolordosis of the lower cervical spine and hyperlordosis of the upper cervical spine.

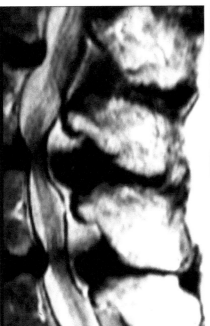

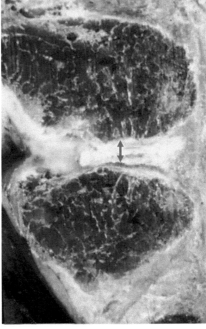

Fig. 3.19 Hypertrophy of the laminae and spinous process in the aging spine.

the horizontalization of the gaze becomes impossible (▶ Fig. 3.23c). The neck is forced into P1 protraction. The line of gravity then falls in front of the base of support. An anterior support becomes indispensable (▶ Fig. 3.23c).

Osteoarthritic stenosis of the spinal canal will lead to more symptoms in extension (or lordosis) than in flexion (or kyphosis), because regardless of the level of the spinal canal, the AP diameter decreases in extension and increases in flexion. At the same time, according to nerve root dynamics, the rootlets and roots advance toward the vertebral bodies and disks in flexion and move backward toward the posterior arch in extension (▶ Fig. 3.24, ▶ Fig. 3.25). This explains the exacerbation of compressive osteoarthritic neck and arm pain in extension of the neck and the improvement of neurogenic claudication caused by lumbar stenosis in flexion or lumbar kyphosis. Standing radiographs in extension without (▶ Fig. 3.25) or with injection of contrast (myelography; ▶ Fig. 3.26) demonstrate this dynamic compression.

The kyphotic changes of the vertebral column may cause compression of the neurological elements, primarily the cauda equina in the narrow lumbar canal. Neurogenic claudication following stenosis is aggravated in extension. Some cases of anterior imbalance can be improved by simple root decompression.

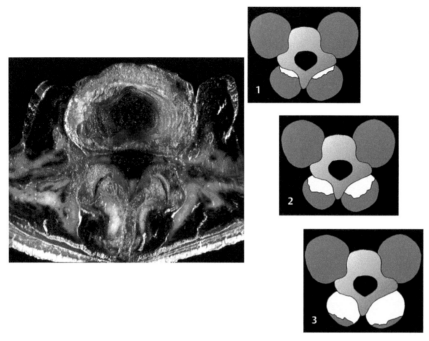

Fig. 3.20 Muscular fatty degeneration with the three stages of Hadar.

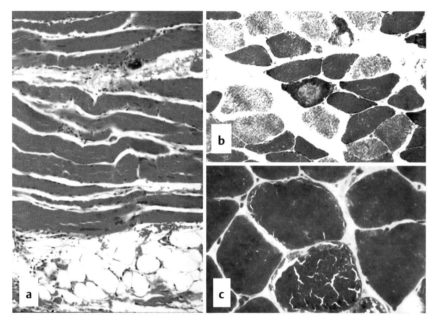

Fig. 3.21 Fibroadiposis (a), targetoid/core fiber (b), and ragged red fiber (c).

3.3 Evaluation of the Static Standing Position

3.3.1 EOS System

Developed by Charpak, the EOS radiological system based on the principle of planar sensors, allows 2D and 3D data acquisition of the entire skeleton in standing position, from head to feet, on AP and lateral views. The irradiation is 8 to 10 times lower than that of simple radiographs in 2D EOS imaging and 100 to 1000 times lower than CT scanning in 3D EOS imaging.

The positioning of the patient must be perfectly controlled to obtain reproducible images. If there is no sagittal imbalance, the knees are extended. The position of the head is controlled by a mirror in which the subject looks into his or her own eyes (▶ Fig. 3.27). Indeed, Solow and Tallgren et al[15] and Peng and Cooke[16] have studied the reproducibility of the natural position of the head in the standing subject. They advocate the use of the mirror as it can be applied at the level of the panel of the EOS system located in front of the subject. Sugrue et al[17] proposed verifying the position of the head by placing the nasion–inion line (external occipital protuberance) horizontally (▶ Fig. 3.28). This technique requires repeat films to make sure the proper position of the head. The present authors prefer the use of the mirror. It should be noted that this reference position of the head on the images corresponds to a horizontal gaze in contrast to the ergonomic reference position with the gaze directed 30°

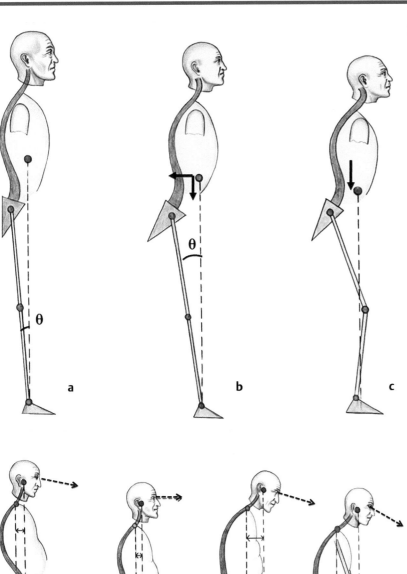

Fig. 3.22 Different strategies: ankle (**a**), hip (**b**), and inferior limb flexion (**c**).

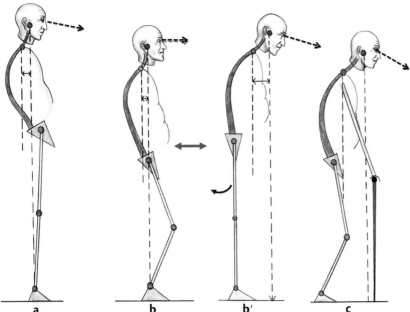

Fig. 3.23 Compensatory phenomena.

downward. The hands are placed on the cheeks rather than on the clavicles (position proposed by the Scoliosis Research Society), to better see the cervicothoracic junction. If there is an anterior imbalance, it is possible to compare the "natural" position of the patient with flexion of the knees that displaces the trunk posteriorly and corrects the anterior imbalance with the "corrected" position, knees in extension, which evaluates the true anterior imbalance.

3.3.2 Radiological Landmarks of the Skull

Vital and Sénégas[18] have extensively studied the center of gravity of the skull. The so-called suspension method was applied to six cadaveric pieces of three women and three men weighing between 3 kg 671 g and 5 kg 213 g, with cranial index

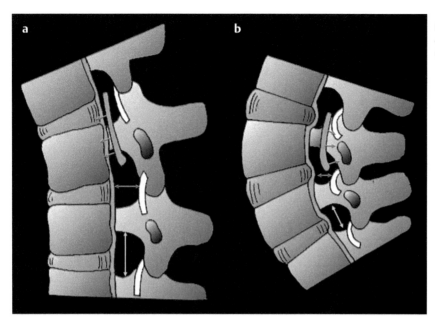

Fig. 3.24 Displacement of the nerve roots and evolution of the spinal canal dimensions in flexion (a) and extension (b).

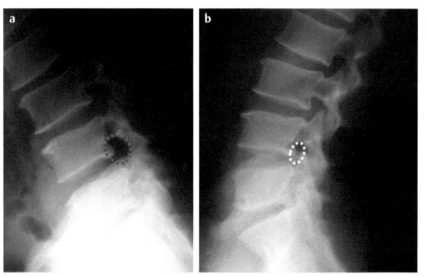

Fig. 3.25 Comparison of the intervertebral foraminal dimensions in flexion (a) and extension (b).

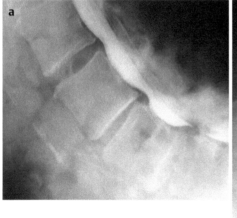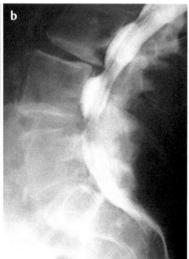

Fig. 3.26 Decrease in size of the central canal in L3L4 and L4L5. on saccoradiculography in extension (b) compared to flexion (a).

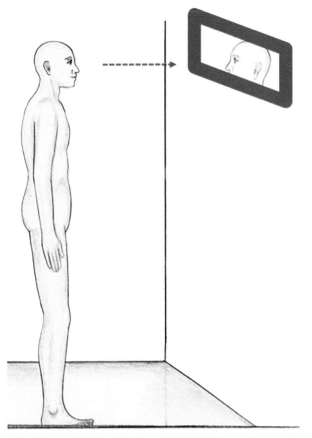

Fig. 3.27 Control of head positioning with a mirror.

ranging from 72 (dolichocephalic) to 85 (brachycephalic). The penetration points of Gardner tongs, which were used to establish the center of gravity of the head, were all on an area of 1 cm² situated above the tragus. Radiologically, the center of gravity fell in the middle of the nasion–inion line (external occipital protuberance), slightly posterior to the sella turcica and directly above the external auditory canal (EAC) (▶ Fig. 3.28, ▶ Fig. 3.29, ▶ Fig. 3.30, ▶ Fig. 3.31).

Next to the EAC, there are other cranial radiological landmarks (▶ Fig. 3.31). The McGregor line is the most classic landmark of the skull. It connects the hard palate to the opisthion (posterior edge of the great occipital foramen). The sella turcica is easy to find, being situated slightly in front of the EAC, which are more difficult to localize. It is important to remember that the EAC is always situated vertically above the tip of the dens.

3.3.3 Angles Measured in the Cervical Spine

Recently, many articles have focused on cervical spine sagittal balance. The position of the head may be controlled with a mirror, as mentioned above, and various angles can be investigated (▶ Fig. 3.32, ▶ Fig. 3.33, ▶ Fig. 3.34):

- The occipito-C2 angle exists between McGregor's line and the line passing through the lower endplate of C2. This angle is useful in evaluating the occipito-C1 and C1-C2 joints.
- The C1-C2 angle occurs between the line joining the anterior and posterior arches of the atlas and the line passing through the lower endplate of C2. It is used to evaluate the C1-C2 joint and is much higher than the C3-C7 angle (24° to 25° on average).

Fig. 3.28 Description of the suspension method.

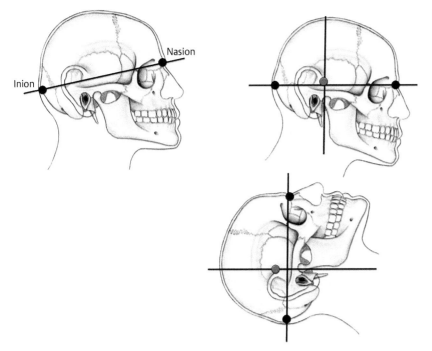

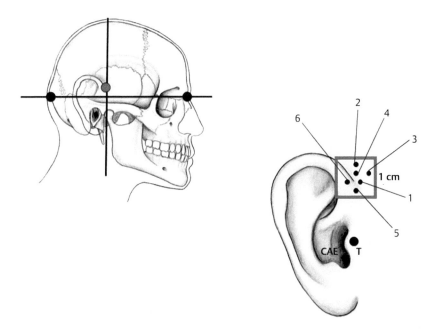

Fig. 3.29 Projection on six cadaver specimens of the centers of the gravity.

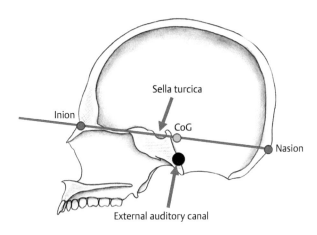

Fig. 3.30 Projection on a skull X-ray of the center of gravity.

- Aside from these two angles that explore the upper cervical spine, the C1-C7 angle between the axis of C1 and superior endplate of C7 explores the entire cervical spine (30° on average) and the C3-C7 angle explores the lower cervical spine (only 6°).
- The slope of C7 is measured between a horizontal line and the upper endplate of C7. This angle determines the amount of cervical lordosis that rebalances the head to maintain the gaze horizontal. Vidal and Marnay[19] noted in 1984 that a small slope of C7 was associated with a small cervical lordosis, in some cases even a cervical kyphosis. In contrast, a large slope of C7 was associated with cervical hyperlordosis (▶ Fig. 3.35).
- The cranial tilt is measured between a vertical line drawn downward from the middle of the body of C7 and the line that joins this point and the EAC. This angle can be used to distinguish protraction (associating lower cervical kyphosis and upper cervical lordosis) and retraction (associating lower cervical lordosis and upper cervical kyphosis) of the neck.

To conclude on these cervical angles, one should remember that lower cervical lordosis (C3-C7), much less marked than upper cervical lordosis (C1-C2), is very dependent on the slope of C7. To maintain the gaze horizontal, the upper cervical spine behaves like an inverted pendulum and its lordosis changes inversely with the lordosis of the lower cervical spine.

3.3.4 Angles Measured in the Thoracic and Lumbar Spine

Thoracic kyphosis and lumbar lordosis are not measured between T1 and T12 for the thorax or between L1 and S1 for the lumbar region, but between the most tilted vertebrae, which might not correspond to theoretical anatomical limits. The angles of thoracic kyphosis and lumbar lordosis are closely correlated with the angle of PI described by Duval-Beaupère et al[3] according to the formula: lumbar lordosis = PI ± 9°. In 1953, Delmas and Depreux[20] introduced the notion of dynamic spinal morphotypes, with marked cervical and thoracic curves, and static morphotypes, with smaller curves, and consequently a flatter column. Much more recently, Roussouly et al[21] described four types of spinal morphotypes, from 1 (with low PI) to 4 (with high PI and marked spinal curves). In the lower lumbar region there are important "regional rules" to be retained, especially in lumbar and lumbosacral arthrodesis: 40% of lumbar lordosis is in the L5-S1 segment, 25% in L4-L5, and two-thirds of lumbar lordosis is between L4 and S1.

3.3.5 Angles Measured in the Pelvic Ring

The pelvic ring is considered by Jean Dubousset as an intermediate vertebra between the vertebral column and the lower limbs.

Duval-Beaupère et al[3] described three angles on lateral X-rays:
- The PI angle is calculated between a line joining the middle of the FHs and the middle of the endplate of S1 and a line perpendicular to that endplate drawn down from the middle

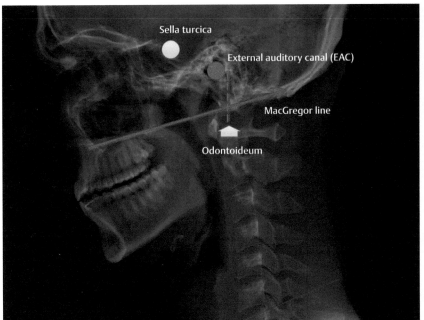

Fig. 3.31 Main radiological landmarks of the skull.

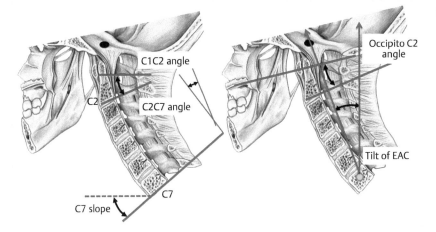

Fig. 3.32 Main craniocervical and cervical angles.

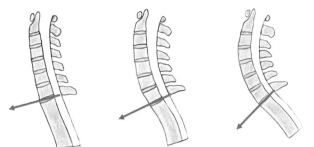

Fig. 3.33 Relationship between C7 slope and cervical lordosis.

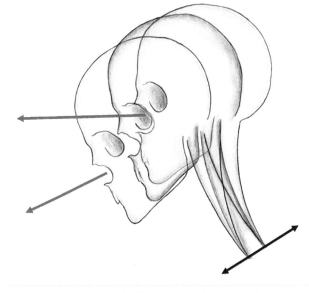

Fig. 3.34 Cervical spine works like an adjustment rod upward to maintain horizontal gaze and downward depending on the thoracic kyphosis (C7 slope).

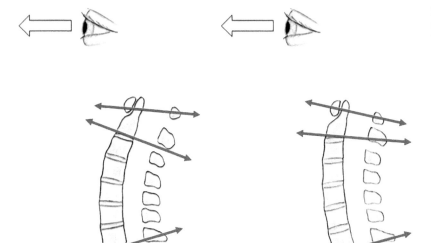

Fig. 3.35 Compensation of the upper cervical spine above the lower cervical spine to maintain the gaze horizontal.

of it. This angle characterizes the shape and more precisely the width of the pelvis in the anteroposterior direction and determines the spinal curves, notably lumbar lordosis. It increases during growth[22] and is determined genetically. It does not vary with the position of the pelvis and theoretically does not vary with aging. Indeed, recent research[23] showed that PI can increase with age, because of the laxity of the sacroiliac joint, which is situated between the FHs (or acetabulum) and the sacrum.

- The pelvic tilt is calculated between a vertical line passing through the center of the FH and the line joining the FH to the center of the endplate of S1. This positional angle increases when the pelvis is in retroversion, as this is an automatic correction of anterior imbalance, and decreases during anteversion of the pelvis.
- The T9 sagittal overhang is calculated between a vertical line through the FH and the line joining the FH to the middle of T9, that is the center of gravity of the trunk according to Duval-Beaupère. This angle positions the trunk, not the pelvis, the position of which is characterized by the pelvic tilt. The T9 sagittal overhang remains constant for long periods of time and can decrease or even reverse itself in case of severe anterior imbalance.

3.3.6 Angles Measured in the Lower Limbs

Like Duval-Beaupère angles, Itoi[24] described complementary angles in a series of osteoporotic patients, and also a femorotibial angle between the axes of the femoral and tibial diaphysis. It is positive as soon as the knees bend, that it is the second means of compensation for severe anterior imbalance. Mangione and Sénégas[25] described the femoropelvic angle between the axis of the femoral diaphysis and the line from the centers of the FH to the middle of the sacral endplate: it measures hip extension (and not hip flessum) in severe anterior imbalance.

More recently, Hovorka et al[26] and Lazennec et al[27] studied the reserve of hip extension by rear slot radiographs to evaluate the capacity of the coxofemoral joint to authorize a substantial retroversion of the pelvis in cases of severe anterior imbalance.

3.3.7 Mechanisms of Compensation for Anterior Imbalance

In this chapter describing the balance from the head to the feet, one cannot be satisfied with the measurement of the C7 plumb line, as it may imply evaluating a "decapitated" subject. It seems to be important to integrate the skull and pelvis in this overall study by examining the line that connects the EAC (center of gravity of the skull) and the centers of the FH, which are almost in the center of the pelvis. Gangnet et al[28] demonstrated the vertical alignment of these two points (EAC and FH) in healthy subjects with normal pelvic version and extended knees (perfect balance), but also in patients with an equilibrium that is compensated first by retroversion, which pushes the FH forward under the EAC, then by the knee flessum that displaces the trunk backward, and finally by flattening of the thoracic spine, sometimes with retrolisthesis in upper lumbar segments. The capacity of retroversion is greater in subjects with large PI. Sénégas et al[15] described the strategy of hyperextending the ankles to uncomfortably correct anterior imbalance.

Sometimes, despite all these processes that are often difficult for the patient to bear, the vertical axis lowered from the EAC falls in a natural position, in front of the FH, and we designate this as anterior imbalance.

The EAC–FH vertical alignment, which may persist for a long time in certain disorders, led the present authors to define upward or downward alignment that can be applied regarding segments that are still flexible, primarily in the cervical spine.

An upward alignment explains the cervical kyphosis observed in idiopathic scoliosis that often presents a flat thoracic spine (► Fig. 3.36). Other demonstrations of upward alignment are the increased cervical lordosis in large osteotomies for lumbar kyphosis (► Fig. 3.37, ► Fig. 3.38), the decrease in cervical lordosis in the surgical treatment of thoracic Scheuermann disease, and the reappearance of thoracic kyphosis and the shortening of lumbar lordosis in surgical corrections of lumbosacral kyphosis accompanying dysplastic spondylolisthesis (► Fig. 3.39, ► Fig. 3.40).

A downward alignment, that is rarer, may be observed with very severe cervical kyphosis as a result of neurofibromatosis with underlying thoracic flat back (► Fig. 3.41).

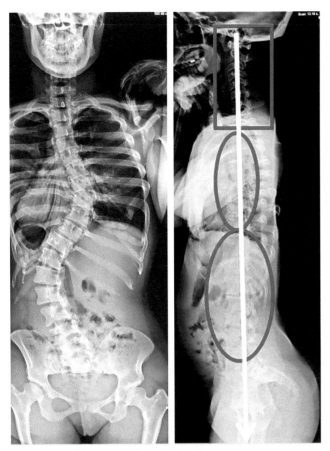

Fig. 3.36 "Upward alignment" with cervical kyphosis above flattened spine as a result of idiopathic scoliosis.

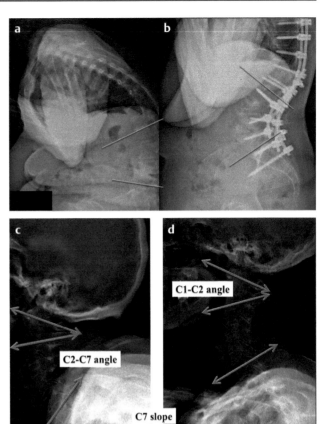

Fig. 3.37 "Upward alignment" in a case of lumbar subtraction osteotomy: preoperative lumbar X-ray (a), postoperative lumbar X-ray (b), preoperative cervical X-ray (c), and postoperative cervical X-ray (d). There is a great decrease in the C2-C7 angle but also a small decrease in the C1-C2 angle

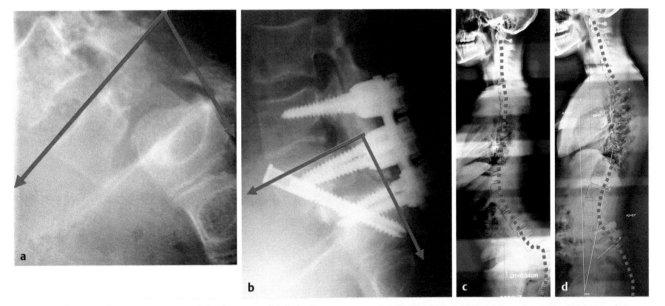

Fig. 3.38 "Upward alignment" in a case of dysplastic spondylolisthesis surgery; preoperative lumbosacral X-ray (a), postoperative lumbosacral X-ray (b), global preoperative X-ray (c), and global postoperative X-ray (d).

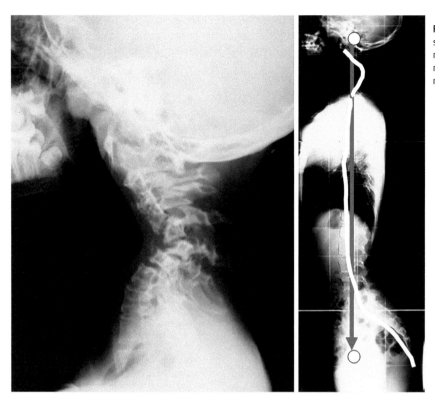

Fig. 3.39 "Downward alignment" in case of severe cervical kyphosis in neurofibromatosis; note the flattening of the thoracic spine to maintain optimal alignment between the external auditory canal and the femoral head.

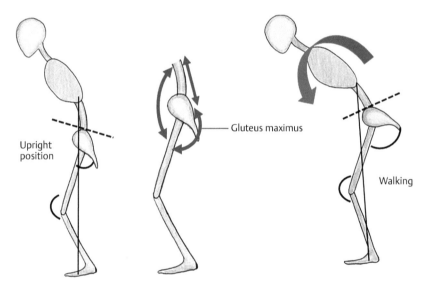

Upright position

Gluteus maximus

Walking

Fig. 3.40 During ambulation, there is an increase in sagittal imbalance because the gluteus maximus cannot maintain pelvic retroversion.

3.4 Assessment of Walking

Static radiographs of the entire spine do not represent the phenomena encountered during movement. Lee et al[29] have shown that the anterior imbalance in patients with postoperative flat back was much more evident in walking than on static lateral images. Muscular insufficiency of the gluteus maximus, which fails to maintain extreme retroversion of the pelvis during ambulation is a possible explanation. Compensatory phenomena are pushed to the maximum in static studies, but they fail to function in dynamic studies.[30]

There are patients with imbalance with hyperretroversion. They "sit on their pelvis," with the plumb line from the EAC behind the FH, tilting forward during walking. These patients improve significantly with lumbar osteotomies (▶ Fig. 3.40).

The dynamic analysis of the spine during walking is highly complex. It involves a combination of measuring the positioning of the segments in space by means of a kinematic analysis associated with an analysis of the activity of the trunk muscles (erector spinae and abdominalis) and gluteus (mainly gluteus maximus).

The kinematic analysis is carried out by means of reflective sensors (set markers) placed on reference bone surfaces chosen

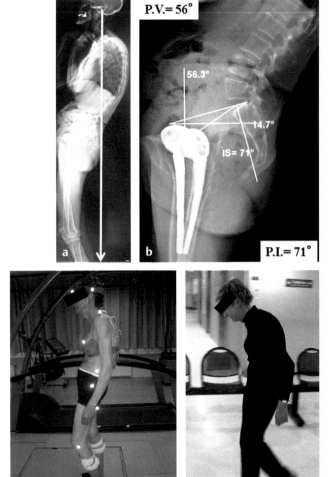

Fig. 3.41 Posterior static imbalance (**a**), in patient with large pelvic incidence and large compensatory retroversion (**b**). Gait evaluation (**c**), to confirm the severe sagittal imbalance when the patient is walking (**d**).

by the experimenter. Their position is permanently recorded by a series of infrared cameras and analyzed by dedicated software to precisely describe their position in the three orthogonal planes of space (x, y, z). In addition to the amplitudes of movement; one may determine a walking cycle, which starts with the heel contact and ends with the contralateral heel contact. Thus, it is also possible to determine walking parameters such as speed, width, length, and regularity of the step.

Muscular analysis is performed using surface electromyography. The sensors are coupled to the kinematic analysis' sensors to facilitate the association between movement and muscular activity of a dedicated group.

Corrective surgery has a positive impact on walking parameters, and notably a positive correlation with the restoration of spinal balance in the sagittal plane.[31] Nevertheless, their walking remains different from that of healthy subjects, despite surgery. Ambulation deteriorates even more in the patients who have revision surgery for sagittal imbalance.[32]

The study of postoperative walking parameters is an objective marker of the effects of the intervention, complementary to the complete radiological evaluation as described above.[33]

References

[1] Luboga SA, Wood BA. Position and orientation of the foramen magnum in higher primates. Am J Phys Anthropol. 1990; 81(1):67–76

[2] Tardieu C, Bonneau N, Hecquet J, et al. How is sagittal balance acquired during bipedal gait acquisition? Comparison of neonatal and adult pelves in three dimensions. Evolutionary implications. J Hum Evol. 2013; 65(2): 209–222

[3] Duval-Beaupère G, Schmidt C, Cosson P. A barycentremetric study of the sagittal shape of spine and pelvis: the conditions required for an economic standing position. Ann Biomed Eng. 1992; 20(4):451–462

[4] Morvan G, Wybier M, Mathieu P, Vuillemin V, Guerini H. Clichés simples du rachis: statique et relations entre rachis et bassin [in French]. J Radiol. 2008; 89(5 Pt 2):654–663, quiz 664–666

[5] Schlösser TPC, Janssen MMA, Vrtovec T, et al. Evolution of the ischio-iliac lordosis during natural growth and its relation with the pelvic incidence. Eur Spine J. 2014; 23(7):1433–1441

[6] Abitbol MM. Evolution of the lumbosacral angle. Am J Phys Anthropol. 1987; 72(3):361–372

[7] Marty C, Boisaubert B, Descamps H, et al. The sagittal anatomy of the sacrum among young adults, infants, and spondylolisthesis patients. Eur Spine J. 2002; 11(2):119–125

[8] Goff CW, Landmesser W. Bipedal rats and mice; laboratory animals for orthopaedic research. J Bone Joint Surg Am. 1957; 39-A(3):616-6–22

[9] Aylott CEW, Puna R, Robertson PA, Walker C. Spinous process morphology: the effect of ageing through adulthood on spinous process size and relationship to sagittal alignment. Eur Spine J. 2012; 21(5):1007–1012

[10] Hadar H, Gadoth N, Heifetz M. Fatty replacement of lower paraspinal muscles: normal and neuromuscular disorders. AJR Am J Roentgenol. 1983; 141(5):895–898

[11] Cruz-Jentoft AJ, Baeyens JP, Bauer JM, et al. Sarcopenia: European consensus on definition and diagnosis: report of the European Working Group on Sarcopenia in Older People. Age Ageing. 2010; 39(4):412–423

[12] Fortin M, Videman T, Gibbons LE, Battié MC. Paraspinal muscle morphology and composition: a 15-yr longitudinal magnetic resonance imaging study. Med Sci Sports Exerc. 2014; 46(5):893–901

[13] Vital JM, Gille O, Coquet M. Déformations rachidiennes: anatomopathologie et histoenzymologie [in French]. Rev Rhum. 2004; 71:263–264

[14] Sénégas J, Bouloussa H, Liguoro D, Yoshida G, Vital JM. Evolution morphologique et fonctionnelle du rachis vieillissant. In: Anatomie de la Colonne Vertébrale: Nouveaux Concepts (in French). Montpellier, France: Sauramps Médical; 2016:111–155

[15] Solow B, Tallgren A. Natural head position in standing subjects. Acta Odontol Scand. 1971; 29(5):591–607

[16] Peng L, Cooke MS. Fifteen-year reproducibility of natural head posture: A longitudinal study. Am J Orthod Dentofacial Orthop. 1999; 116(1):82–85

[17] Sugrue PA, McClendon J, Jr, Smith TR, et al. Redefining global spinal balance: normative values of cranial center of mass from a prospective cohort of asymptomatic individuals. Spine. 2013; 38(6):484–489

[18] Vital JM, Sénégas J. Anatomical bases of the study of the constraints to which the cervical spine is subject in the sagittal plane. A study of the center of gravity of the head. Surg Radiol Anat. 1986; 8(3):169–173

[19] Vidal J, Marnay T. Sagittal deviations of the spine, and trial of classification as a function of the pelvic balance (in French). Rev Chir Orthop Repar Appar Mot. 1984; 70 Suppl 2:124–126

[20] Delmas A, Depreux R. Spinal curves and intervertebral foramina (in French). Rev Rhum Mal Osteoartic. 1953; 20(1):25–29

[21] Roussouly P, Gollogly S, Berthonnaud E, Dimnet J. Classification of the normal variation in the sagittal alignment of the human lumbar spine and pelvis in the standing position. Spine. 2005; 30(3):346–353

[22] Mangione P, Gomez D, Sénégas J. Study of the course of the incidence angle during growth. Eur Spine J. 1997; 6(3):163–167

[23] Jean L. Influence of age and sagittal balance of the spine on the value of the pelvic incidence. Eur Spine J. 2014; 23(7):1394–1399

[24] Itoi E. Roentgenographic analysis of posture in spinal osteoporotics. Spine. 1991; 16(7):750–756

[25] Mangione P, Sénégas J. Sagittal balance of the spine (in French). Rev Chir Orthop Repar Appar Mot. 1997; 83(1):22–32

[26] Hovorka I, Rousseau P, Bronsard N, et al. Extension reserve of the hip in relation to the spine: Comparative study of two radiographic methods (in French). Rev Chir Orthop Repar Appar Mot. 2008; 94(8):771–776

[27] Lazennec JY, Charlot N, Gorin M, et al. Hip–spine relationship: a radio-anatomical study for optimization in acetabular cup positioning. Surg Radiol Anat. 2004; 26(2):136–144

[28] Gangnet N, Pomero V, Dumas R, Skalli W, Vital JM. Variability of the spine and pelvis location with respect to the gravity line: a three-dimensional stereoradiographic study using a force platform. Surg Radiol Anat. 2003; 25(5)(–)(6):424–433

[29] Lee CS, Lee CK, Kim YT, Hong YM, Yoo JH. Dynamic sagittal imbalance of the spine in degenerative flat back: significance of pelvic tilt in surgical treatment. Spine. 2001; 26(18):2029–2035

[30] Shiba Y, Taneichi H, Inami S, Moridaira H, Takeuchi D, Nohara Y. Dynamic global sagittal alignment evaluated by three-dimensional gait analysis in patients with degenerative lumbar kyphoscoliosis. Eur Spine J. 2016; 25(8):2572–2579

[31] Yagi M, Kaneko S, Yato Y, Asazuma T, Machida M. Walking sagittal balance correction by pedicle subtraction osteotomy in adults with fixed sagittal imbalance. Eur Spine J. 2016; 25(8):2488–2496

[32] Engsberg JR, Bridwell KH, Reitenbach AK, et al. Preoperative gait comparisons between adults undergoing long spinal deformity fusion surgery (thoracic to L4, L5, or sacrum) and controls. Spine. 2001; 26(18):2020–2028

[33] Engsberg JR, Bridwell KH, Wagner JM, Uhrich ML, Blanke K, Lenke LG. Gait changes as the result of deformity reconstruction surgery in a group of adults with lumbar scoliosis. Spine. 2003; 28(16):1836–1843, discussion 1844

4 Modeling of the Spine

Carl-Eric Aubin and Xiaoyu Wang

Abstract

The pelvis and vertebral column have a complex anatomical structure providing segmental motions, posture control, and functional loads bearing. Sagittal balance is critical for the maintenance of proper functions of the musculoskeletal system. Angle measurements on radiographs, pelvic parameters, and C7 plumb line are clinical indices to assess sagittal balance. The main treatment option for severe spinal imbalance remains surgical instrumentation. The results of this procedure depend on many patient-specific factors and surgical techniques that vary from surgeon to surgeon. Studies on the sagittal balance are mostly focused on geometric parameters; the biomechanics of sagittal balance is not yet fully understood. This chapter aims to present biomechanical modeling techniques and selected examples with emphasis on those adapted to be applied in a clinical setup to complement clinical analysis and for preoperative surgical planning. 3D geometry was built with biplanar radiographs and 3D multiview reconstruction techniques and used in finite element models (FEMs) and multibody models (MBMs). The MBM is based on theories of the dynamics of multibody systems. To build an MBM, vertebrae from T1 through L5 and the pelvis were modeled as rigid parts; intervertebral tissues and connections were modeled using multiple flexible elements with appropriate mechanical properties. Osteotomy procedures were modeled by removing the modeling elements involved in the procedure. Surgical instrumentation and correction maneuvers were modeled with kinematics joints and applied displacements and forces. FEM is a numerical method for solving complex problems based on variational formulation, discretization strategy, solution algorithms, and postprocessing procedures. To build a FEM, geometries of the intervertebral disks, ligaments, and facet joints from a previously built generic model were registered into the patient-specific model such that vertebral and pelvic geometries of the generic model matched the reconstructed patient-specific geometries using 3D dual kriging. A bony component was modeled as a trabecular core enveloped by a cortical bone layer. Mechanical properties of the intervertebral disks, ligaments, and facet joints were calibrated using experimental results reported in the literature. The models have been calibrated and validated to perform biomechanical analysis of spinal instrumentation for kyphotic deformity, proximal junctional kyphosis, and spinopelvic parameters. The developed techniques allow subject-specific biomechanical modeling of the spine and pelvis in a clinical setup. The MBM and FEM can be used to investigate the biomechanical behaviors of the pathological versus asymptomatic spine. Simulations using the MBM allow the prediction of the biomechanical results of surgical strategies and postoperative function movements. FEM allows the analysis at stress and strain levels of the spinal biomechanics. The techniques are also of high value in a research and development context. They can be used to evaluate patient positioning, new treatment concepts, construct designs, and optimize treatment and design parameters. The combination of MBM and comprehensive FEM gives rise to a hybrid modeling approach enabling highly efficient analysis of the pathomechanisms of spinal imbalance and its treatment.

Keywords: biomechanical modeling, biomechanics, deformity, instrumentation, sagittal balance, spine

4.1 Introduction

The spine and pelvis have complex structure and biomechanics providing segmental motions, functional load bearing, and posture control. Sagittal balance is critical for the maintenance of proper biomechanical functions of the musculoskeletal system.[1] Angle measurements on radiographs,[2] pelvic parameters,[3] and a plumb line drawn onto full-length radiographs[4] are geometric indices used in clinics to assess the geometric components of sagittal balance.

The main treatment option for severe spinal imbalance remains surgical instrumentation to restore posture balance.[5] The result of this procedure depends on numerous factors; some of them are inherent to the particular pathology of each individual patient such as preoperative sagittal balance and spinopelvic parameters, while others pertain to construct design, instrumentation configuration, and surgical techniques. Great variation persists in preoperative planning and instrumentation designs between surgeons for a given case; consensus on the most appropriate surgical strategies has yet to be reached for optimal results. Studies on the sagittal balance are most focused on its geometric descriptors and their correlations[6,7]; the biomechanics of sagittal balance (e.g., characteristics of the forces to attain mechanical equilibrium and stability of the spine) are not yet fully understood.

Computer biomechanical models can play an important role for the understanding of the pathomechanisms and the evaluation of treatment concepts. It is relevant to assess stress, strain, and motion within the anatomical structure as well as muscle forces actively stabilizing the spine. Finite element models (FEMs) have been reported to estimate trunk muscle forces,[8] load-sharing along the ligamentous spine,[9] and residual motion within the instrumented spine.[10] Different patient-specific FEMs were developed to predict deformity correction and overall loads in the spine and pelvis[11,12] and analyze at a detailed level stress and strain associated with different conditions.[13,14,15]

This chapter aims to present biomechanical modeling techniques of the spine and selected examples from the authors' experience with emphasis on those adapted to be applied in a clinical setting to complement clinical analysis and for preoperative surgical planning.

4.2 Patient-Specific Computational Biomechanical Modeling of the Spine and Instrumentation

Multibody modeling (MBM),[16,17] FEM techniques,[11,15] and their combination (hybrid)[18] have been used for the biomechanical modeling of the spine and pelvis. FEM is a numerical method for solving complex problems based on variational formulation, discretization strategy, solution algorithms, and postprocessing procedures. It allows the investigation of stress and strain within each component of the spine and pelvis, such as vertebral body, facet joint, and intervertebral ligament. MBM technique is based on theories of the dynamics of multibody systems and focuses on the resultant forces, moments, and displacements among different components. Compared to MBM, patient-specific FEM creation, calibration, and simulation are significantly longer and more complex processes and require more computation resources. The process for MBM is less complex and time consuming, but with fewer details for each individual component of the spine and pelvis.

4.2.1 3D Geometric Model Reconstruction of the Spine

The first modeling step is to acquire the geometry of the anatomy to be included in the model, which is generally based on medical imaging techniques (i.e., coronal and sagittal radiographs),[19,20] computed tomography (CT) scan,[21,22] and magnetic resonance imaging (MRI).[23] A CT-scan is a 3D imaging method with high accuracy of bony structure, but it induces a high radiation dose for the patient. Methods based on MRI do not have the problem of high radiation dose, but are more for soft tissues than for bony structures; they are more expensive and not appropriate for patients with implants of ferromagnetic materials. The modeling technique presented in this chapter used patient-specific 3D data of the spine and pelvis from biplanar radiographs acquired for routine clinical assessment of spinal pathologies.

3D spine geometry is built using coronal and lateral plain radiographs and 3D multiview reconstruction techniques.[19] On the two digital radiographs acquired with patients wearing a calibration object, key anatomical landmarks on the spine and pelvis (e.g., pedicles, vertebral endplate middle and corner points, transverse and spinous process extremities, femoral head centers, and iliac crests) are identified and their 3D coordinates are computed using an optimization algorithm.[19] The reconstruction process was completed by registering detailed vertebral models using a free-form deformation technique.[19] Average reconstruction accuracies for pedicles and vertebral bodies were 1.6 mm (SD 1.1 mm) and 1.2 mm (SD 0.8 mm), respectively.[24] Reconstruction variations for a given patient are 0.8° or less (Cobb angles), 5.3° or less (sagittal curves), and 4°–8° (vertebral axial rotation), which are within the error levels reported for equivalent 2D measurements used by clinicians.[24,25]

4.2.2 Multibody Modeling of the Spine

MBMs have been developed to investigate the biomechanics of the spine. In our long-standing experience, MBMs were developed to particularly assess biomechanical indices, such as spinal balance, deformity corrections, and forces at the bone–implant interface. The MBM of the spine and pelvis was built using their reconstructed geometries. Vertebrae from T1 through L5 and the pelvis were modeled as rigid parts, and intervertebral tissues and connections were modeled using multiple flexible elements with appropriate mechanical properties. For each functional spinal unit (FSU), six cable-like elements, two 6D general springs, and one primary general spring were defined to connect a pair of vertebrae (▶ Fig. 4.1). The cable-like elements represent the anterior longitudinal ligament, posterior longitudinal ligament, ligamentum flavum, intertransverse ligament, and the combined effect of the interspinous ligament (ISL) and the supraspinous ligament. The biomechanical behavior of the facet joints is more complex compared to the other intervertebral ligaments[26]; they were represented by two 6D springs. The primary general spring represents the intervertebral disk also incorporating the combined effect of all elements not explicitly modeled (e.g., the rib cage and surrounding muscles and their interconnections).

Stiffness of model component was defined in four complementary processes. In the first method, the stiffness of cable-like elements was defined based on experiments on cadaveric specimens[27,28]; the stiffness matrices of the three general springs were defined such that the load-displacement simulations reproduced the reported load displacements.[29,30] In the second approach, the stiffness of the modeling elements was

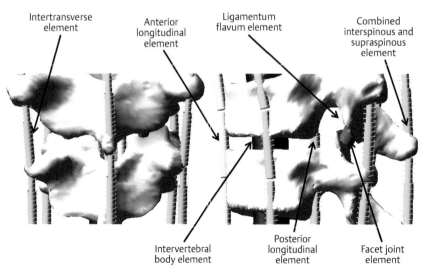

Fig. 4.1 Illustration of modeling elements of intervertebral connections.

Intertransverse element

Anterior longitudinal element

Ligamentum flavum element

Combined interspinous and supraspinous element

Intervertebral body element

Posterior longitudinal element

Facet joint element

Posteroanterior view

Lateral view

modified to adjust their percent contribution to the overall stiffness of the FSU using data from biomechanical tests.[31,32,33,34] In the third method, a weighting factor was applied to the stiffness matrix of the primary general spring to account for the contribution of the rib cage to the overall stiffness of the thoracic spine (i.e., 40%, 35%, and 31%, respectively, in flexion/extension, lateral bending, and axial rotation).[35] Finally, all model element stiffness could be further adjusted such that side bending (or traction) simulations reproduced the Cobb angles measured on the patient's side bending (or traction or supine) radiographs using an optimization technique reported in Refs. 17 and 36. Osteotomy procedures were modeled by removing the modeling elements involved in the procedure.

4.2.3 Multibody Modeling of Spinal Instrumentation and Postoperative Physiological Loads

The intraoperative surgical position of the patient was modeled by applying boundary conditions such that the pelvis had a fixed position and T1 was constrained on a caudocranially oriented line and free to rotate in all directions. The rods were modeled as flexible beams whose definitions were based on their geometry and material properties. Hooks and fixed-angle screws (monoaxial screws) were modeled as single-component rigid bodies; uniaxial and multiaxial (polyaxial) screws were modeled as two-component rigid bodies whose components were connected through hinge joint and ball-socket joint, respectively. Implant models were positioned and aligned with the anchoring vertebrae according to the respective surgical techniques.[37] The implant–vertebra connection was modeled as a nonlinear general spring (represented with a flexible connector available on the computer-aided engineering platform Adams/View, Version MD Adams 2010). These springs used parametric force-displacement and moment-angle curves to relate the implant-vertebra relative displacement to the implant-vertebra load. Mechanical properties acquired from experimental tests on instrumented cadaveric vertebrae were used to define these parametric curves.[17,38] The commonly used deformity correction maneuvers were modeled, which included rod reduction, rod derotation, vertebral derotation, compression/distraction, and set-screw tightening. This was done by applying appropriate forces, moments, and kinematic constraints on and between the instrumentation constructs.[38]

Change from an intraoperative position to a postoperative upright position was modeled by applying new boundary conditions for an upright position. The T1 plumb line and pelvic tilt (PT) were estimated using linear regression equations reported in Ref. 39 ($\Delta PT = -0.185\Delta LL - 7.299$ and $\Delta SVA = -1.52\Delta LL - 11.45$, where ΔPT is PT change [°], ΔLL is L1-S1 lumbar lordosis change [°], and ΔSVA is sagittal balance change [mm]). The T1 plumb line and the pelvis were repositioned using the estimations and the pelvis was fixed. A downward force was applied to each vertebra whose magnitude was determined based on the weight of the specific body section at each vertebral level, as reported in Pearsall's anthropometric model.[40] The application point was positioned anteriorly with respect to the vertebral center of mass as reported by Kiefer et al.[41] Between each pair of adjacent vertebrae, follower loads were applied between the

transverse and spinous processes, respectively, and their magnitudes were determined such that gravity forces were balanced at the estimated T1 plumb line position.

Functional flexion/extension, side bending, and transverse plane rotation were simulated with forward/backward, side translation of T1 plumb line, and T1 rotation in the transverse plane; additional external force and/or moment were simulated by applying force and/or moment on T1. Validation works of the modeling techniques have been done by simulating surgical spinal instrumentations and comparing the simulation results with the actual surgery results, with the former being ±5° to the latter in terms of Cobb angles in the coronal and sagittal planes.[17]

4.2.4 Patient-Specific Finite Element Models

Using the reconstructed 3D geometry of the spine, pelvis, and rib cage combined with the trunk external surface acquired through surface topography, a FEM of the patient's trunk can be created. The model allows the biomechanical evaluation of spinopelvic and balance parameters,[42] the biomechanical effects of spinal fusion on the sacral loading,[12] and the correction of custom-fit braces.[43] A spinal growth model was developed and incorporated in the FEM to enable biomechanical simulation and analysis of deformity correction using fusionless correction devices.[44] Including the lower limbs, the FEM can be exploited to examine the impact of intraoperative lower limb positions.[45] The spinal cord was also modeled for the assessment of the neurological impact of deformity correction.[13]

4.2.5 Hybrid Patient-Specific Finite Element Models

Detailed FEM linked to an MBM can be built to exploit the advantages of each approach. For instance, stress and strain throughout each component of the spine and pelvis can be analyzed using the detailed FEM with outputs from the MBM as boundary and loading conditions. The geometry of the pelvis, vertebrae, intervertebral disks, ligaments, and facet joints from a previously built generic spine model were first registered such that vertebral geometries from the generic model matched the reconstructed patient-specific vertebral geometries using 3D dual kriging.[46] Each of the bony components was then modeled as a trabecular core enveloped by a cortical bone layer with its thickness locally adapted from data reported in Refs. 47 and 48. Both parts were meshed using four-node tetrahedral elements between 0.4 mm (close to the bone–implant interface and areas of high surface curvatures) and 1.5 mm characteristic length. An elastoplastic material law was employed to simulate the vertebral bone viscoelastic and failure behaviors.[49] The cortical and trabecular bones were considered as homogeneous isotropic materials and their properties were derived using an inverse FEM and simulation technique.[49] The mechanical properties of the intervertebral disks, ligaments, and facet joints were calibrated such that the intervertebral load-displacement simulation results with different levels of ligament dissection corresponded to experimental data.[50] Implant models can be incorporated into the FEM and bone–implant interface established using techniques reported in Ref. 18.

4.3 Selected Applications to Computationally Model Sagittal Plane Balance and Biomechanics

4.3.1 Biomechanical Analysis of Spinal Instrumentation for Kyphotic Deformity

Ponte (PO) and pedicle subtraction osteotomy (PSO) are commonly used osteotomies to restore sagittal balance.[51] PO allows 5° to 15° correction per osteotomy level while one-level PSO allows 25° to 35° correction.[51] The objective of this study was to analyze deformity corrections, change in balance, and biomechanical loads within the instrumented spine with different PO and PSO scenarios.

Seven patients operated on with PO were selected from a medical center under institutional review board approval. Preoperative T2-T12 kyphosis were 82° ± 11°. Three alternative surgical strategies with different osteotomy types and levels and postoperative 30° functional flexion were simulated for each patient: (a) single-level PSO at the apex, (b) three-level PO around the apex, and (c) six-level PO around the apex. Results were analyzed with regard to three biomechanical indices on the osteotomy site: vertebra–implant force, rod moment, and spinal compressive force.

Simulated corrections with multilevel PO were close to those with one-level PSO. In an upright position, average implant forces were from 225 N to 280 N and rod-bending moments were ~ 10 Nm with no significant difference among the three strategies ($p > 0.05$). In simulations of 30° flexion, rod-bending moments increased by 38%, 2%, and 8% and implant forces increased by 28%, 23%, and 26% for the one-level PSO, three-level PO, and six-level PO, respectively. Correction per vertebral level was smaller than the maximum correction allowed by PO and PSO.

Based on the simulation results, multilevel PO can provide similar kyphosis correction to single-level PSO in spinal deformities with mixed indications for PO and PSO. Under postoperative functional loading, loads on the instrumentation constructs in PSO were higher than multilevel PO. The highest loads were located more often on the osteotomy sites. The kyphotic shape of the rods on the osteotomy sites in the thoracic region was not compatible with the achievement of maximum correction per osteotomy level. The rod shape may be adapted to the anticipated, significantly increased correction on the osteotomy sites (e.g., less curved or straight in the osteotomy zone for thoracic kyphosis deformities).

4.3.2 Biomechanical Analysis of Proximal Junctional Kyphosis

One of the undesirable consequences of spinal instrumentation is proximal junctional kyphosis (PJK).[52,53] PJK is an abnormal kyphotic deformity between the upper instrumented vertebra (UIV) and the UIV + 2 greater than or equal to 10°, and 10° greater than the preoperative value.[53,54] Posterior element disruptions, fusion levels, change of sagittal balance, and implant types were reported as potential risk factors of PJK.[53,55,56] The objective of this study was to assess the biomechanical effects of independent instrumentation variables involved in PJK. The

study was performed through numerical simulations of spinal instrumentations and postoperative functional loadings of six adult scoliosis patients (females, average 37.5 years). Four patients had thoracolumbar scoliosis and two thoracic scoliosis. Fusion levels ranged between 8 and 14 (average 11.3). The preoperative proximal junctional (PJ) angle was 2° ± 2° (from 0° to 5°) while the postoperative PJ angle was 14° ± 2° (from 11° to 16°). The biomechanical effects of independent instrumentation variables were assessed:

- Postoperative sagittal balance: (1) actual surgical postoperative sagittal balance (B1), and (2) actual postoperative sagittal balance shifted by 20 mm posteriorly (B2).
- Proximal fusion level: (1) actual surgical proximal fusion level (FL1), and (2) actual surgical proximal fusion level −1 (FL2).
- Three implant types at UIV: fixed angle pedicle screw, multi-axial pedicle screw, and transverse process hook.
- Four different levels of intervertebral elements dissections on the PJ FSU: (1) intact FSU, (2) bilateral complete facetectomy of the inferior facets of UIV + 1 (BCF), (3) posterior supraspinous and ISL dissection between UIV and UIV + 1 (posterior ligament dissection [PLD]), and (4) BCF with PLD.
- Four rod curvatures: 10°, 20°, 30°, and 40° measured in the thoracic region.
- Two proximal rod diameters between the last two proximal instrumented vertebral levels: the diameter was reduced from 5.5 mm to 4 mm, or was kept at 5.5 mm.

The assessment was done by evaluating four PJ biomechanical-dependent variables: the PJ angle, thoracic kyphosis, flexion moment, and extension force on the proximal noninstrumented vertebrae.

The PJ angle, proximal moment, and force were reduced by 18%, 25%, and 16%, respectively, when one more proximal vertebra was included in the fusion. When posteriorly shifting the sagittal balance by 20 mm, the PJ angle, proximal moment, and force increased by 16%, 22%, and 37%, respectively. BCF, posterior ligaments resection, and the combination of the two resulted in an increase of the PJ angle (by 10%, 28%, and 53%, respectively), flexion forces (by 4%, 12%, and 22%, respectively), and proximal moments (by 16%, 44%, and 83%, respectively). Transverse process hooks at UIV allowed about 26% lower PJ angle and flexion loads. The use of proximal transition rods with proximal diameter reduced from 5.5 to 4 mm, slightly reduced PJ angle, flexion force, and moment (less than 8%). The increase in sagittal rod curvature from 10° to 40° increased the PJ angle (from 6% to 19%), flexion force (from 3% to 10%), and moment (from 9% to 27%).

Based on the simulation results, sagittal balance and proximal fusion level had significant effects on PJ angle, proximal bending moment, and proximal extensor force. A posteriorly situated T1 plumb line, as compared with an anteriorly situated one, was associated with higher PJ angle and proximal bending moment. Instrumenting more proximal vertebrae allowed lower PJ angle and proximal bending moment, resulting in lower mechanical risk of PJK. Avoiding posterior shift of the sagittal balance, reasonably extending instrumentation proximally, preserving PJ intervertebral elements, and using more flexible proximal anchorage, helps reduce the biomechanical risks of PJK. Studies of the combined effects of more independent variables on an extended number of cases will be needed to acquire comprehensive knowledge on the risk control of PJK.

4.3.3 Biomechanical Analysis of Spinopelvic Parameters

The pelvis plays an important role in bearing and transferring loads from the upper body to the lower limbs and maintaining postural balance. Changes in spinopelvic alignment are thought to be involved in the spinal pathophysiology, but how the transferred load between the spine and pelvis is related to the spinal deformity is not well understood. Personalized FEMs of the spine and pelvis were constructed for 11 right main thoracic, 23 left thoracolumbar/lumbar adolescent idiopathic scoliosis, and 12 asymptomatic controls.[42] Stress distribution on the sacrum endplate was computed. The position of the stress distribution barycenter on the sacrum superior endplate with respect to the central hip vertical axis was projected on the transverse plane and compared between scoliotic subgroups and controls.

The difference was significant between the scoliotic subgroups and controls with regard to the mediolateral positions of the stress distribution barycenters on the sacrum superior endplate ($p < 0.05$). The stress distribution barycenter was located on the right of the central hip vertical axis in 82% of the right main thoracic patients and to the left in 91% of the left thoracolumbar/lumbar patients. Findings on the transferred load to the sacrum provided insight into the biomechanical spinopelvic interaction in 3D, showing that a thoracolumbar/lumbar scoliotic curve has an increased influence on sacral loads when compared to a main thoracic scoliotic curve.

4.3.4 Assessment of Stresses in the Spine Associated with Different Types of Sagittal Spinal Alignments

One of the surgical objectives for the treatment of sagittal deformity is to restore normal sagittal balance. A wide variation exists in sagittal spinal alignments, which are clinically considered as normal; knowledge on how mechanical stresses are distributed in spines of normal alignment is essential to determine patient-specific surgical strategies.[57]

Biomechanical models of three of the four types of spinal alignments according to the Roussouly classification[57,58] are presented in ▶ Fig. 4.2. Finite element analyses revealed similar stress patterns in the main thoracic region for the three types of spinal alignments. For type 1 alignment, higher compressive stresses were found in the anterior part of the proximal lumbar region, whereas higher compressive stresses were found in the posterior part of the distal lumbar spine. In the lumbar region, type 4 alignment had slightly higher compressive stresses in the posterior part than type 2 alignment. High shearing stresses were found in thoracolumbar and lumbosacral junctions. Typical results of stress distribution from finite element analyses in the spine are provided in ▶ Fig. 4.3.

4.4 Discussion

The 3D biomechanical models of the spine and pelvis, based on patient-specific biplanar radiographs, were found useful to characterize the spinopelvic alignment and assess surgical scenarios. Compared to traditional clinical evaluations based on radiographs and solely on geometric parameters, 3D models provide more insight into the nature of the spinal deformity, such as torsion of the spine in the transverse plane and forces and stresses within the anatomical structures and instrumentation.

The various biomechanical modeling techniques have different computation costs (from a few minutes for an MBM to many hours or days for a comprehensive FEM); the required level of model details has to be carefully adapted while ensuring the capability of evaluating biomechanical indices of clinical importance. This made it possible for the techniques to be used in clinical practices.

One of the advantages of computational model is to help overcome the inability in clinical studies to test different surgical solutions on the same patient. In a clinical study,

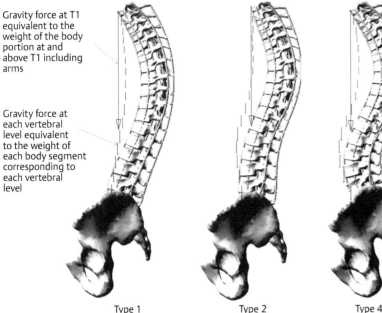
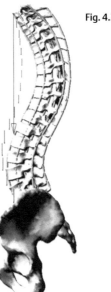

Gravity force at T1 equivalent to the weight of the body portion at and above T1 including arms

Gravity force at each vertebral level equivalent to the weight of each body segment corresponding to each vertebral level

Type 1   Type 2   Type 4

Fig. 4.2 Three variations of spinal alignments.

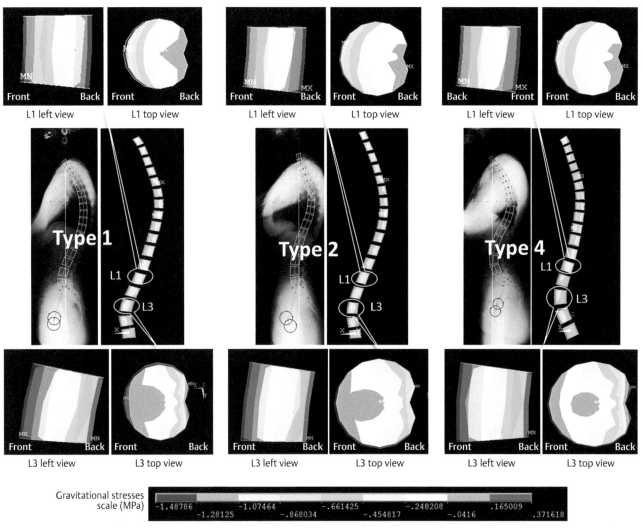

L1 left view   L1 top view   L1 left view   L1 top view   L1 left view   L1 top view

L3 left view   L3 top view   L3 left view   L3 top view   L3 left view   L3 top view

Gravitational stresses scale (MPa)

Fig. 4.3 Stress distribution (changes of stresses from compression to tension are represented by colors from blue to red).

surgical solutions have to be compared among different patients, and the impact of a surgical solution cannot be isolated from the impact of the particularity of the individual patient. There is a high heterogeneity among spinal pathologies, spinal mechanical properties of different patients, instrumentation construct designs, and surgical techniques, all of them have different effects on the outcomes of the spine surgery. This may explain why great variation continues to exist in surgical strategies among surgeons for a given case, and consensus has yet to be reached for optimal results. Using the developed modeling techniques, it is possible to preoperatively test different surgical solutions and compare the results to find the one with the most potential to achieve optimal outcomes with a rationalized number of implants.[59,60] Systematic studies may also be conducted on a large number of patients having a wide variety of spinal pathologies or similar pathologies but treated with different surgical solutions. Data acquired from such studies could be valuable for surgeons and biomedical engineers to make progress in developing new surgical treatments using new instrumentation construct designs.

In a research and development context, the modeling techniques can be used to investigate the biomechanical behaviors of pathological spine versus asymptomatic spine, such as geometric and internal mechanical load characteristics in various conditions and functional movements. As shown in Section 4.3.4, the results of finite element analyses of stresses in the spines of different Roussouly types were in support of clinical assertions that degenerative evolution in a spinal region was correlated with Roussouly's type of the spine. Depending on the Roussouly type, high stresses were located forward on the disk or backward on the facets in different spinal regions, and correspondences were found between the stress distribution patterns and locations of the degenerative evolutions. This is useful to study the pathomechanisms and progression of spinal pathology as well as treatment concepts. The techniques can be used for design evaluation in product development.

To lower the computation costs, the biomechanical model was sometimes simplified (e.g., vertebrae were modeled as rigid body); intervertebral disk, ligaments, and intervertebral articulations were respectively modeled using a single elastic element without considering their viscoelasticity. This may be considered as having a minor effect if the model is used for comparative studies with a focus on major clinical geometric indices and resultant forces and moments in spinal instrumentation. The modeling techniques can be adapted and improved by substituting mechanical property definition of each modeling element with a new definition, incorporating time-dependent mechanical behaviors. The multibody modeling techniques can be complemented by FEM to develop a hybrid modeling approach. With the relatively low computation costs, the multibody technique is used to evaluate the geometries and resultant forces and moments for a large number of loadings and instrumentation scenarios; the results provide boundary and loading conditions for a highly detailed FEM to analyze, at stress and strain levels, the biomechanics of the spine using multiple dedicated computing servers and days of solving times.

Further studies on the modeling of the spine and pelvis should be conducted on posture control, especially the balance in the sagittal plane. Depending on the needs of the biomechanical analysis to be performed, the posture control may be simplified as applying boundary conditions, such as displacement constraints on the pelvis and proximal end of the spine; it may also be necessary to model the behavior of the complex neuromuscular system of the subject in controlling their posture. Substantial efforts should be made to acquire, in vitro and in vivo, comprehensive biomechanical data to improve model calibration and validation, and make the modeling of the spine play an even more important role in studies on the biomechanics of the spine.

4.5 Conclusion

The presented modeling techniques allow subject-specific biomechanical modeling of the pelvis and spine in a clinical setup. The level of MBM detail is adequate for the assessment of geometric indices used by clinicians to evaluate deformity and balance of the spine. Resultant forces and moments of clinical interest, such as those at the bone–implant interface and intervertebral disks, can be evaluated using the MBM. The MBM combined with the modeling of spinal instrumentation allows the prediction of the biomechanical results of an instrumentation strategy. The MBM can therefore be used in preoperative planning to assist surgeons in comparing different surgical strategies and find solutions for the best clinical outcomes. The subject-specific FEM can be used to investigate the biomechanical behaviors of pathological spine versus asymptomatic spine, such as geometric and internal mechanical load characteristics in various conditions and functional movements. The presented techniques are also of high value in a research and development context. They can be used to evaluate patient posture, new treatment concepts, and construct designs and optimize treatment and design parameters. The combination of MBM and comprehensive FEM gives rise to a hybrid modeling approach enabling to further analyze, with reasonable modeling time and computational costs at stress and strain level, the pathomechanisms of spinal imbalance and its treatment.

References

[1] Lafage V, Schwab F, Skalli W, et al. Standing balance and sagittal plane spinal deformity: analysis of spinopelvic and gravity line parameters. Spine. 2008; 33(14):1572–1578

[2] Jackson RP, McManus AC. Radiographic analysis of sagittal plane alignment and balance in standing volunteers and patients with low back pain matched for age, sex, and size. A prospective controlled clinical study. Spine. 1994; 19(14):1611–1618

[3] During J, Goudfrooij H, Keessen W, Beeker TW, Crowe A. Toward standards for posture. Postural characteristics of the lower back system in normal and pathologic conditions. Spine. 1985; 10(1):83–87

[4] Mac-Thiong JM, Transfeldt EE, Mehbod AA, et al. Can C7 plumbline and gravity line predict health related quality of life in adult scoliosis? Spine. 2009; 34(15):E519–E527

[5] Ames CP, Scheer JK, Lafage V, et al. Adult spinal deformity: epidemiology, health impact, evaluation, and management. Spine Deform. 2016; 4(4):310–322

[6] Labelle H, Roussouly P, Berthonnaud E, et al. Spondylolisthesis, pelvic incidence, and spinopelvic balance: a correlation study. Spine. 2004; 29(18):2049–2054

[7] Rajnics P, Templier A, Skalli W, Lavaste F, Illés T. The association of sagittal spinal and pelvic parameters in asymptomatic persons and patients with isthmic spondylolisthesis. J Spinal Disord Tech. 2002; 15(1):24–30

[8] Rohlmann A, Bauer L, Zander T, Bergmann G, Wilke HJ. Determination of trunk muscle forces for flexion and extension by using a validated finite element model of the lumbar spine and measured in vivo data. J Biomech. 2006; 39(6):981–989

[9] Naserkhaki S, Jaremko JL, Adeeb S, El-Rich M. On the load-sharing along the ligamentous lumbosacral spine in flexed and extended postures: finite element study. J Biomech. 2016; 49(6):974–982

[10] Bono CM, Khandha A, Vadapalli S, Holekamp S, Goel VK, Garfin SR. Residual sagittal motion after lumbar fusion: a finite element analysis with implications on radiographic flexion-extension criteria. Spine. 2007; 32(4):417–422

[11] Zhang H, Hu X, Wang Y, et al. Use of finite element analysis of a Lenke type 5 adolescent idiopathic scoliosis case to assess possible surgical outcomes. Comput Aided Surg. 2013; 18(3–4):84–92

[12] Pasha S, Aubin CE, Labelle H, Parent S, Mac-Thiong JM. The biomechanical effects of spinal fusion on the sacral loading in adolescent idiopathic scoliosis. Clin Biomech (Bristol, Avon). 2015; 30(9):981–987

[13] Henao J, Aubin CE, Labelle H, Arnoux PJ. Patient-specific finite element model of the spine and spinal cord to assess the neurological impact of scoliosis correction: preliminary application on two cases with and without intraoperative neurological complications. Comput Methods Biomech Biomed Engin. 2016; 19(8):901–910

[14] Wang W, Aubin CE, Cahill P, et al. Biomechanics of high-grade spondylolisthesis with and without reduction. Med Biol Eng Comput. 2016; 54(4):619–628

[15] Filardi V, Simona P, Cacciola G, et al. Finite element analysis of sagittal balance in different morphotype: forces and resulting strain in pelvis and spine. J Orthop. 2017; 14(2):268–275

[16] Jalalian A, Tay FEH, Arastehfar S, Liu G. A new method to approximate load-displacement relationships of spinal motion segments for patient-specific multi-body models of scoliotic spine. Med Biol Eng Comput. 2017; 55(6):1039–1050

[17] Aubin CE, Labelle H, Chevrefils C, Desroches G, Clin J, Eng AB. Preoperative planning simulator for spinal deformity surgeries. Spine. 2008; 33(20):2143–2152

[18] Fradet L, Wang X, Lenke LG, Aubin CE. Biomechanical analysis of proximal junctional failure following adult spinal instrumentation using a comprehensive hybrid modeling approach. Clin Biomech (Bristol, Avon). 2016; 39:122–128

[19] Cheriet F, Laporte C, Kadoury S, Labelle H, Dansereau J. A novel system for the 3-D reconstruction of the human spine and rib cage from biplanar X-ray images. IEEE Trans Biomed Eng. 2007; 54(7):1356–1358

[20] Rehm J, Germann T, Akbar M, et al. 3D-modeling of the spine using EOS imaging system: inter-reader reproducibility and reliability. PLoS One. 2017; 12(2):e0171258

[21] Bonnier L, Ayadi K, Vasdev A, Crouzet G, Raphael B. Three-dimensional reconstruction in routine computerized tomography of the skull and spine. Experience based on 161 cases. J Neuroradiol. 1991; 18(3):250–266

[22] Breau C, Shirazi-Adl A, de Guise J. Reconstruction of a human ligamentous lumbar spine using CT images—a three-dimensional finite element mesh generation. Ann Biomed Eng. 1991; 19(3):291–302

[23] Simons CJ, Cobb L, Davidson BS. A fast, accurate, and reliable reconstruction method of the lumbar spine vertebrae using positional MRI. Ann Biomed Eng. 2014; 42(4):833–842

[24] Delorme S, Petit Y, de Guise JA, Labelle H, Aubin CE, Dansereau J. Assessment of the 3-D reconstruction and high-resolution geometrical modeling of the human skeletal trunk from 2-D radiographic images. IEEE Trans Biomed Eng. 2003; 50(8):989–998

[25] Labelle H, Dansereau J, Bellefleur C, Jéquier JC. Variability of geometric measurements from three-dimensional reconstructions of scoliotic spines and rib cages. Eur Spine J. 1995; 4(2):88–94

[26] Jaumard NV, Welch WC, Winkelstein BA. Spinal facet joint biomechanics and mechanotransduction in normal, injury and degenerative conditions. J Biomech Eng. 2011; 133(7):071010

[27] Myklebust JB, Pintar F, Yoganandan N, et al. Tensile strength of spinal ligaments. Spine. 1988; 13(5):526–531

[28] Pintar FA. The Biomechanics of Spinal Elements (Ligaments, Vertebral Body, Disc) [PhD thesis]. Ann Arbor, MI: Marquette University; 1986

[29] Panjabi MM, Brand RA, Jr, White AA, III. Three-dimensional flexibility and stiffness properties of the human thoracic spine. J Biomech. 1976; 9(4): 185–192

[30] Panjabi MM, Oxland TR, Yamamoto I, Crisco JJ. Mechanical behavior of the human lumbar and lumbosacral spine as shown by three-dimensional load-displacement curves. J Bone Joint Surg Am. 1994; 76(3):413–424

[31] Holewijn RM, Schlösser TPC, Bisschop A, et al. How does spinal release and Ponte osteotomy improve spinal flexibility? The law of diminishing returns. Spine Deform. 2015; 3(5):489–495

[32] Pal GP, Routal RV. A study of weight transmission through the cervical and upper thoracic regions of the vertebral column in man. J Anat. 1986; 148:245–261

[33] Wiemann J, Durrani S, Bosch P. The effect of posterior spinal releases on axial correction torque: a cadaver study. J Child Orthop. 2011; 5(2):109–113

[34] Yang KH, King AI. Mechanism of facet load transmission as a hypothesis for low-back pain. Spine. 1984; 9(6):557–565

[35] Watkins R, IV, Watkins R, III, Williams L, et al. Stability provided by the sternum and rib cage in the thoracic spine. Spine. 2005; 30(11):1283–1286

[36] Petit Y, Aubin CE, Labelle H. Patient-specific mechanical properties of a flexible multi-body model of the scoliotic spine. Med Biol Eng Comput. 2004; 42 (1):55–60

[37] Kim YJ, Lenke LG, Bridwell KH, Cho YS, Riew KD. Free hand pedicle screw placement in the thoracic spine: is it safe? Spine. 2004; 29(3):333–342, discussion 342

[38] Wang X, Aubin CE, Crandall D, Parent S, Labelle H. Biomechanical analysis of 4 types of pedicle screws for scoliotic spine instrumentation. Spine. 2012; 37 (14):E823–E835

[39] Liu H, Li S, Wang J, et al. An analysis of spinopelvic sagittal alignment after lumbar lordosis reconstruction for degenerative spinal diseases: how much balance can be obtained? Spine. 2014; 39(26 Spec No.):B52–B59

[40] Pearsall DJ, Reid JG, Livingston LA. Segmental inertial parameters of the human trunk as determined from computed tomography. Ann Biomed Eng. 1996; 24(2):198–210

[41] Kiefer A, Shirazi-Adl A, Parnianpour M. Stability of the human spine in neutral postures. Eur Spine J. 1997; 6(1):45–53

[42] Pasha S, Aubin CE, Parent S, Labelle H, Mac-Thiong JM. Biomechanical loading of the sacrum in adolescent idiopathic scoliosis. Clin Biomech (Bristol, Avon). 2014; 29(3):296–303

[43] Cobetto N, Aubin CE, Parent S, et al. Effectiveness of braces designed using computer-aided design and manufacturing (CAD/CAM) and finite element simulation compared to CAD/CAM only for the conservative treatment of adolescent idiopathic scoliosis: a prospective randomized controlled trial. Eur Spine J. 2016; 25(10):3056–3064

[44] Clin J, Aubin CE, Parent S. Biomechanical simulation and analysis of scoliosis correction using a fusionless intravertebral epiphyseal device. Spine. 2015; 40(6):369–376

[45] Driscoll C, Aubin CE, Canet F, Labelle H, Horton W, Dansereau J. Biomechanical study of patient positioning: influence of lower limb positioning on spinal geometry. J Spinal Disord Tech. 2012; 25(2):69–76

[46] Wagnac E, Arnoux PJ, Garo A, Aubin CE. Finite element analysis of the influence of loading rate on a model of the full lumbar spine under dynamic loading conditions. Med Biol Eng Comput. 2012; 50(9):903–915

[47] Silva MJ, Wang C, Keaveny TM, Hayes WC. Direct and computed tomography thickness measurements of the human, lumbar vertebral shell and endplate. Bone. 1994; 15(4):409–414

[48] Hirano T, Hasegawa K, Takahashi HE, et al. Structural characteristics of the pedicle and its role in screw stability. Spine. 1997; 22(21):2504–2509, discussion 2510

[49] Garo A, Arnoux PJ, Wagnac E, Aubin CE. Calibration of the mechanical properties in a finite element model of a lumbar vertebra under dynamic compression up to failure. Med Biol Eng Comput. 2011; 49(12):1371–1379

[50] Heuer F, Schmidt H, Klezl Z, Claes L, Wilke HJ. Stepwise reduction of functional spinal structures increase range of motion and change lordosis angle. J Biomech. 2007; 40(2):271–280

[51] Diebo B, Liu S, Lafage V, Schwab F. Osteotomies in the treatment of spinal deformities: indications, classification, and surgical planning. Eur J Orthop Surg Traumatol. 2014; 24 Suppl 1:S11–S20

[52] Daubs MD. Sagittal alignment changes and proximal junctional kyphosis in adolescent idiopathic scoliosis. Spine J. 2016; 16(6):784–785

[53] Kim YJ, Bridwell KH, Lenke LG, Glattes CR, Rhim S, Cheh G. Proximal junctional kyphosis in adult spinal deformity after segmental posterior spinal instrumentation and fusion: minimum five-year follow-up. Spine. 2008; 33 (20):2179–2184

[54] Kim YJ, Bridwell KH, Lenke LG, Kim J, Cho SK. Proximal junctional kyphosis in adolescent idiopathic scoliosis following segmental posterior spinal instrumentation and fusion: minimum 5-year follow-up. Spine. 2005; 30 (18):2045–2050

[55] Lonner BS, Ren Y, Newton PO, et al. Risk factors of proximal junctional kyphosis in adolescent idiopathic scoliosis—the pelvis and other considerations. Spine Deform. 2017; 5(3):181–188

[56] Yagi M, King AB, Boachie-Adjei O. Incidence, risk factors, and natural course of proximal junctional kyphosis: surgical outcomes review of adult idiopathic scoliosis. Minimum 5 years of follow-up. Spine. 2012; 37(17):1479–1489

[57] Roussouly P, Nnadi C. Sagittal plane deformity: an overview of interpretation and management. Eur Spine J. 2010; 19(11):1824–1836

[58] Roussouly P, Gollogly S, Berthonnaud E, Dimnet J. Classification of the normal variation in the sagittal alignment of the human lumbar spine and pelvis in the standing position. Spine. 2005; 30(3):346–353

[59] Le Navéaux F, Larson AN, Labelle H, Wang X, Aubin CE. How does implant distribution affect 3D correction and bone-screw forces in thoracic adolescent idiopathic scoliosis spinal instrumentation? Clin Biomech (Bristol, Avon). 2016; 39:25–31

[60] Wang X, Larson AN, Crandall DG, et al. Biomechanical effect of pedicle screw distribution in AIS instrumentation using a segmental translation technique: computer modeling and simulation. Scoliosis Spinal Disord. 2017; 12:13

5 Sagittal Balance: The Main Parameters

João Luiz Pinheiro-Franco and Pierre Roussouly

Abstract:
While corrective surgeries that modify sagittal alignment and spinopelvic balance are highly complex and may remain the realm of specialized surgeons for the foreseeable future, a thorough understanding of these underlying concepts has become requisite for all spine surgeons to prevent iatrogenic deformities, even with very short fusions.

In humans, due to our bipedal posture and inherent pathophysiology of disk degeneration, sagittal imbalance has been determined to be a common and clinically relevant problem—termed adult degenerative spinal deformity (ADSD). A concise evaluation of spinal balance in most adults can be thus divided in the assessment of pelvic parameters, spinal parameters and global sagittal balance.

Among the most important compensation mechanisms of sagittal balance, there is the ability to position the pelvis in rotation around the femoral heads. Pelvises with smaller Pelvic Incidence (PI) have less ability to retrovert over the femoral heads. Therefore, morphology defines the functional ability of the pelvis to rotate more or less, and to provide for an adequate or inadequate sagittal imbalance compensation.

Understanding that there is a great variability of PI, and that analyses of compensatory mechanisms should not be based exclusively on absolute values of Pelvic Tilt (PT), it is paramount not to assume absolute PT values to define if the spine is balanced or not.

Historically, the human spine was divided into a lumbar lordosis, a thoracic kyphosis and a cervical lordosis. In opposition to this old anatomical segmentation of the spine, there have been different proposals for a functional segmentation, arguing that it is the orientation of the successive vertebrae that defines the curvatures: lordosis represents the area where the successive vertebrae are in extension, and kyphosis in flexion. This functional segmentation allows a true sagittal measurement to be made using the Cobb method. Several authors have tried to combine those parameters in order to define the limits between balanced and unbalanced status. Some formulae as PI-LL seemed to cover a large range of situations, but we know now that pathological evolutions are not unique but mainly depending on the various shapes linked to PI value.

Keywords: pelvic incidence, pelvic tilt, sacral slope, lumbar lordosis, thoracic kyphosis, C7 plumb line, sagittal vertical axis, Barrey ratio, sagittal balance, pelvic parameters, spinal parameters, global spine balance, spino-sacral angle, distal spinal lordosis, functional spinal lordosis, methods of measurement of sagittal balance

5.1 Introduction

The concept of the spine having a "normal" alignment and that any deviation from this "norm" is not simply an anatomical variation but a fundamental problem, has been intrinsic to medicine since ancient times. Historic medical literature is rife with examples from Greek, Roman, and Arab sources of early attempts to manipulate or modify spinal alignment. Certain types of deformities that had been studied throughout the ages were instrumental in spurring the development of spine surgery since its inception in the early 19th and 20th centuries, particularly postinfectious (tuberculous), pediatric, and syndromic deformities. Nonetheless, a more comprehensive understanding of sagittal alignment and degenerative spinal deformity came into focus much later and may be considered the most valuable breakthrough in spinal degenerative pathology in the past 30 years. Whereas corrective surgeries that modify sagittal alignment and spinopelvic balance are highly complex and may remain the realm of specialized surgeons for the foreseeable future, a thorough understanding of these underlying concepts has become requisite for all spine surgeons to prevent iatrogenic deformities, even with very short fusions.

Ideal spinal alignment may be defined as the harmonious balance of the trunk over the pelvis, one which requires minimal energy expenditure to place the weight-bearing axis in a balanced physiological position.[1] In humans, because of our bipedal posture and inherent pathophysiology of disk degeneration, sagittal imbalance has been determined to be a common and clinically relevant problem, termed adult degenerative spinal deformity (ADSD). A concise evaluation of spinal balance in most adults can be thus divided into the assessment of pelvic parameters, spinal parameters, and global sagittal balance.

5.2 Methods of Measurement

The study of the sagittal balance of the spine is dependent on radiographs in a standardized fashion. The Cobb method may be used: a lateral radiograph of the spine is made with vertical 30- to 90-cm film with a constant 72-in distance from the radiographic source. The knees and hips must be in a natural position (full extension is not required). Be mindful that there are controversies about the arm positions. To avoid radiological superposition of arms and spine, a forward position of arms is necessary. Two main options are possible: fist on clavicle and arms on support. In a study by Mac-Thiong et al,[2] for two main French institutions, subjects stood with shoulders flexed 30° to 45° with hands resting on supports, whereas the remaining subjects recruited in North American institutions adopted the fist-on-clavicle position.[3] Vedantam et al[4] found that elevating the arms from 30° to 90° in standing lateral radiographs shifted the sagittal vertebral axis (SVA) 10 mm posteriorly in subjects with previous spinal fusion, which was not significant in subjects without spinal fusion. They also found that thoracic and lumbar curvatures were not affected by arm position in both subjects. For some weak patients (aging, neuromuscular), prolonged immobility without support is difficult to obtain and may induce artifacts. Marks et al[5] affirmed that shoulder flexion of 45° is the best position to use when a lateral radiograph is made for repeated SVA measuring.

Recently, the EOS system has been developed, which allows for full-spine standing imaging with minimal irradiation. When using EOS, the sliding sources system needs only 6 to 10 seconds for image capture but requires a highly stable patient positioning during the full procedure to avoid artifacts.

The main rule for positioning the patient is the standardization of the radiography procedure to allow for the comparison two different images. The radiograph must show the femoral heads (FHs) and at least the skull base. Radiographs need be digitized, and all measurements should be performed using specialized software, such as Surgimap or KEOPS (SMAIO, Lyon, France). Such software permits rapid and precise measurements of all angular parameters on digitized radiographs. Using a computerized software, the intraobserver and interobserver reliability is very high and the results are similar to those obtained by manual measurement.[6,7] Other reports have evaluated the intra- and interobserver reliability of measuring pelvic incidence (PI) using manual methods on digitized radiographs.[8,9] Dimar et al[9] obtained low intraclass correlation coefficients (ICCs) of intra- and interobserver reliability for manual measurements of PI even among experienced spinal surgeons (0.69 and 0.41, respectively). Dimar et al recommended computer-assisted method for measuring PI with high reliability.[9] Yamada et al[10] used a computer-assisted method obtaining exceptionally high agreement of intra- and interobserver ICC of Full Spine (FS)-PI (0.84 and 0.79, respectively) and correlation coefficient of 0.81 between FS-PI and Computed Tomography (CT)-PI. These authors[10] noted that the error of measuring PI is not mainly a result of the difficulty in precisely identifying the bicoxofemoral axis but a result of the difficulty in identifying the sacral endplate in cases with lumbar scoliosis, obesity, and elderly patients with possible osteoporosis. Legaye et al[11] observed, especially in situations with a dome-shaped sacrum, that the inaccurate visualization of the superior plate of S1 does not allow an exact measurement of PI.

Whatever the employed technique, it is mandatory and essential to obtain good radiographs with perfectly readable landmarks. In case of doubtful situations where radiological landmarks are missing or are not visible, the analyzed case must be rejected.

5.2.1 Pelvic Parameters

Central to the concept of global spinal balance is the idea that the sacrum, as the basis of spine building, is almost a contiguous and fully mobile element of the spine: the "pelvic vertebra" as it is referred to by Jean Dubousset (▶ Fig. 5.1). The sacrum is part of the pelvic ring through the sacroiliac joints (SIJs), a diarthrodial joint with minimal movement thus comprising a single functional unit with the pelvis, articulating with the FHs through the acetabulum. The relationship between the sacrum and the acetabulum is thought to remain stable during most of an adult's life, with changes usually as a consequence of trauma or surgery with consequent alterations to the SIJ or a suggested very slow and small increase as a result of aging.[12] Effective hip and pelvic balance are necessary to provide the spinal and pelvic muscles an optimal alignment that effectively supports the spinal column, which consequently is crucial to maintain a standing erect posture.

These concepts came to light in the late 1980s not only as a result of an enhanced understanding of the normal aging of the spine but also of increased perception of iatrogenic spinal deformities following spinal fusions.[11,13] Although some anatomists such as Delmas in France had previously described variations in the sacral anatomy, it was only in 1986 that During et al[14] presented a new pelvis morphometry that demonstrated a variability in the pelvis anatomy that influenced the pelvis orientation and the spinal shape. During et al proposed a skeletal outline of the spinopelvic complex defining morphological and positional angles. It was suggested that "aberrations of posture" might cause low back pain as a result of patterns of stress concentrations. This concept was very advanced for the

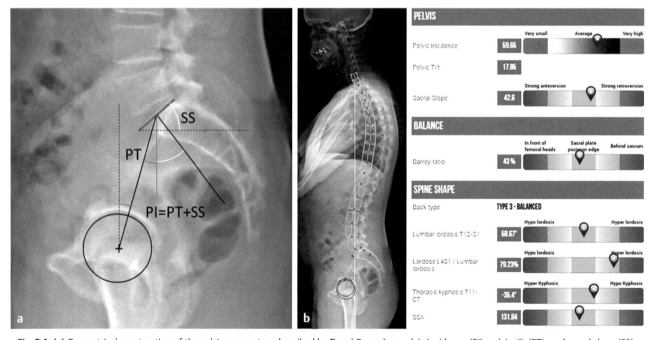

Fig. 5.1 (a) Geometrical construction of the pelvic parameters described by Duval-Beaupère: pelvic incidence (PI), pelvic tilt (PT), and sacral slope (SS). **(b)** Sagittal reconstruction of the spine using KEOPS software.

time and even the term "sagittal balance" was never mentioned. During's system of arcs of circle were to become the cradle to the classification of lordosis types by Roussouly et al.[15] Duval-Beaupère et al[16] clarified a pelvic morphological evaluative method defining the PI as the angle linking the anatomical and functional relations between the sacrum and the hips joints. These relationships between hip-pelvis and spine may be exemplified mathematically and radiologically by three angles, collectively termed pelvic parameters.

5.2.2 The Morphological Pelvic Parameter

PI is the main angle and demonstrates the anatomical relationship between the acetabulum and the S1 endplate. PI is the morphological angle representing the mature morphology of the pelvis. It is considered to grow from childhood until reaching the maximal value. PI is the angle between two lines: the line perpendicular to the midpoint of the sacral endplate and the line drawn by the union of two points: the midpoint of the sacral endplate and the center of the bifemoral axis (or the midpoint of a line connecting both FHs if they are misaligned) (▶ Fig. 5.1). As mentioned above, PI was once thought to remain stable during adulthood but there is increasing evidence that aging will lead to a gradual increase in PI through modification of SIJ anatomy.[17,18]

Anatomists have never described variations in pelvic shape with consideration of PI. In asymptomatic populations, there is a large range of PI values between 35° and 85° with extremes of less than 20° until 95° in pathology.[15] What is the morphological significance of such variations? Roughly in cases of small PI (< 45°), the sacral plateau is just over the FH, the sacrum is long, and the sacral plateau horizontal projection is close to the iliac crest. In cases of high PI, the sacrum is shorter as if a part of the sacral vertebra was missing and is positioned more posteriorly regarding the FH center. The sacral plateau is far below the projection of the iliac crest. A pelvis with small PI is referred to as a narrow pelvis, whereas one with high PI represents a large pelvis. However, it is uncertain whether this hypothesis is correct. It has been supposed that there exist anatomical variations of iliac bone orientation: more frontal in small PI and more sagittal in high PI. This hypothesis needs to be considered

in the evolution of the bipedal acquisition, as large apes have a more frontal iliac bone orientation compared to the human pelvis. Pelvic shape in *Homo sapiens*, on the other hand, has poor variation in the iliac bones, whereas changes in PI are mainly a result of the sacral morphology. Debate exists whether PI is higher in human females or whether there is no difference according to gender. Likewise, there is discussion of whether there are regional or ethnic variations[19,20] as well.

To accurately measure PI, the physician may be faced with several difficulties. The sacral endplate with anterior and posterior limits is usually easy to identify. Inversely, determination of the FH center may be confounding because it is difficult to have both FH centers superimposed when using classical radiographs with a fixed source. Two situations may occur:

1. The FHs are shifted on the vertical axis (▶ Fig. 5.2). This is because of the X-ray beam inclination to lower limb length difference. Using the midpoint of the line between both centers of FH is therefore acceptable for measuring PI.
2. The FHs are shifted on the horizontal axis (▶ Fig. 5.3). This should be unacceptable when this situation interferes with the correct analysis of the sagittal balance. This may happen because of a horizontal rotation of the pelvis. The image is no longer a true lateral view and if the shift is too great, the important PI measurement will be compromised, and the radiograph needs to be rejected.

When using the EOS system for spinal balance analysis, the perfect horizontal alignment of the beams at each level may allow for the perfect superposition of FH except for lower limb inequality. However, a rotational position of the pelvis with a horizontal shift remains possible and PI measurements have yet to be rejected when the shift overpasses the half diameter of FH.

Sometimes the identification of the sacral endplate may be difficult. In high-grade dysplastic spondylolisthesis, the sacral endplate is no longer flat, and its rounded contour is referred to as "dome"-shaped. In these cases, PI measurement is impossible. In cases of junctional L5-S1 abnormalities, when L5 is sacralized, the L5-S1 vestigial disk must be used for PI measurement when clearly visible. When S1 is part of the lumbar spine, the upper plate of S1 may be used (▶ Fig. 5.4). Sometimes, in the case of strong ambiguity, the general aspect of the spine may be a guide for the choice of vestigial disk for PI

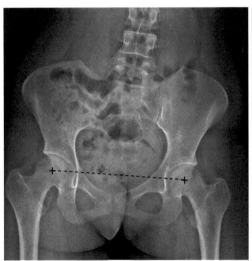
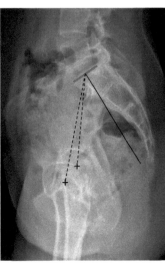

Fig. 5.2 Vertical femoral head misalignment as a result of inequality of lower limbs: poor change in pelvic incidence (PI) measurement.

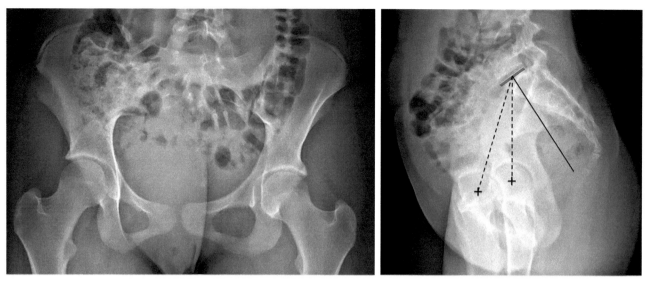

Fig. 5.3 Horizontal FH misalignment as a result of pelvic rotation: high change in pelvic incidence (PI) measurement, risk of error in PI evaluation.

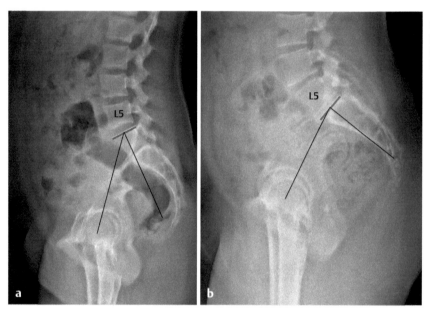

Fig. 5.4 Lumbosacral junctional anomaly: **(a)** S1-S2 vestigial disk, using S1 plateau for pelvic incidence (PI) identification. **(b)** Sacralization of L5, using S1 plateau below L5 to measure PI.

measurement. In every case, when it is impossible to identify the sacral endplate, PI measurement should be rejected.

5.2.3 The Functional Pelvic Parameters

The pelvis has the freedom to rotate on the sagittal plane over the FH, so there is a true relationship between sacral plate orientation and pelvic rotation (► Fig. 5.5). This is evaluated by the two composite angles of the PI, that is, pelvic tilt (PT) and sacral slope (SS). There is a fine tuning of the pelvis sagittal orientation in space to maintain the erect position with a minimum of energy expenditure by using the back muscles. To obtain an economic sagittal balance, the position of the hips and sacrum may change from a more horizontal to a more vertical sacrum.

PT indicates the rotational positioning of the pelvis around FH. PT is the angle between two lines: the line formed by the union of the midpoint of the FH with the midpoint of the sacral plate and the vertical line originating from the center of the FH.

Mean PT is 13° ± 6°.[20] A value of 20° or lower has been considered the reference range for a "normal" PT in the Schwab classification for ADSD.[21] Understanding that there is a great variability of PI, and that analyses of compensatory mechanisms should not be based exclusively on absolute values of PT, it is paramount not to assume absolute PT values to define whether the spine is balanced or not. A PT of 20° in a PI of 70° may be normal, whereas a PT of 20° with a PI of 45° will probably represent a compensated condition. On the contrary, when PT is less than 5°, this could indicate a hyper anteverted pelvic situation because of an inadequate, too high lordosis. Values and formulas should be analyzed in a more global context, by convention, when the midpoint of the sacral endplate is aligned with the vertical line (PT = 0°). If the pelvis rotates backward, PT increases. If the pelvis rotates forward, PT decreases.

PT angle is directly connected to hip motion. In a fixed standing position, when the femur is vertical, PT measures the position of the hip joints to balance the pelvis-spine system. If

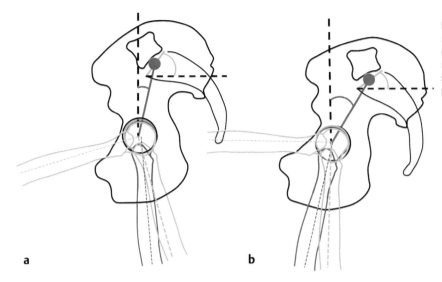

Fig. 5.5 Hip range of motion and positioning regarding the pelvis orientation and pelvic tilt. **(a)** Pelvis in neutral position: hips move between maximal flexion (in yellow) and maximal extension (in green). **(b)** Retroverted pelvis: decreasing possibility of hips extension.

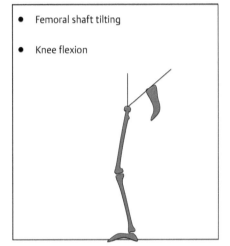

- Femoral shaft tilting

- Knee flexion

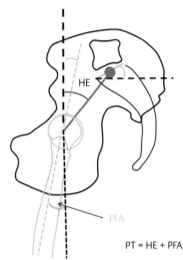

Fig. 5.6 When pelvic tilt (PT) increases, hip extension is overpassed and knees flexum allows PT to increase. PFA, Proximal femoral angle.

PT = HE + PFA

the balance needs more PT, hip extension (HE) increases. If PT increases, needing more HE, hip positioning in extension may be overpassed; in this case, the femoral shaft must tilt through flexion of the knees. As such, PT is no longer a result of the hips but of the addition of the femoral tilt and HE. Mangione and Sénégas have described the proximal femoral angle (PFA) as being between the femoral shaft axis and the vertical line.

When the knee flexion is required for adjusting PT, it may be written PT = PFA + HE. (▶ Fig. 5.6). When PT decreases after surgical treatment, PFA decreases until PT = HE and the knee compensation disappear spontaneously. Because the midpoint of the sacral endplate was chosen by convention, PT has no real significance regarding hip positioning. It is difficult to define when the hips are in a neutral position. Likewise, it is difficult to establish an ideal or neutral PT value.

SS is a positional angle and may change throughout life, according to sagittal balance requirements. The SS is the angle between two lines, namely, the line of the sacral endplate and a horizontal line. The orientation of SS directly guides the orientation of L5 and the whole spine above. This parameter is the direct link between the pelvis and the lumbar lordosis (LL). In normal situations, SS is always tilted forward with positive increasing values. In pathological situations, SS may even reach

the horizontal line (SS = 0°). Negative SS values, always indicating pathology, are exceptional. In the seating position, SS may be negative.

5.3 Influence of PI Variation on Positional Parameters PT and SS

PI, SS, and PT are linked by the geometrical equation PI = PT + SS. When SS tends to reach 0°, PT tends to equal PI. Pelvic anteversion (lower PT, increased SS) or retroversion (higher PT, lower SS) are physiologic strategies that enable humans to assume a bipedal posture in a more energy-efficient manner. This ability to position the pelvis in rotation around FH is one of the most important compensation mechanisms of sagittal balance. Pelvic retroversion (increasing PT) allows both decreasing SS to adapt to the loss of lordosis, by bringing the trunk backward to fight against forward gravity displacement. The ability to do so is mathematically higher in patients with a large PI pelvis.[22] (▶ Fig. 5.7). In other words, there are increased possibilities for pelvic retroversion when PI is high. The ability to retrovert the pelvis is an important evaluation tool in ADSD. Pelvises with smaller PI have less ability to retrovert over the

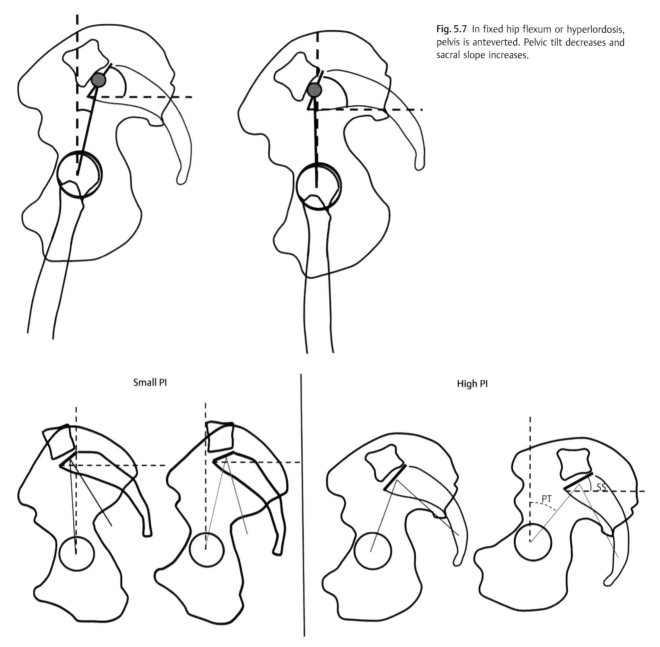

Fig. 5.7 In fixed hip flexum or hyperlordosis, pelvis is anteverted. Pelvic tilt decreases and sacral slope increases.

Fig. 5.8 Difference in pelvic tilt range regarding the value of pelvic incidence (PI). Note that in smaller PI, the sacral plateau is higher over the femoral head (FH) close to the projection of the iliac crest. With higher PI, the sacrum looks smaller; the sacral plateau is in the lower position compared to the iliac crest level and posterior to FH.

FHs (▸ Fig. 5.8). Therefore, morphology defines the functional ability of the pelvis to rotate more or less and to provide for an adequate or inadequate sagittal imbalance compensation.

The orientation of the sacral endplate, more or less tilted (as the L5-S1 disk), influences the sagittal alignement of the whole spine. The greater the PI, the greater the SS, and the greater LL.[22]

5.4 Sagittal Regional Parameters— Spinal Parameters

Over time, there have been many different methods to measure and report normative values for cervical lordosis (CL), thoracic

kyphosis (TK), and LL. Initially, these measures were derived from purely morphological studies and a myriad of angles and measurements that were described with uncertain clinically significant terms that provided overlapping information at best.[23] In addition, population-based normative studies carried with them the intrinsic problem of age and ethnic variation. With the advent of an important multicenter data registry and the recognition of the value of standardized measurement techniques to compare results, certain measurement parameters began to gain more acceptance.[24,25]

Most mammals have a long kyphosis in the thoracic and lumbar areas. Acquisition of lordosis was the adaptation that allowed bipedalism in humans. From embryology, it is known that the normal human spine possesses one primary (thoracic curvature) and two secondary (cervical and lumbar) curves. The thoracic curve is termed primary because it is initially developed while still in an embryo as the secondary curves are not present at birth; with normal neuromuscular development, CL develops by 3 months and LL by 1 year.

Historically, the human spine was divided into an LL, a TK, and a CL. This segmentation first described by Hippocrates, assigned for each anatomical segment of the spine a particular orientation: convex forward from L5-S1 to T12-L1, convex backward from T1 to T12-L1, and convex forward in the cervical spine. Even with using long-standing X-rays into more modern times, this anatomical segmentation remained. Initially, most authors described LL as the angle between the L1 superior endplate and L5 inferior endplate. More recently, there has been consensus to extend LL to the S1 plate. In the thoracic area, because of the difficulty in visualizing the upper thoracic vertebrae, the classical measurement of TK has been between T5 and T12.

In opposition to this old anatomical segmentation of the spine, there have been different proposals for a functional segmentation, arguing that it is the orientation of the successive vertebrae that defines the curvatures: lordosis represents the area where the successive vertebrae are in extension and kyphosis in flexion. This functional segmentation allows a true sagittal measurement to be made using the Cobb method. The representation and construction of the functional lordosis has been studied and demonstrated by different geometrical methods: arc of circle[26] and quadrant of an ellipse.[27] The

ellipsoidal construct is extremely complex to be used in routine practice.[1] Berthonnaud et al.[26] defined a mathematical design of the lordotic curve (▶ Fig. 5.9). It was proposed to define lordosis using the Cobb method as the curve between the sacral endplate and the inflection point where lordosis bends into kyphosis. Berthonnaud et al[26,27] proposed this segmentation model of the spine, suggesting the inflection point where lordosis turns into kyphosis, without reference to a specific anatomical landmark. Accordingly, the lordosis curvature is divided into two tangent arcs of a circle at the apex. The lower arc is located between the sacral plateau line and the horizontal line passing through the apex. The upper arc is the angle defined by the horizontal line through the apex and the perpendicular to the tangent passing on the inflection point. A particular geometrical property is the strict equality between the lower arc of lordosis and SS. This same segmentation may be obtained at the thoracic level for TK. Lordosis area and kyphosis are linked by a relation of equality between the upper arc of lordosis and the lower arc of kyphosis (▶ Fig. 5.9).

Because of a possible confusion between both anatomical and functional definitions of LL, it is proposed here to use LL for the lordosis between T12-L1 and the sacral plateau, and distal spinal lordosis (DSL) for the lordosis between the inflection point and the sacral plateau (▶ Fig. 5.10). In the first case, only one angle is needed to define LL; in the second case, one angle and the number of included vertebrae are necessary (▶ Fig. 5.10).

At the cervicothoracic level, the same segmentation model may be used through the cervicothoracic inflection point; TK is

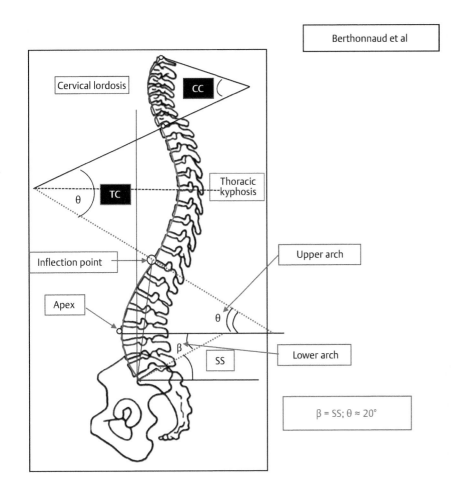

Berthonnaud et al

Fig. 5.9 Spinal segmentation according to Berthonnaud et al.[26] CC, Cervical curve; SS, sacral slope; TC, thoracic curve.

Cervical lordosis

CC

Thoracic kyphosis

TC

θ

Inflection point

Upper arch

Apex

θ

β

SS

Lower arch

$\beta = SS; \theta \approx 20°$

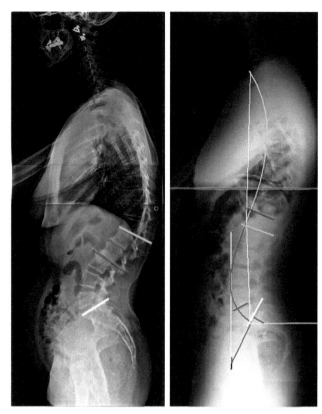

Fig. 5.10 Comparison between classic lumbar lordosis definition and new distal spinal lordosis (DSL). Note the effects on the length of lordosis. The yellow line is the S1 endplate, the green line is the superior L1 endplate, and the red line refers to the DSL. Note that in these two situations, there are strong biomechanical differences between two different DSL (on the left, DSL is small, and on the right, DSL is large).

defined between the two inflection points and CL may be defined from C3 to the proximal inflection point under proximal spinal lordosis. As radiological techniques (numerical or EOS) have allowed better visualization of T1, the orientation of T1 superior plate has taken on a greater importance. T1 slope is the angle between the superior plate of T1 and the horizontal line. This may offer useful information for cervical orientation.

In fuctional segmentation, there is a double reciprocity between TK and DSL: first in length, when TK increases in length, DSL decreases and vice versa. Second in angles, the lower arc of TK is equal to the upper arc of DSL. There is a therapeutic consequence: when, by surgical procedure, the length and angle of DSL is increased by artificially increasing the upper arc; TK consequentially increases and may induce proximal junctional kyphosis (PJK).

5.5 Is There a Relation between PI, SS, and DSL?

As it has been explained, the lower arc of DSL is equal to SS. Chapter 6 discusses how the upper arc of DSL in asymptomatic populations is almost always constant. However, there is a strong correlation between SS and the global angle of DSL ($R = 0.86$). It is important to note that the wide variation of DSL stays inside SS. As PI varies closely with SS, it seems evident

that DSL varies with PI. A strong PI correlates with a large DSL or LL and vice versa. This observation (and the use of PI-LL mismatch to clinically assess the balance) might be correct in numerous cases but as will be seen in the next chapter, it is not a rule to be applied in every case.

5.6 Global Assessment of Sagittal Balance

The aim of global balance identification is to relate the top of the cervicothoracolumbar spine with the shape and/or the position of the pelvis. Classically, the well-identifiable middle of the C7 vertebral body was chosen. In Chapter 3, Vital et al proposed the internal ear conduct, including the cervical spine and the skull for global balance evaluation.[11] Other studies focused on the T1 vertebral body that is more visible now with digitized radiographs. Because of its approximation to the level of the global center of gravity, T9 has been used mainly in France with Duval-Beaupère.[28] Distally, the anatomical landmarks were essentially the sacral endplate (limits and midpoint) and FH (center, bifemoral axis). Different parameters have been described either as distance or as angles.[1]

Distance analyses may be confounding. A precise measurement of a distance between two points needs an accurate calibration of radiographs that is not always done with perfection. The second problem is the size ratio: is it possible to compare distance in a tall man with a small woman? Ratio of distances is a more appropriate method to avoid the two causes of uncertainty. It allows the positioning of one point relative to two other points; there is no need for calibration and it allows for ignoring the size ratio.

Calibration of radiographs is not mandatory with angle comparison, but size ratio may bring to light very different offsets for a same angle. With very small angles and very small variations, artificially good correlations may be obtained. An angle drawn between two anatomical intrinsic lines is a morphological or shape angle; one measured between an anatomical line and a directional reference (vertical or horizontal) is a positional angle (▶ Fig. 5.11). The addition of 90° or 180° to a previously described angle does not change the angle meaning but sometimes it may help for a better geometrical understanding.

The global balance of the spine has been studied extensively and several forms of descriptions have arisen:

1. T9 tilt: Duval-Beaupère defined this parameter to indicate the sagittal balance through the body center mass.[16,20] T9 tilt is the angle between two lines, namely, the vertical line passing through the center of T9 and the line uniting the center of the FH and the center of T9. Reflecting the sagittal balance of the spine, it is dependent on three factors: a linear combination of the PI, LL, and SS; the PT; and the TK.

2. C7 plumb line: The readability of the C7 vertebral body is possible in most whole-spine lateral radiographs. A review of the literature has validated this parameter as a reliable and stable indicator of global sagittal balance.[29] For measuring the C7 plumb line, a vertical line is drawn from the center of C7 vertebra, and the physician must study the distance from this vertical line in relation to the posterior end of the sacral plate. As T1 vertebra is sometimes not visible on FS radiographs, the C7 plumb line is a preferrable method.

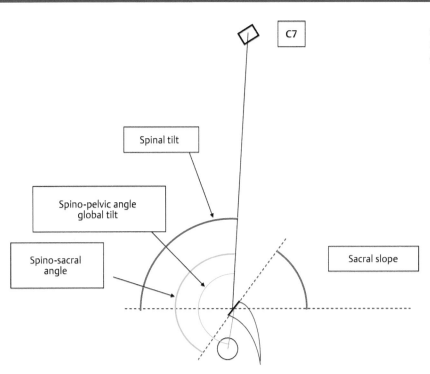

Fig. 5.11 Spinal balance through C7 assessment using angles. In red are positioning angles, and in green, shape angles.

Global radiological assessment of the spine begins by analyzing whether the radiographs are adequately performed, that is, the position of the arms, face, and hips. C7 is marked out and a plumb line drawn from the center of its vertebral body, perpendicular to the ground.

There are three methods of using the C7 plumb line in evaluating sagittal balance:

1. Distance measurement: The SVA is widely used as a method to evaluate global sagittal balance. SVA is the distance from the C7 plumb line to the posterior end of the sacral plate. Schwab et al[30] defined 5 cm as an indicator of sagittal imbalance. However, it is well known that radiographic measurements are prone to errors. An imprecise calibration will lead one to perform an error analysis. SVA is considered positive when the C7 plumb line is anterior to the posterosuperior corner of the sacrum and negative when the C7 plumb line is posterior from the posterosuperior corner of the sacrum.

2. Angles measurement: Utilizing a line drawn from the center of C7 to the center of the sacral endplate, two angles can be defined:

   • C7 tilt is a positional parameter. The angle is quite constant in an asymptomatic population with approximately 3° to 5° backward.

   • Spinosacral angle (SSA) is a morphological parameter consisting of the angle formed by two lines named the sacral endplate line and the line from the C7 centroid to the midpoint of sacral endplate, as described by Roussouly et al.[31] It defines the total kyphosis of the thoracolumbar spine, not taking into account the cervical spine. There is a robust association between SSA and SS in asymptomatic individuals, implicating body efforts to balance C7 plumb line over the sacrum in normal situations. SSA gives a value of the global kyphosis of the spine and decreases when the spine gains kyphosis. This provides a good evaluation of global change of the spine after a pedicle subtraction osteotomy (PSO) procedure.

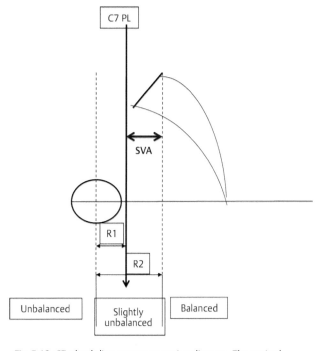

Fig. 5.12 C7 plumb line assessment using distance. The sagittal vertical axis is a direct distance measured in mm. Barrey ratio R1/R2 allows a relative position of C7PL.

   • Spinopelvis angle (SPA), first decribed by Roussouly then more recently by Obeid as global tilt (GT) (GT = 180° − SPA), is described as a line from C7 to the midpoint of the sacral plate, and FH to the middle of the sacral plate. GT = PT + C7 tilt.[32] Obeid has demonstrated a good correlation with global balance.

3. Distance ratio (► Fig. 5.12) was described by Barrey[1] as the ratio between the horizontal distance from the C7 plumb line

to the posterior end of sacral plate, and the horizontal distance from C7 plumb line to the center of FH. The ratio allows the analysis of the position of C7 plumb line relative to these morphological landmarks. This ratio describes an adimensional value determining the position of the C7 plumb line relative to vertical lines passing through FH and the posterior end of S1:

- When the C7 PL is located behind the posterior end of the sacral endplate, the ratio is higher than 1 and the spine is balanced.
- If C7 PL is located between the FH and posterior end of sacral endplate, the ratio is between 0 and 1 and balance is compromised.
- If C7 PL is anterior to FH, the spine is unbalanced.

The author prefers to use angles or distance ratio, as these are not prone to calibration errors commonly found in radiographs. Furthermore, to obviate some of these problems, several measurements have been described, yet lately one method has been gaining more acceptance: the T1 pelvic angle (T1PA), measured from the center of the T1 vertebral body to the center of the FH and then to the midpoint of the S1 endplate. Its angular components are the PT and the T1 spinopelvic angle. Although obviating the need for calibration, it may be difficult to detect small variations of the T1PA and not nearly as much evidence has been accumulated supporting it as the SVA.[3,33]

5.7 Final Considerations

No single radiological parameter objective of surgery should outweigh the clinical objectives of maintaining an erect posture with as little effort as possible and with comfortable horizontal gaze. In summary, these goals are best accomplished if the spine is within the cone of energy. However, surgeons will realize, early in in their careers, that attempting to attain alignment parameters typical of a young spine in an elderly patient is not only a dangerous and lengthy process, but it may also be inadequate and nonphysiologic, predisposing patients to additional problems such as PJK. There is considerable evidence supporting the restoration or improvement in sagittal balance results in fortuitous postoperative outcomes and better quality of life.[21,25] However, procedures designed primarily to restore sagittal thoracolumbar balance are fraught with complications whether performed in a conventional or so-called "minimally invasive" manner, with major complication rates as high as 70% and significant mortality.[34,35]

Measurements with important clinical correlations have recently been summarized in the SRS-Schwab Adult Spinal Deformity Classification: PI-LL mismatch, SVA, and PT.[21] The authors found that restricting evaluation to only these parameters may occasionally fail to adequately demonstrate cervicothoracic deformity and always stress the importance of a thorough clinical exam. Restoration of global alignment may in some specific cases be obviated or delayed in the case of very frail or osteoporotic patients and in a diametrically opposite population, that of very active, younger adults in the fifth or sixth decade for whom a long fusion may have significant implications because of rigidity. As usual, sagittal balance should still be considered and patients along with their surgeon should adjust their expectations accordingly and plan for postoperative surveillance[36] (▶ Fig. 5.13).

5.8 Conclusion

This is not intended to be an "all-inclusive" review of the history of ADSD but a concise review and practical guide to assessment and surgical planning. With that goal in mind, we have willfully omitted certain measurements and concepts with undeniable historical and morphological significance, which some surgeons may individually favor. However, as clinical evidence accumulates from clinical registries and are disseminated through scientific publications, it becomes a self-fulfilling prophecy—more trainees become aware of certain measurements favored by these groups and put them into practice, making them more popular. These measurements in use today will certainly evolve and may not be in use in 5 or 6 years, especially as more advanced imaging is developed, and more surgeons recognize and overcome this problem.

The important message is that awareness of sagittal balance is necessary for every spinal surgeon even if not treating ADSD—one must absolutely avoid transforming the ADSD patient into an iatrogenic deformity case, which is much harder to address. Even if a "short" or "small" treatment is planned, which may be very adequate depending on the circumstance, expectations must be adjusted accordingly.[36] While surgery for ADSD may remain a specialized realm with significant regional variations for the foreseeable future because of the cost, resource utilization, and surgical skill necessary, every single patient must have his or her balance assessed, even the "simple" lumbar disk herniation or one-level spondylolisthesis case from which many T2-pelvis fusions for iatrogenic deformity started many years before. A stern final word of caution is also necessary to remind surgeons of the origin of some of these concepts—whether from asymptomatic populations or from surgical databases—is to understand that global sagittal alignment has large variations in the normal population and that a stooped forward patient may

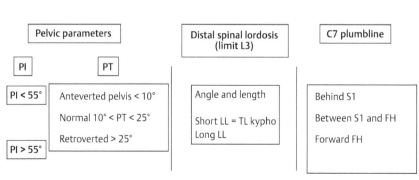

Fig. 5.13 Sagittal balance algorithm. Method of using sagittal balance parameters: (1) pelvic incidence level, (2) pelvic tilt level, (3) lumbar lordosis length and angle, and (4) C7PL position regarding femoral head and sacral plateau.

not necessarily be a problem. Once again, as always, an accurate patient interview and clinical assessment are not only key but perhaps more important than any single or group of radiological measurements.

References

[1] Barrey C. Equilibre Sagittal Pelvi-Rachidien et Pathologies Lombaires Degeneratives [these doctorat], Université Claude-Bernard, Lyon, France; 2004

[2] Mac-Thiong J-M, Pinel-Giroux F-M, de Guise JA, Labelle H. Comparison between constrained and non-constrained Cobb techniques for the assessment of thoracic kyphosis and lumbar lordosis. Eur Spine J. 2007; 16 (9):1325–1331

[3] Mac-Thiong J-M, Roussouly P, Berthonnaud E, Guigui P. Sagittal parameters of global spinal balance: normative values from a prospective cohort of seven hundred nine Caucasian asymptomatic adults. Spine. 2010; 35(22): E1193–E1198

[4] Vedantam R, Lenke LG, Bridwell KH, Linville DL, Blanke K. The effect of variation in arm position on sagittal spinal alignment. Spine. 2000; 25(17): 2204–2209

[5] Marks MC, Stanford CF, Mahar AT, Newton PO. Standing lateral radiographic positioning does not represent customary standing balance. Spine. 2003; 28 (11):1176–1182

[6] Rillardon L, Levassor N, Guigui P, et al. Validation of a tool to measure pelvic and spinal parameters of sagittal balance (in French). Rev Chir Orthop Reparatrice Appar Mot. 2003; 89(3):218–227

[7] Bari JT, Hallager DW, Tøndevold N, et al. Moderate inter-rater and substantial intra-rater reproducibility of the Roussouly Classification System in patients with adult spinal deformity. Spine Deform. 2019; 7(2):312–318. doi: 10.1016/j.jspd.2018.08.009.

[8] Vialle R, Ilharreborde B, Dauzac C, Guigui P. Intra and inter-observer reliability of determining degree of pelvic incidence in high-grade spondylolisthesis using a computer assisted method. Eur Spine J. 2006; 15(10):1449–1453

[9] Dimar JR, II, Carreon LY, Labelle H, et al. Intra- and inter-observer reliability of determining radiographic sagittal parameters of the spine and pelvis using a manual and a computer-assisted methods. Eur Spine J. 2008; 17(10): 1373–1379

[10] Yamada K, Aota Y, Higashi T, Ishida K, Nimura T, Saito T. Accuracies in measuring spinopelvic parameters in full-spine lateral standing radiograph. Spine. 2015; 40(11):E640–E646

[11] Legaye J, Duval-Beaupère G, Hecquet J, Marty C. Pelvic incidence: a fundamental pelvic parameter for three-dimensional regulation of spinal sagittal curves. Eur Spine J. 1998; 7(2):99–103

[12] Lee J-H, Na K-H, Kim J-H, Jeong H-Y, Chang D-G. Is pelvic incidence a constant, as everyone knows? Changes of pelvic incidence in surgically corrected adult sagittal deformity. Eur Spine J. 2016; 25(11):3707–3714

[13] Duval-Beaupère G, Robain G. Visualization on full spine radiographs of the anatomical connections of the centres of the segmental body mass supported by each vertebra and measured in vivo. Int Orthop. 1987; 11(3):261–269

[14] During J, Goudfrooij H, Keessen W, Beeker TW, Crowe A. Toward standards for posture. Postural characteristics of the lower back system in normal and pathologic conditions. Spine. 1985; 10(1):83–87

[15] Roussouly P, Gollogly S, Berthonnaud E, Dimnet J. Classification of the normal variation in the sagittal alignment of the human lumbar spine and pelvis in the standing position. Spine. 2005; 30(3):346–353

[16] Duval-Beaupère G, Schmidt C, Cosson P. A barycentremetric study of the sagittal shape of spine and pelvis: the conditions required for an economic standing position. Ann Biomed Eng. 1992; 20(4):451–462

[17] Jean L. Influence of age and sagittal balance of the spine on the value of the pelvic incidence. Eur Spine J. 2014; 23(7):1394–1399

[18] Skalli W, Zeller RD, Miladi L, et al. Importance of pelvic compensation in posture and motion after posterior spinal fusion using CD instrumentation for idiopathic scoliosis. Spine. 2006; 31(12):E359–E366

[19] Janssen MMA, Drevelle X, Humbert L, Skalli W, Castelein RM. Differences in male and female spino-pelvic alignment in asymptomatic young adults: a three-dimensional analysis using upright low-dose digital biplanar X-rays. Spine. 2009; 34(23):E826–E832

[20] Vialle R, Levassor N, Rillardon L, Templier A, Skalli W, Guigui P. Radiographic analysis of the sagittal alignment and balance of the spine in asymptomatic subjects. J Bone Joint Surg Am. 2005; 87(2):260–267

[21] Terran J, Schwab F, Shaffrey CI, et al. The SRS-Schwab adult spinal deformity classification: assessment and clinical correlations based on a prospective operative and nonoperative cohort. Neurosurgery. 2013; 73(4):559–568

[22] Le Huec JC, Aunoble S, Philippe L, Nicolas P. Pelvic parameters: origin and significance. Eur Spine J. 2011; 20 Suppl 5:564–571

[23] Roussouly P, Pinheiro-Franco JL. Biomechanical analysis of the spino-pelvic organization and adaptation in pathology. Eur Spine J. 2011; 20 Suppl 5:609–618

[24] Ames CP, Smith JS, Eastlack R, et al. Reliability assessment of a novel cervical spine deformity classification system. J Neurosurg Spine. 2015; 23(6): 673–683

[25] Schwab FJ, Blondel B, Bess S, et al. Radiographical spinopelvic parameters and disability in the setting of adult spinal deformity: a prospective multicenter analysis. Spine. 2013; 38(13):E803–E812

[26] Berthonnaud E, Dimnet J, Roussouly P, Labelle H. Analysis of the sagittal balance of the spine and pelvis using shape and orientation parameters. J Spinal Disord Tech. 2005; 18(1):40–47

[27] Roussouly P, Berthonnaud E, Dimnet J. Geometrical and mechanical analysis of lumbar lordosis in an asymptomatic population: proposed classification (in French). Rev Chir Orthop Reparatrice Appar Mot. 2003; 89(7):632–639

[28] Boulay C, Tardieu C, Hecquet J, et al. Sagittal alignment of spine and pelvis regulated by pelvic incidence: standard values and prediction of lordosis. Eur Spine J. 2006; 15(4):415–422

[29] Kuntz C, IV, Levin LS, Ondra SL, Shaffrey CI, Morgan CJ. Neutral upright sagittal spinal alignment from the occiput to the pelvis in asymptomatic adults: a review and resynthesis of the literature. J Neurosurg Spine. 2007; 6(2): 104–112

[30] Schwab FJ, Hawkinson N, Lafage V, et al. Risk factors for major peri-operative complications in adult spinal deformity surgery: a multi-center review of 953 consecutive patients. Eur Spine J. 2012; 21(12):2603–2610

[31] Roussouly P, Gollogly S, Noseda O, Berthonnaud E, Dimnet J. The vertical projection of the sum of the ground reactive forces of a standing patient is not the same as the C7 plumb line: a radiographic study of the sagittal alignment of 153 asymptomatic volunteers. Spine. 2006; 31(11):E320–E325

[32] Obeid I, Boissière L, Yilgor C, et al. Global tilt: a single parameter incorporating spinal and pelvic sagittal parameters and least affected by patient positioning. Eur Spine J. 2016; 25(11):3644–3649

[33] Protopsaltis T, Schwab F, Bronsard N, et al. The T1 pelvic angle, a novel radiographic measure of global sagittal deformity, accounts for both spinal inclination and pelvic tilt and correlates with health-related quality of life. J Bone Joint Surg Am. 2014; 96(19):1631–1640

[34] Haque RM, Mundis GM, Jr, Ahmed Y, et al. Comparison of radiographic results after minimally invasive, hybrid, and open surgery for adult spinal deformity: a multicenter study of 184 patients. Neurosurg Focus. 2014; 36(5):E13

[35] Smith JS, Shaffrey CI, Glassman SD, et al. Clinical and radiographic parameters that distinguish between the best and worst outcomes of scoliosis surgery for adults. Eur Spine J. 2013; 22(2):402–410

[36] Fontes RB, Fessler RG. Lumbar radiculopathy in the setting of degenerative scoliosis: MIS decompression and limited correction are better options. Neurosurg Clin N Am. 2017; 28(3):335–339

6 Spinal Curves Segmentation and Lumbar Lordosis Classification

Amer Sebaaly and Pierre Roussouly

Abstract

Since Hippocrates, spinal sagittal curvatures were described with an anatomical segmentation limiting the curves in cervical lordosis (CL), thoracic kyphosis, lumbar lordosis (LL), and sacral kyphosis. Recently, there has been a trend to use functional segmentation based on the concept of inflection point where curve orientation changes. Instead of only angle variation in the first anatomical concept, curves vary in angle, length, and apex positioning. We propose to name curves of this new disposition spinal kyphosis (SK) and lordosis (SL). Berthonnaud and others proposed, for each curve, a segmentation from a horizontal line through the apex. This undersegmentation introduces a geometrical proximal angles reciprocity: the lower arc of SL is equal to the sacral slope (SS), and the upper arc of SL is equal to the lower arc of SK. Based on this geometrical segmentation, Roussouly proposed a classification of four normal shapes in asymptomatic populations based on the strong correlation between SS and SL: (1) type 1: $SS < 35°$, short $SL < 3$ levels, low apex $< L4$, SK extended to the thoracolumbar area; (2) type 2: $SS < 35°$, longer LL, higher apex $= L4$, lower angle, global flat back; (3) type 3: $35° < SS < 45°$, apex $= L4$, harmonious SL; and (4) type 4: $SS > 45°$, SL increases in angle and length, apex $=$ L4-L3, most curved back. Based on the apex segmentation, SL varies with SS mainly; the upper arc remains almost constant (average 21°) in every type, allowing the equation: $SL = SS + 21°$. Because of the strong relation between SS and pelvic incidence (PI), there is a reciprocity between PI and the types: types 1 and 2 are found with lower PI ($< 50°$) and types 3 and 4 with higher PI ($> 45°$). Laouissat demonstrated an exception in the anteverted pelvis, allowing the possibility of type 3 with low PI. This segmentation may permit the description of the degenerative evolution, inducing local intervertebral changes and curve variations. Restoration of curves orientation regarding PI could be the basis of treatment strategy of spinal deformities.

Keywords: lumbar lordosis, Roussouly's classification, spinal curves, thoracic kyphosis

6.1 Introduction

As discussed in previous chapters, human bipedalism is an exclusive, vertical, stable, and ergonomic posture. This upright position adoption has resulted in the pelvis being more vertical and, in the same way, in the appearance of characteristic spinal curves.[1] These spinal curves are unique to *Homo sapiens* and resulted in a better energy-sparing morphology for the transition to the above-described upright posture. The interest in spinal shapes and segmentation started since ancient Greece with Hippocrates of Kos (460–370 BC). Hippocrates, regarded as the father of medicine, was the first to describe the normal spinal curvatures with their anatomical limits and orientation. Hippocrates also realized, by observation of cadavers on the battlefield, that the spine was held together by means of

intervertebral disks, ligaments, and muscles.[2] Therefore, since Hippocrates, then Galen, the spinal curvatures are classically segmented in sacral kyphosis, lumbar lordosis (LL), thoracic kyphosis (TK), and cervical kyphosis (▶ Fig. 6.1).

Despite this ideal segmentation in anatomical well-established limits, recently, some authors tend to use a functional segmentation dictated by the intervertebral orientation in the sagittal plane (▶ Fig. 6.2). This chapter provides an overview of the spinal curve segmentation leading to LL classification. A modern knowledge of the principles of sagittal spine segmentation is pivotal to understand spinal pathology and to implement a surgical strategy. This understanding is intended to provide optimum outcomes when treating spinal disorders. Hippocrates had recognized, a long time ago, the importance of the spine as stated in his famous manuscript *On Joints*: "One should first get a knowledge on the structure of the spine; this is also a requisite for many diseases."[3]

6.2 Classical Spinal Segmentation: Kyphosis and Lordosis

The term "lordosis" comes from the Greek word lordos (λόρδος) meaning "bent forward," while "kyphosis" originates

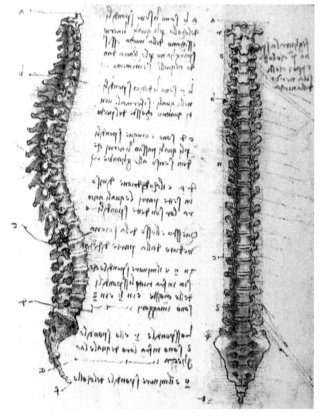

Fig. 6.1 Natural spinal curvatures as designed by Leonardo da Vinci.

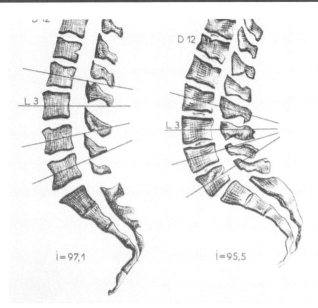

Fig. 6.2 From Delmas: on the left "static" lordosis with a higher (vertical) sacrum and more horizontal sacral plate; on the right "dynamic" lordosis with a lower sacrum and a more tilted sacral plateau.

from Greek kyphos (κυφός) meaning "hump." It seems that "lordos" was used for normal curvature, whereas "kyphos" was used for pathological curves. In his book *On Articulations and Mochlikon*, Hippocrates described the classical anatomical teaching on the spinal curvatures with consecutive lordosis and kyphosis going from the cervical spine to the sacrum. He described three categories of vertebrae: the cervical vertebrae located above the clavicle and going from C2 to the "great vertebra" (C7 or T1), the thoracic vertebrae, and the lumbar vertebra. The normal alignment of the lumbar vertebrae was termed "ithiscolios," that means that the spine is straight in the coronal but curved in the sagittal plane.[2]

This succession of curvature is of primary importance for an economical bipedal gait of *H. sapiens*. In fact, dorsal kyphosis is the only sagittal curvature present at birth (▸ Fig. 6.3).[4] The development of CL is caused by the lifting of the head and horizontal gaze allowing economical load transmission from the skull to the pelvis. In addition, the human cervical spine is unique by being perpendicular to the cranial base and the foramen magnum being more anteriorly (or less posteriorly) placed as compared to other mammals.[5] On the other hand, the lumbar curve acquires its lordosis with the acquisition of standing and walking (▸ Fig. 6.4). It is characterized, in humans, by being long and mobile allowing a fixed position of the upper spine and the cranium (fixed horizontal gaze) when the pelvis rotates during walking. As mentioned above, sagittal spinal curves increase resistance to vertical loads by directing deformations into preordered directions, which can be quickly controlled by the fast intervention of muscle contraction.[4] Compared to the quadrupeds in which the sacrum is positioned forward, the femoral heads, the vertical erected human has the sacrum backward, the femoral heads with a retroverted pelvis (▸ Fig. 6.5). This position combined with the LL allows the balance of the body weight above the pelvis generating an economical bipedal gait.[6]

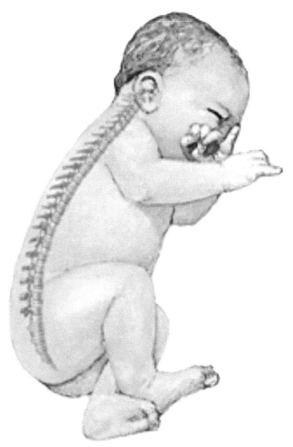

Fig. 6.3 The newborn has a C-shaped spine. The first lordotic curvature to appear is the cervical lordosis with crawling (to maintain horizontal gaze). Acquisition of lumbar lordosis allows walking.

The SRS-Schwab classification (and subsequent North American publications) define LL as the angle between the upper endplate of S1 and the upper endplate of L1.[7] TK was defined as the angle between the lower endplate of T12 and the upper endplate of T1 (▸ Fig. 6.6). Because T1 vertebra is frequently overshadowed by the humeral head and rib cage on the lateral films, and the reliability of measuring T1-T5 kyphosis is low, many authors recommend the measurements of the T4-T12 angle.[8] This segmentation of the thoracic and lumbar spine is anatomical and divides the spine into 12 thoracic and 5 lumbar vertebrae. The main problem with the anatomical segmentation is that a fixed limit (T12 or L1) does not take into account the kyphotic and lordotic curvatures with respective lengths and magnitudes. Therefore, there is the importance of the application of the functional segmentation to the spine (▸ Fig. 6.6).

6.3 Functional Segmentation of the Spine

There is no unanimity for the exact angular definition of LL. Galen of Pergamon (130–210 AD) described the anatomy of the spine stating that Nature formed the structure of the spine: "Nature creates nothing without a purpose." He insisted that vertebral body shapes provide the harmony in spinal motion.[2] Nineteen centuries later, the relationship between pelvic and

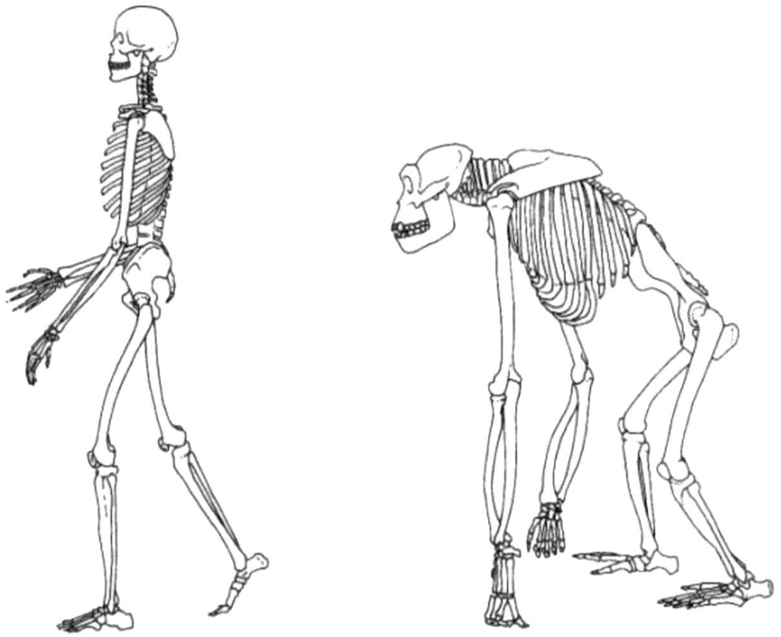

Fig. 6.4 Comparison of spinal curvatures between the big ape and human.

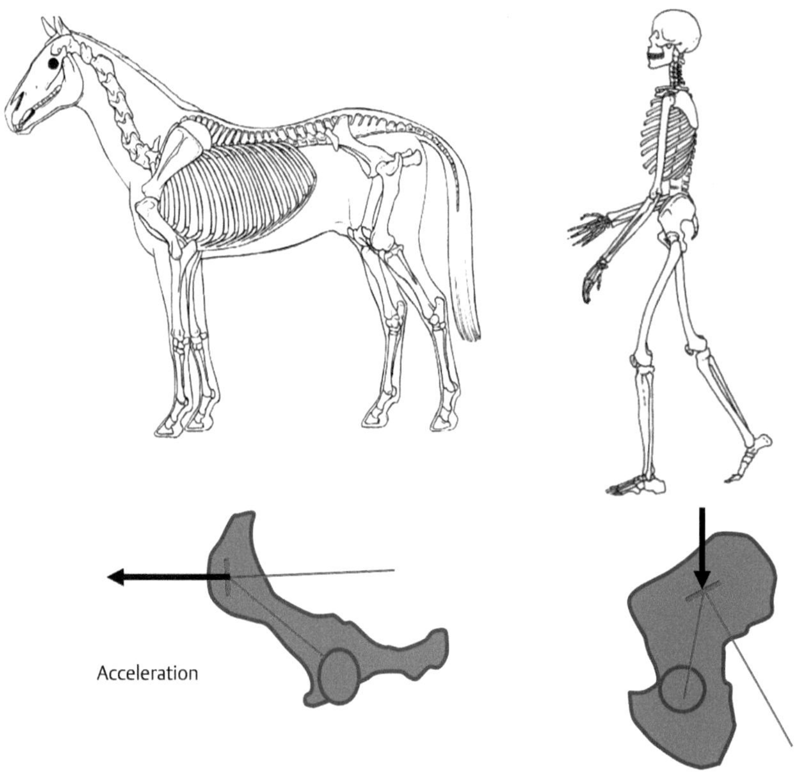

Fig. 6.5 Comparison of pelvis orientation: quadruped versus human. In quadrupeds, the pelvis is tilted forward with a vertical sacral plateau to provide horizontal force and acceleration. In humans, the pelvis is tilted backward to support vertical body weight.

Acceleration

spinal parameters was initially approached by Delmas in 1953 (▶ Fig. 6.2). He described an array of variation of normal spine ranging from "static" curved back to "dynamic" flat back, with high and low sacral slope (SS), respectively. To better understand the problematic definition of LL, it is necessary to review the different possibilities for measuring this important parameter.

Based on the studies of Delmas, and later, Stagnara et al,[9] Dimnet and Berthonnaud[10] described the "inflection point" in 2005. In fact, the spine represents a dynamic chain where the curves change direction at a specific point: the inflection point (▶ Fig. 6.7). In this articulating chain, each anatomical segment orientation and shape relates to and influences the adjacent segment in maintaining an upward posture with a minimum of energy expenditure.[10] The change of the orientation or the shape of one segment will induce a change or orientation of another segment, with the "inflection point" being the fulcrum of this change. Moreover, at the inflection point, the thoracic and lumbar curves are both tangents to a line of its limited vertebrae.

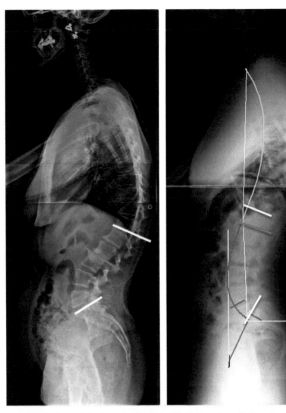

Fig. 6.6 Effect of the length of lordosis as observed in whole spine lateral radiographies. On the left, there is a short spinal lordosis (SL), with the angle being concentrated in a few vertebrae. Note that the upper end of the lordotic curve is in L3. On the right, there is a longer SL.

In the functional segmentation of the spine, the limits of LL and TK are based on the individual sagittal shape of the spine. In other words, the upper limit of LL would not be fixed at L1, and LL would be measured from the upper endplate of the sacrum to the upper limit vertebra in a similar way to the coronal Cobb angle of the scoliosis (▶ Fig. 6.6).[11] The LL spans the vertebrae from the upper sacral endplate to the inflection point where TK begins. Likewise, the TK spans the vertebrae from the inflection point with the LL to the inflection point marking the limit with CL. The conventional method of delineating TK from LL based on anatomical landmarks such as the thoracolumbar junction is overly simplistic. The advantage of this new method is that the segments are defined by the change in spatial relationships between the vertebrae at the inflection point. The present method gives a more accurate definition of each sagittal curve and the number of vertebral bodies in kyphosis and lordosis.

The analysis of the spinal curves comprises other concepts. The angle arc of a curvature of the spine (i.e., LL) may be divided into two arches limited by the apex of the curve, which determines a horizontal line (▶ Fig. 6.7). Berthonnaud et al[10] defined two tangent arcs of a circle, delimited by the apex of the curve with each arch being tangential to the vertical axis at the apex of the curve. The radius and length of each arc are independent and are determined by two critical points: the apex of the curve and the upper inflection point (▶ Fig. 6.7). Thus, the length of the upper arc of LL is localized between the apex of the LL and the inflection point. Likewise, the length of the lower

arc of the LL curve is located between the apex of the LL and the sacral endplate. In the same manner, the TK is divided into two arcs: the upper arc of TK and the lower arc of TK. The upper arc of TK is localized between the apex of the TK and the inflection point of the CL. The length of the lower arc of the TK curve is located between the apex of the TK and the inflection point between LL and TK.

Several mathematical characteristics rule these different angles. The lower arch of the LL is geometrically equal to the SS as they are corresponding angles. The upper arch of LL and the lower arch of the TK are also equal for the same reason. This could explain that an increase in LL would be followed by an increase of TK, maintaining the "spinal harmony." Even more, in a study on a cohort of asymptomatic individuals, Roussouly et al[12] found the upper arch of LL to be constant and to have a value of ~ 21.5°. As the lower arch of LL and SS are equal, LL could be predicted by the formula LL = SS + lower arc. Then by replacing each arch by its corresponding value, we have the relation LL = SS + 21°. This feature confirms the strong correlation found between SS and LL ($R = 0.86$) and indicates that the lordosis is directly dependent on SS.

6.4 Relationship between Pelvic Parameters and Spinal Parameters

The concept that pelvic parameters play an important role in spinal balance has been stressed by Dubousset,[13] who proposed the nomenclature "the pelvic vertebra" for the sacrum. Several attempts have been made to correlate pelvic and spinal parameters. Schwab et al[14] found that restoring the anatomical LL value according to formula LL = PI ± 9° was correlated to better surgical outcomes and better quality of life scores (PI = pelvic incidence). Even though this "rule of thumb" is helpful for novice spinal surgeons, it has several limitations. First, PI is a constitutional parameter and does not vary during adulthood. On the other hand, LL is a positional and very variable parameter during someone's life. Associating these two parameters with a mathematical formula seems logically unfounded. Second, albeit this formula would fit medium range PI, in other situations with PI values in the extremes (< 35 and > 70), applying this formula for correction would result in overcorrection in a low PI group and undercorrection in a high PI group. This "miscorrection" would thus lead to various surgical complications and bad results. This will be further discussed later in this book (Chapter 24).

Few studies compared the anatomic segmentation of the spine (always L1-S1) and the functional segmentation approach. In 2005, Vialle et al[15] published a cornerstone study correlating spinal and pelvic parameters. They found that "anatomic segmentation LL" was correlated to SS ($R = 0.76$) and to a lesser extent to PI ($R = 0.6$) and to pelvic tilt (PT) ($R = 0.24$). On the other hand, "functional segmentation of LL" (also nominated "maximal LL") was better correlated to SS ($R = 0.86$)—a similar result was found by Roussouly et al[12]—and to a lesser extent to PI ($R = 0.6$) and to PT ($R = 0.26$). They recommended the use of maximal LL as a value for LL and proposed that the calculation method for all the sagittal parameters be based on correlation (▶ Table 6.1). In the same manner, Berthonnaud et al found high correlations between cervical lordosis (CL) and

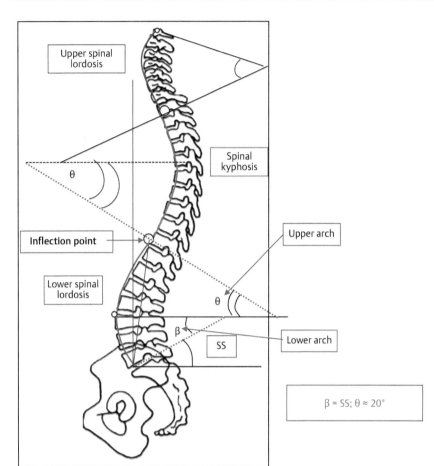

Upper spinal lordosis

Spinal kyphosis

Inflection point

Upper arch

Lower spinal lordosis

θ

β

SS

Lower arch

$\beta = SS; \theta \approx 20°$

Fig. 6.7 The geometric relationships between the lower arc of spinal lordosis (SL) and the sacral slope (sacral slope is equal to the lower arc of lumbar lordosis) as well as the upper arch of the SL and the lower arch of spinal kyphosis. The location of the inflection point between kyphosis and lordosis, position of the apex, and the degrees of curvature of the lower arc of lordosis are important determinants of sagittal morphology.

Table 6.1 Formulas for calculation of the spinal and pelvic parameters

$$SS = 7.3 + 0.63 * PI$$

$$PT = -7 + 0.37 * PI$$

$$MLL = -16 - 1.06 * SS$$

$$MLL = -2.72 - 1.1 * PI + 1.1 * PT - 0.31 * MTK$$

Abbreviations: SS, Sacral slope; PI, pelvic incidence; PT, pelvic tilt; MLL, maximal lumbar lordosis (referred to in this chapter as lower spinal lordosis); MTK, maximal thoracic kyphosis (referred to in this chapter as spinal kyphosis).
Source: Adapted from Vialle et al.[12]

LL to pelvic parameters (PT, SS, and PI) but low correlations to TK. The authors demonstrated a chain of interactions between pelvis parameters and LL ($p = 0.54$), then LL and TK ($p = 0.46$), and then TK and CL ($p = 0.58$). These stronger correlations observed between shape and orientation parameters occur at highly mobile areas of the spine—the lumbar and cervical areas —whereas the less mobile thoracic spine does not appear to react and compensate as easily as the mobile spine.[10]

6.5 Remark

The term LL is probably confusing, and, for the majority of authors, it is difficult to accept that lordosis may overpass or be shorter than the lumbar area. We think it is necessary to propose a new nosology: spinal lordosis (SL) for the segment of the spine

where the vertebrae are in extension (increasing angle between two successive inferior endplates) and spinal kyphosis (SK) where vertebrae are in flexion (decreasing angle between two successive inferior endplates) (▶ Fig. 6.7). According to this nomenclature, the normal spine would have three curvatures: the upper SL (USL) in the cervical (and or thoracic area), the SK in the thoracic (with possible extension to cervical and lumbar areas) and lower SL (LSL) in the lumbar area (with possible extension to the thoracolumbar spine). In the remaining parts of this chapter, SL (USL and LSL) and SK nosology will be used.

6.6 Why It Is Necessary to Determine this Curve Segmentation?

Recently, many authors have recommended surgical strategies by controlling the LL correction. Angle correlations or formulas based on the relation between PI and LL were employed. Their idea was to provide a simple method to determine an ideal angle for LL corresponding to PI. On the other hand, based on the concept of inflection point and the two arches theory, the present authors believe that the LSL should be strategically planned and constructed with its maximum in the lower arch. The best example for this recommendation is shown in ▶ Fig. 6.8. In the initial situation, a "normal type 3" lordosis is presented with the sagittal apex of the lordosis on the L3-L4 disk with the maximum extension (i.e., lordosis) occurring

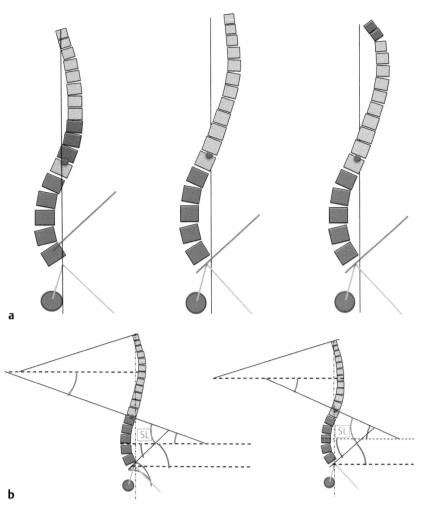

a

b

Fig. 6.8 (a) (1) Normal alignment of a type 4. (2) Same spine after L4-L5 and L5-S1 disk collapsing and distal lordosis loosening. Simulation of correction by increasing lordosis on L3-L4, L2-L3, and L1-L2 (upper arc). Global angle of lordosis is the same as in the previous situation. To maintain the same global balance (C7PL), thoracic kyphosis has to increase by correspondence between the upper lordosis arc and the lower kyphosis arc. **(b)** (1) As described in ▶ Fig. 6.8a (2), the new junctional kyphosis segment, because of a too-proximal correction of kyphosis, may be the origin of a proximal junctional kyphosis (PJK) T11, T10 when the proximal instrumented vertebra is T12 or T11. (2) If, with the same disposition, fusion and instrumentation are extended proximally on T3, T4, reducing the distal kyphosis, the proximal spine is projected backward (C7PL behind the sacrum). (3) This situation may induce a proximal PJK by mechanism of kyphosis restitution. SL, Spinal lordosis.

between L4 and S1. With degenerative changes, the extension at L4-S1 is decreased. If restoration of LL is done by increasing extension of the upper angle of lordosis, we could obtain the same LL angle value as the theoretical value. Nonetheless, by geometrical correlation between the upper angle of lordosis and the lower angle of kyphosis, a synchronous increase of the lower angle of kyphosis is to appear at level T8-T11, explaining the T8-T10 proximal junctional kyphosis (PJK) if instrumentation stops at T10. If an extension of the instrumentation to T3 is done for this PJK and if it does not respect this kyphosis compensation and a flattening of the lower arch of TK is done, the resulting backward projection of T3 may induce a cervicothoracic PJK. Therefore, it is necessary to respect not only the angle of lordosis but at the same time to respect the distal distribution of the intervertebral extension. This "theory" was recently confirmed in a large adult spinal deformity cohort. The authors found a 4.6 reduction of the risk of PJK if the sagittal apex of the lordosis is matched with the patient's PI.[16]

6.7 Theoretical Variability of Lower Spinal Lordosis

Based on the theory of inflection point and the sagittal apex of the lordosis, Roussouly et al proposed the classification of spinopelvic morphotypes by studying a group of 160 asymptomatic individuals. Prior to this study of Roussouly et al,[12] there was no classification to describe the shapes of the asymptomatic spine. It is obvious that there are wide variations on what is considered normal (▶ Fig. 6.6). Considering that the LSL is formed by two arches—one lower arch that equals the SS and one quasi constant upper arch—Roussouly et al defined four types of LSL based on the SS and the extent of LSL (▶ Fig. 6.9).[12] With lower SS values, there are two options: the radius of the lower arch of LSL tends to reduce (type 1), or the radius of the lower arch increases, close to a straight line (type 2). With higher SS values, the lower arch of LSL increases in angle and length with a higher apex of LSL (types 3 and 4) (▶ Fig. 6.9). The different types of lordosis could be defined as follows:

- Type 1 lordosis (▶ Fig. 6.10): characterized by low SS (< 35°), the LSL is short. The apex of the LL is located in the center of the L5 vertebral body. The inflection point is low and posterior and does not exceed the L2-L3 level, creating a short lordosis with a maximum of three vertebrae in LSL. The upper spine has a significant kyphosis spanning the thoracolumbar junction and thorax.
- Type 2 lordosis (▶ Fig. 6.11): characterized by low SS (< 35°). The apex of the LL is located at the base of the L4 vertebral body. The inflection point is higher and more anterior creating a longer but flat LSL (over three levels), close to a straight

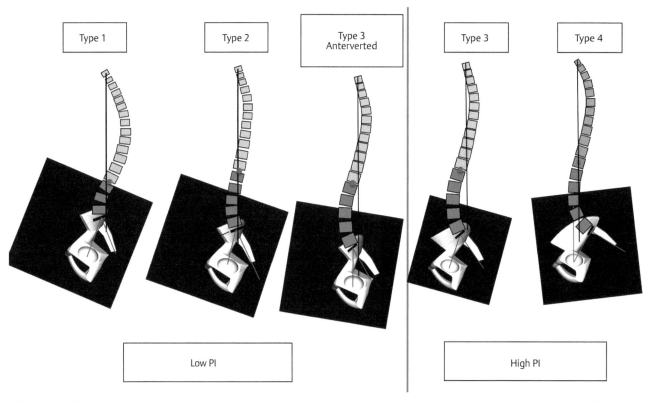

Fig. 6.9 The different types of the Roussouly classification. Note that types 1, 2, and the anteverted type are associated with low pelvic incidence (PI) values and types 3 and 4 are associated with higher PI values.

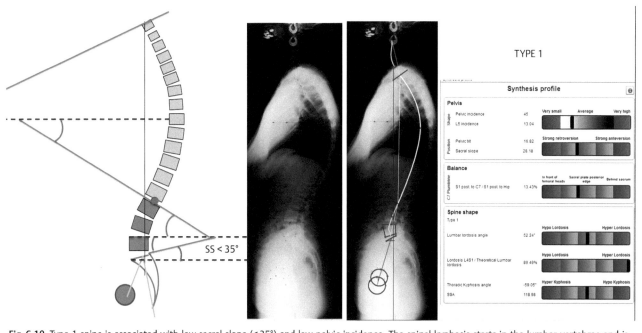

Fig. 6.10 Type 1 spine is associated with low sacral slope (< 35°) and low pelvic incidence. The spinal kyphosis starts in the lumbar vertebrae and is associated with long thoracolumbar kyphosis.

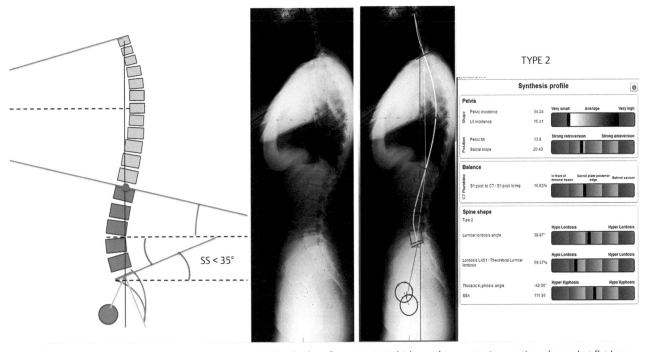

Fig. 6.11 Type 2 spines characterized by low sacral slope (SS) (<35°). The inflection point is higher and more anterior, creating a longer but flat lower spinal lordosis (over three levels), close to a straight line. The entire spine is relatively hypolordotic and hypokyphotic. It is a harmonious flat back.

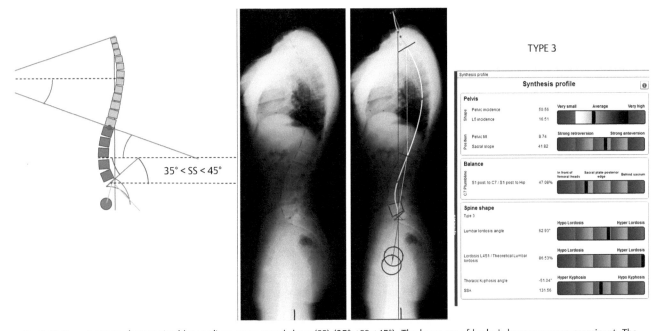

Fig. 6.12 Type 3 spines characterized by medium range sacral slope (SS) (35°≤SS≤45°). The lower arc of lordosis becomes more prominent. The inflection point is at the thoracolumbar junction with a well-balanced lumbar lordosis between its two arches. It is a well-balanced harmonious spine.

line. The entire spine is relatively hypolordotic and hypoky-photic. This is the harmonious flat back.

- Type 3 lordosis (▶ Fig. 6.12): characterized by medium range SS (35°≤SS≤45°). The apex of LL is in the center of the upper L4 vertebral body or the L3-L4 disk. The lower arc of lordosis becomes more prominent. The inflection point is at the thoracolumbar junction with a well-balanced

LL between its two arches. Type 3 is a well-balanced harmonious spine.

- Type 4 lordosis (▶ Fig. 6.13): characterized by high SS (greater than 45°). The apex of the LL is located at the base of the L3 vertebral body or higher. The number of vertebrae in a lordotic orientation is equal or greater than 5, and a state of segmental hyperextension exists.

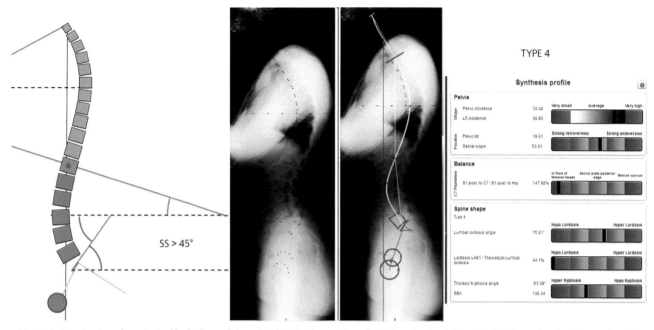

Fig. 6.13 Type 4 spines characterized by high sacral slope (SS) (>45°). The number of vertebrae in a lordotic orientation is greater than five, and a state of segmental hyperextension exists.

6.8 Role of Pelvic Incidence and Definition of Anteverted Types

The originality of Roussouly's classification is the introduction of a geometrical relation between SS and the lower arc of lordosis (between the S1 plateau and the horizontal line through the LSL apex) and thus with the construction of the whole spinal shape over the pelvis fulcrum represented by SS. With subtype analysis, types 1 and 2 were shown to have a low PI (< 50°), whereas types 3 and 4 had high PI values (> 50°).

Although several studies demonstrated a strong correlation between SS and PI,[17] the geometrical relation, PI = PT + SS, allows for the possibility of high SS with smaller PI if PT is small or negative (e.g., PI = 40°, PT = 0°, and SS = 40°). Thus, the original Roussouly's classification could have missed a spinal shape type where SS is high (>35°) and PT is nearly zero or negative. Laouissat et al[18] recently published an updated revision of the original classification and included this missed type. They termed it the anteverted type 3 as it has the same characteristics of the classical type 3 (35° < SS < 45°) but with a low PT (PT ≤ 5°) (▶ Fig. 6.14). The authors noted that these anteverted types had low PI.[18] Thus, there is a possibility of higher-than-expected SS with small PI. As LL correlates with SS, type 3 LL may be found associated with small PI when the pelvis is anteverted (small or negative PT). This situation is not exceptional: 16% of the population could be characterized as having "anteverted type 3."[18]

These findings have important implication in spinal pathology. In fact, a patient lordosis with sagittal imbalance with a PI < 50° must have been types 1 and 2 or anteverted type 3, whereas if PI > 50°, the original spinal alignment would be type 3 or 4 and never type 1 or 2. In addition, this classification helps in determining the high local stress zones in the spine: the more the lumbar spine is curved, the more contact force there is on the posterior elements (facet joints in particular). On the contrary, the lower the lumbar curvature or flat back, the higher the impact on the disks.[19] We may summarize this assertion that a "pathological" or degenerated spine had previously a normal shape and the only morphological signature of this original shape is the PI.

6.9 Implication of Normal Spinal Curves in Pathological Situations

The apparent problem with Roussouly's classification is that it was established in asymptomatic populations and was unusable in pathological conditions. Yet, the physiological curves of the spine also affect the response to various pathological conditions. As mentioned above and detailed in Chapters 9 and 10, the spinal sagittal morphotype determines the areas of maximum contact pressure. This contact pressure is higher in the disk area in the low PI morphotypes, whereas it is higher in posterior elements in patients with higher PI morphotypes. This is associated with magnetic resonance degenerative findings in the posterior elements of the spine, mainly facet joints. An anatomical study found that degenerative disk disease was associated with low SS and low PI, whereas high SS and high PI determined higher incidences of isthmic and degenerative spondylolisthesis.[20] This classification is important as it will constitute the basis of the development of degenerative spine classification discussed in Chapter 10.

One of the most valuables concepts of the functional segmentation of the spine is the reciprocity between the upper arch of the LL and the lower arch of the TK around the inflection point. This important concept has several implications in the surgical corrective strategy of spinal deformities. In fact, the higher the inflection point between lordosis and kyphosis, the lesser the space for the kyphosis to be constructed. This lack of room for kyphosis in the thoracic area pushes the flexion area in the proximal thoracic spine. As there is a short area in flexion to

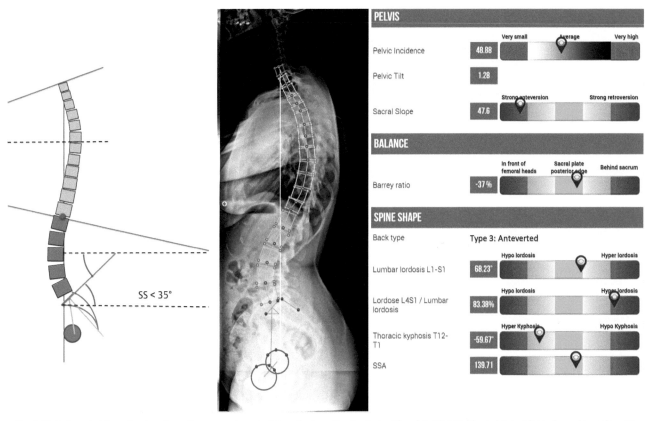

Fig. 6.14 Anteverted type 3 spines have the same characteristics of a type 3 spine but with pelvic tilt < 5°. The pelvic incidence has a low value. SS, Sacral slope.

counteract the long lordosis, the only way for balancing is an increasing angle of kyphosis. This is in evidence in the long concave back when the cervical spine is in kyphosis. This may explain a PJK occurring over too much of a lordotic correction of the lumbar spine.

Another concept presented by Roussouly is the apex of the curves. Low PI curves have a low lordosis apex, whereas higher PI curves have a higher apex. This implies the need to the restitution of the normal apex when treating deformity and thus affects the level of osteotomy.[21] In fact, Lafage el al[22] recommended the use of L3 osteotomy as it yields the same corrective results with fewer complication profiles. Nonetheless, when performing a pedicle subtraction osteotomy in patients with low PI and a type 1 shape, the lordosis becomes nonharmonious with a high apex by reducing the thoracolumbar kyphosis inducing a type 3 lordosis that rotates the pelvis in an anteverted position. In types 3 and 4, when correcting the lordosis in the upper arc instead of the lower arc, it changes the global disposition of the lordosis that may directly affect the lower arch of kyphosis, because of the reciprocity of both arches (upper lordosis and lower kyphosis).

Another implication of this classification is the response of the spine to traumatic forces. Within the kyphosis, a certain vertebra is distant from the body's anterior–posterior balance axis, which normally passes through the external auditory canals, the interspaces C7-D1 and L5-S1, and the center of the femoral heads) and is subjected to eccentric loads.[4] Eccentric axial loads create anterior load displacement with higher lever arms and bending moments in the anterior part of the bodies.

In a trauma setting, this favors the occurrence of wedge compression fractures.[4] In the lordotic segments, concentric loads are applied to the vertebra with forces running through the middle and posterior elements. The forces are more evenly distributed on the endplates and, according to Newton's third law, it favors the occurrence of central or burst fractures.[4] Thus, patients with low PI have an increased risk of burst fractures in the more concentrically loaded vertebra in the upper lumbar areas.

Recently, the Roussouly classification was applied in a cohort of adolescent idiopathic scoliosis. The authors found that Roussouly types 3 and 4 patients showed more severe scoliosis with higher LL and TK. They also found that Roussouly type 1 patients demonstrated a significantly higher incidence of low-grade scoliosis, whereas groups 3 and 4 had a higher incidence of high-degree scoliosis.[23] In another study, Kharrat et al[24] found that Roussouly's classification was correlated to scoliosis type and apical vertebral rotation: Roussouly types 1 and 2 were associated with Lenke 5 curves, whereas Roussouly's types 3 and 4 were associated with Lenke types 1 and 2 curves.

Bakouny et al[25] correlated gait parameters to Roussouly's morphotypes. These authors found that type 2 subjects had significantly more mean pelvic retroversion with less PT during gait compared to types 3 and 4 subjects and a significantly larger range of motion of the pelvic obliquity compared to type 4 subjects. Type 2 subjects presented with larger maximal hip extension. The association of both hip extension and pelvic retroversion could predispose to posterior femoroacetabular impingement and, consequently, osteoarthritis.

6.10 Conclusion

Spinal sagittal segmentation in various curvatures was known since Hippocrates respecting anatomical divisions. With a functional segmentation, it is possible to propose a classification of normal variations of human spinal sagittal curvatures. From this analysis, we may conclude that curvature definition is not only a matter of angle reciprocity, but shape and angle are required to characterize spinal curves and sagittal balance.

References

[1] Berge C. Heterochronic processes in human evolution: an ontogenetic analysis of the hominid pelvis. Am J Phys Anthropol. 1998; 105(4):441–459

[2] Vasiliadis ES, Grivas TB, Kaspiris A. Historical overview of spinal deformities in ancient Greece. Scoliosis. 2009; 4:6

[3] Marketos SG, Skiadas P. Hippocrates. The father of spine surgery. Spine. 1999; 24(13):1381–1387

[4] Izzo R, Guarnieri G, Guglielmi G, Muto M. Biomechanics of the spine. Part I: spinal stability. Eur J Radiol. 2013; 82(1):118–126

[5] Morvan G, Wybier M, Mathieu P, Vuillemin V, Guerini H. Plain radiographs of the spine: static and relationships between spine and pelvis. J Radiol. 2008; 89(5, Pt 2):654–663, quiz 664–666

[6] Le Huec JC, Aunoble S, Philippe L, Nicolas P. Pelvic parameters: origin and significance. Eur Spine J. 2011; 20 Suppl 5:564–571

[7] Schwab F, Ungar B, Blondel B, et al. Scoliosis Research Society—Schwab adult spinal deformity classification: a validation study. Spine. 2012; 37(12):1077–1082

[8] Basques BA, Long WD, Golinvaux NS, et al. Poor visualization limits diagnosis of proximal junctional kyphosis in adolescent idiopathic scoliosis. Spine J. 2017; 17(6):784–789

[9] Stagnara P, De Mauroy JC, Dran G, et al. Reciprocal angulation of vertebral bodies in a sagittal plane: approach to references for the evaluation of kyphosis and lordosis. Spine. 1982; 7(4):335–342

[10] Berthonnaud E, Dimnet J, Roussouly P, Labelle H. Analysis of the sagittal balance of the spine and pelvis using shape and orientation parameters. J Spinal Disord Tech. 2005; 18(1):40–47

[11] Vaz G, Roussouly P, Berthonnaud E, Dimnet J. Sagittal morphology and equilibrium of pelvis and spine. Eur Spine J. 2002; 11(1):80–87

[12] Roussouly P, Gollogly S, Berthonnaud E, Dimnet J. Classification of the normal variation in the sagittal alignment of the human lumbar spine and pelvis in the standing position. Spine. 2005; 30(3):346–353

[13] Dubousset J. Treatment of spondylolysis and spondylolisthesis in children and adolescents. Clin Orthop Relat Res. 1997(337):77–85

[14] Schwab F, Patel A, Ungar B, Farcy JP, Lafage V. Adult spinal deformity—postoperative standing imbalance: how much can you tolerate? An overview of key parameters in assessing alignment and planning corrective surgery. Spine. 2010; 35(25):2224–2231

[15] Vialle R, Levassor N, Rillardon L, Templier A, Skalli W, Guigui P. Radiographic analysis of the sagittal alignment and balance of the spine in asymptomatic subjects. J Bone Joint Surg Am. 2005; 87(2):260–267

[16] Sebaaly A, Riouallon G, Obeid I, et al. Proximal junctional kyphosis in adult scoliosis: comparison of four radiological predictor models. Eur Spine J. 2018; 27(3):613–621

[17] Mac-Thiong J-M, Roussouly P, Berthonnaud E, Guigui P. Sagittal parameters of global spinal balance: normative values from a prospective cohort of seven hundred nine Caucasian asymptomatic adults. Spine. 2010; 35(22):E1193–E1198

[18] Laouissat F, Sebaaly A, Gehrchen M, Roussouly P. Classification of normal sagittal spine alignment: refounding the Roussouly classification. Eur Spine J. 2018; 27(8):2002–2011

[19] Roussouly P, Pinheiro-Franco JL. Sagittal parameters of the spine: biomechanical approach. Eur Spine J. 2011; 20 Suppl 5:578–585

[20] Barrey C, Jund J, Noseda O, Roussouly P. Sagittal balance of the pelvis–spine complex and lumbar degenerative diseases. A comparative study about 85 cases. Eur Spine J. 2007; 16(9):1459–1467

[21] Sebaaly A, Kharrat K, Kreichati G, Rizkallah M. Influence of the level of pedicle subtraction osteotomy on pelvic tilt change in adult spinal deformity. Glob Spine J. 2016; 6(1):s-0036-1583071-s-0036-1583071

[22] Lafage V, Schwab F, Vira S, et al. Does vertebral level of pedicle subtraction osteotomy correlate with degree of spinopelvic parameter correction? J Neurosurg Spine. 2011; 14(2):184–191

[23] Hong J-Y, Kim K-W, Suh S-W, Park SY, Yang JH. Effect of coronal scoliotic curvature on sagittal spinal shape: analysis of parameters in mature adolescent scoliosis patients. Clin Spine Surg. 2017; 30(4):E418–E422

[24] Kharrat K, Sebaaly A, Assi A, et al. Is there a correlation between the apical vertebral rotation and the pelvic incidence in adolescent idiopathic scoliosis? Glob Spine J. 2016; 6:s-0036-1583044-s-0036-1583044

[25] Bakouny Z, Assi A, Massaad A, et al. Roussouly's sagittal spino-pelvic morphotypes as determinants of gait in asymptomatic adult subjects. Gait Posture. 2017; 54:27–33

Part III

Normative Values Following Age and Populations

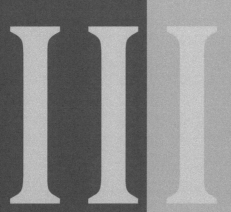

7 Normative Values of Sagittal Balance in Children and Adults

Jean-Marc Mac-Thiong and Fethi Laouissat

Abstract

Knowledge of normal sagittal balance is key when evaluating and treating patients with spinal pathologies. Regional parameters describe the morphology and orientation of the various segments of the human body, while global parameters describe the overall alignment of adjacent segments. Adjacent segments are interdependent, and their relationships result in a stable and balanced posture. Pelvic incidence increases after the acquisition of bipedalism and stabilizes in adulthood. This increase in pelvic incidence mainly results in a proportional increase in pelvic tilt, while sacral slope remains relatively stable. Thoracic kyphosis and lumbar lordosis also tend to increase slightly with growth. C7 plumb line tends to move backward during growth until adulthood where it stabilizes before moving forward when degenerative changes occur, mainly in late middle age. Asymptomatic children and adults stand with a relatively stable global balance, with a narrow range of values for spinosacral angle and spinal tilt. A spinosacral angle between 115° and 149° and a spinal tilt between 84° and 102° are typically expected in 95% of the normal pediatric population. Similarly, it is expected that 95% of normal adults present a spinosacral angle between 114° and 147° and a spinal tilt between 84° and 97°. Overall, 27% of juvenile, 11% of adolescent, and 14% of adult individuals normally stand with a C7 plumb line in front of the sacrum and hip axis. With aging, there is a tendency for retroversion of the pelvis (increasing pelvic tilt and decreasing sacral slope) in adults. The spinosacral angle also tends to decrease while spinal tilt remains stable with aging.

Keywords: adult spine, lumbar lordosis, pediatric spine, pelvis, pelvic incidence, pelvic tilt, sacral slope, sagittal alignment, sagittal balance, spine, thoracic kyphosis

7.1 Introduction

Proper knowledge of normal sagittal balance and underlying concepts is paramount when evaluating and treating patients with spinal pathologies. While postural control and compensatory mechanisms can vary with growth and aging, understanding the differences between children and adults is also important when assessing sagittal balance. In this chapter, references values and key concepts of sagittal balance in normal children and adults are described.

7.2 Parameters of Sagittal Balance

Various parameters have been used to describe normal sagittal balance. Regional parameters typically describe the morphology and orientation of the various segments of the human body: cervical, thoracic and lumbosacral spine, pelvis, and lower extremities. Global parameters are used to describe the overall sagittal alignment for adjacent anatomical segments. When compared to global parameters, regional parameters are

typically associated with larger variability among normal individuals.[1]

It is important to distinguish morphological from orientation parameters of sagittal balance. Morphological parameters such as pelvic incidence describe an anatomical feature that is unaffected—or negligibly affected—by changes in position of the individual. Conversely, orientation parameters are position dependent, and therefore require standardized positioning during radiographic acquisition to ensure adequate reproducibility.

Variations in parameters of sagittal balance can also be amplified by the radiographic and/or measurement techniques that are used. While angular parameters are only slightly influenced by the radiographic and measurement techniques, linear measurements are highly dependent on the radiographic technique and calibration. Angular, adimensional, or qualitative assessments with respect to reference points (▶ Fig. 7.1) are therefore often preferred in an attempt to reduce the errors associated with linear measurements.

7.3 Normal Sagittal Balance: Underlying Concepts

Despite large variations in parameters of sagittal balance, normal individual stand with a balanced posture for which the spine, pelvic, and lower extremities are aligned to minimize the energy expenditure and preserve horizontal gaze. There are basic concepts underlying this principle that need to be considered when evaluating sagittal balance. First and foremost, adjacent anatomical regions are interdependent, and their relationships result in a stable and balanced posture.[2,3] Although normative values of sagittal balance are useful clinical guidelines for evaluating and treating patients with spinal disorders, ensuring and preserving the close relationships between adjacent anatomical regions is of paramount importance. In addition, even if parameters of sagittal balance differ between pediatric and adult subjects, the scheme of correlations between parameters remains similar in the normal pediatric and adult populations.

In the presence of pathology in the spine, pelvis, or lower extremities, compensatory mechanisms to maintain adequate sagittal balance can occur either locally at the level of the pathology and/or remotely in another anatomical region. While regional parameters of sagittal balance can vary widely in the normal population, on some occasions, the presence of an underlying pathology can be reflected only by abnormal relationships among these parameters. When compensatory mechanisms are exceeded to the point where sagittal imbalance occurs, regional parameters of sagittal balance may still remain within normal limits, but parameters of global balance will likely fall outside of normal limits. Accordingly, global parameters of sagittal balance are maintained in a narrow range within the normal population. Clinically, the assessment of global sagittal balance is an important aspect of the evaluation of patients with spinal pathology, of surgical planning, and to

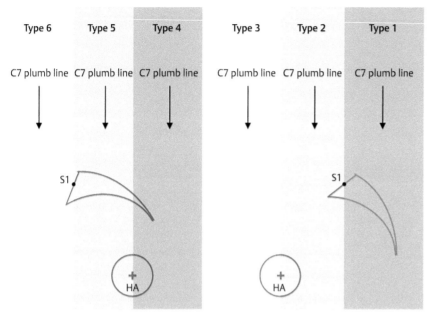

Fig. 7.1 Determination of the global balance type (types 1–6) based on the assessment of the spinopelvic alignment from the position of the C7 plumb line with respect to the center of the upper sacral endplate (S1) and to the hip axis (HA). Types 1–3 refer to cases with HA lying in front of S1, whereas types 4–6 are present when HA is behind S1.

minimize complications such as adjacent segment disease, sagittal imbalance, and pseudarthrosis. The importance of global parameters of sagittal balance is also supported by studies[4,5,6] demonstrating its significant relationship with health-related quality of life in the presence of spinal deformity.

Considering the variability within the normal population, a longitudinal evaluation of sagittal balance is most useful to detect compensatory mechanisms and/or impending sagittal imbalance. In particular, progressive pelvic retroversion, hip and knee flexion, and/or forward displacement of the C7 plumb line should raise a suspicion for an underlying spinal disorder or sagittal imbalance.

7.4 Normal Pediatric Sagittal Balance

Sagittal curvatures of the spine—mainly lumbar lordosis—develop during infancy along with the development of the erect position. Thereafter during growth, the morphology and orientation of the spine, sacrum, and pelvis will change to acquire stable sagittal balance and bipedal gait,[7,8,9] and to accommodate for physiological and morphological changes. To this extent, the pelvis has a central role in the development of a stable sagittal balance as it is the link between the upper and lower body. The sagittal morphology of the pelvis is best measured from the pelvic incidence. Pelvic incidence increases after the acquisition of bipedalism and stabilizes during adulthood.[7,8,9,10] The increase in pelvic incidence with age is small but constant throughout childhood and adolescence.[10] The increase in pelvic incidence mainly results in a proportional increase in pelvic tilt, while sacral slope remains relatively stable. ▶ Table 7.2 presents values of pelvic parameters reported in the literature for different age groups in the normal pediatric population.[7,11]

Table 7.1 Regional parameters of sagittal balance reported for the normal pediatric population in different age groups

Age group	Fetal	Infantile	Juvenile	Adolescent
Age	28.7 ± 6.2 weeks (19–40 weeks)	38.7 ± 23.1 months (12–108 months)	8.1 ± 2.0 years (3–10 years)	13.6 ± 1.9 years (>10 and <18 years)
Pelvic incidence	30.6° ± 5.6° (20°–40°)	39.5° ± 8.9° (22°–64°)	43.7° ± 9.0° (23°–84°)	46.9° ± 11.4° (22°–87°)
Pelvic tilt	—	—	5.5° ± 7.6° (-13°–40°)	7.7° ± 8.3° (-12°–34°)
Sacral slope	—	—	38.2° ± 7.7° (21°–56°)	39.1° ± 7.6° (18°–65°)
Thoracic kyphosis	—	—	42.0° ± 10.6° (8°–65°)	45.8° ± 10.4° (9°–84°)
Lumbar lordosis	—	—	53.8° ± 12.0° (16°–86°)	57.7° ± 11.1° (20°–102°)

Table 7.2 Global parameters of sagittal balance reported for the normal pediatric population

Age group	Juvenile	Adolescent	All
Age	8.1 ± 2.0 years (3–10 years)	13.6 ± 1.9 years (>10 and <18 years)	12.1 ± 3.1 years (>10 and <18 years)
Spinosacral angle	130.4° ± 9.0° (103°–154°)	132.7° ± 8.0° (109°–159°)	132.1° ± 8.4° (103°–159°)
Spinal tilt	92.2° ± 5.7° (76°–107°)	93.5° ± 4.1° (83°–106°)	93.2° ± 4.6° (76°–107°)

Thoracic kyphosis and lumbar lordosis also tend to increase with age (▶ Table 7.2), although the correlations are small.[2,10]

Accordingly, Cil et al[12] observed a tendency for increasing thoracic kyphosis and lumbar lordosis between different age groups. Thoracic kyphosis was 45° ± 11°, 48° ± 11°, 46° ± 11°, and 53° ± 9° in 3–6 year, 7–9 year, 10–12 year, and 13–15 year age groups, respectively. Lumbar lordosis was 44° ± 11°, 52° ± 12°, 57° ± 10°, and 55° ± 10° in 3–6 year, 7–9 year, 10–12 year, and 13–15 year age groups, respectively. Similarly, Voutsinas and MacEwen[13] reported a slight increase in thoracic kyphosis (1.8° mean difference) and lumbar lordosis (4.4° mean difference) from 5 to 20 years old.

The C7 plumb line tends to move backward slightly during growth[11,14] until adulthood where it stabilizes before moving forward when degenerative changes occur. Females also show a tendency for having a slightly more posterior C7 plumb line.[14] Cil et al[11] noted progressive backward displacement of the C7 plumb line with respect to the posterosuperior corner of S1 vertebral body during growth, with mean values of 2.5 ± 4.3 cm, 0.7 ± 4.6 cm, -0.1 ± 4.1 cm, and -0.9 ± 4.4 cm, respectively, for 3–6 year, 7–9 year, 10–12 year, and 13–15 year age groups. However, angular and adimensional parameters of global sagittal balance[15,16] are usually preferred (▶ Fig. 7.1, ▶ Fig. 7.2) because they are less sensitive to variations in the radiographic technique, thereby facilitating comparisons with normative values and between independent studies. Table 7-2 presents global parameters of sagittal spinal balance, while ▶ Table 7.3 shows the typical distribution of global balance types (▶ Fig. 7.1) observed in the normal pediatric population.[16] Overall, asymptomatic children and adolescents tend to stand with a relatively stable global spinal balance, with a narrow range of values for spinosacral angle and spinal tilt. Therefore, a spinosacral angle between 115° and 149°, and a spinal tilt between 84° and 102° are typically expected in 95% of the normal pediatric population. In addition, the line from the center of C7 vertebral body to the center of the upper sacral endplate used to measure the spinal tilt should be very close to the vertical line.[11] Analysis of the global balance type (▶ Fig. 7.1, ▶ Table 7.3) reveals that 27% of juvenile and 11% of adolescent individuals normally stand with a C7 plumb line in front of the sacrum and hip axis (types 3 and 6). This observation suggests that anterior global sagittal balance is not necessarily associated with spinal pathology, particularly in children. For these young individuals, it is assumed that a smaller pelvic incidence will lead to smaller sacral slope and lumbar lordosis, which decreases the ability to position the C7 plumb line behind the sacrum and hip axis.

The most clinically relevant correlations between parameters of sagittal balance involve the lumbosacral–pelvic relationships that highly influence global balance, and that need to be preserved or restored when planning spine surgery. ▶ Fig. 7.3 shows the chain of correlations that is typically observed in the normal pediatric population.[2,14,17]

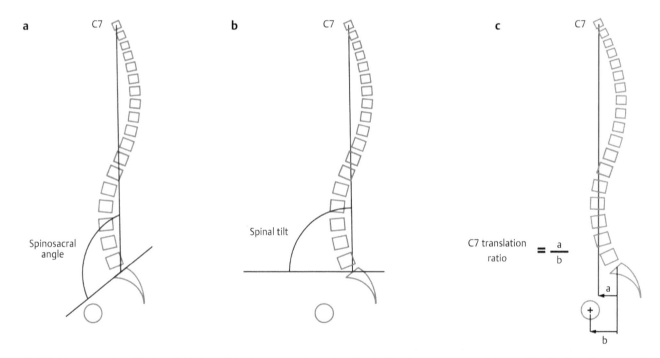

Fig. 7.2 Measurement of global sagittal balance. **(a)** Spinosacral angle: angle subtended by the upper sacral endplate and the line from the center of C7 vertebral body to the center of upper sacral endplate. **(b)** Spinal tilt: angle subtended by the horizontal line and the line from the center of C7 vertebral body to the center of upper sacral endplate. A value greater than 90° indicates that the center of C7 vertebral body is behind the center of the upper sacral endplate, whereas for values less than 90°, the center of the C7 vertebral body is in front of the center of the upper sacral endplate. **(c)** Instead of using a pure distance like SVA (sagittal vertebral axis) that needs precise X-ray calibration, we prefer to use the ratio between two distances (a/b, for example).

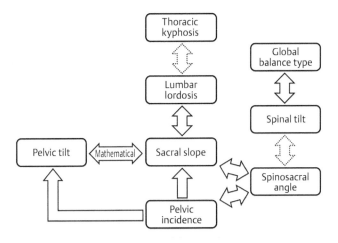

Fig. 7.3 Overview of the chain of correlations between parameters of sagittal balance typically observed in the normal pediatric population. Moderate ($0.3 \leq r < 0.5$) and strong ($r \geq 0.5$) correlations are shown by dotted and full arrows, respectively. The correlation between sacral slope and pelvic tilt is trivial considering that pelvic incidence = pelvic tilt + sacral slope.

7.5 Normal Adult Sagittal Balance

As in the pediatric population, there are variations in parameters of sagittal balance during aging in the normal adult population up to 80 years old (▶ Table 7.4).[16,18] Pelvic incidence remains constant during adulthood.[18] However, there is a tendency for retroversion of the pelvis—and associated decrease in sacral slope—but the changes are small ($r < 0.2$). Similarly, thoracic kyphosis increases slightly with age, especially in late middle age.[19] The slight tendency for the spinosacral angle to decrease with age could be a result of the effort to maintain a normal spinal tilt despite the tendency for increasing pelvic retroversion—and associated decrease in sacral slope—with aging, considering the strong correlation between spinosacral angle and sacral slope ($r = 0.9$).[16] Although spinal tilt is not correlated with age, there is a gradual decrease with aging in the proportion of individuals with type 1 global balance after 50 years old, with reciprocal increase in types 2 and 3 global balance (▶ Table 7.5), suggesting slight forward displacement of the C7 plumb line from late middle age.

Table 7.3 Distribution of global balance types reported for the normal pediatric population

Age group	Type 1	Type 2	Type 3	Type 4	Type 5	Type 6
3–10 years	50.9%	9.0%	19.2%	11.4%	1.8%	7.8%
>10 and <18 years	63.3%	11.9%	7.7%	12.5%	1.0%	3.5%
All	60.1%	11.1%	10.7%	12.2%	1.2%	4.6%

Table 7.4 Parameters of sagittal balance reported for the normal adult population in different age groups

Age group	>18 and <30 years	30–39 years	40–49 years	50–59 years	>60 years	All
Pelvic incidence	52.3° ± 10.9° (22°–88°)	52.1° ± 10.4° (27°–89°)	53.2° ± 9.3° (32°–76°)	53.6° ± 10.3° (25°–85°)	52.7° ± 10.5° (33°–78°)	52.6° ± 10.4° (22°–89°)
Pelvic tilt	12.5° ± 6.7° (-6°–33°)	12.1° ± 6.6° (-7°–28°)	12.8° ± 6.8° (-3°–28°)	14.8° ± 6.7° (0°–32°)	16.1° ± 6.9° (0°–32°)	13.0° ± 6.8° (-7°–33°)
Sacral slope	39.8° ± 8.0° (17°–63°)	40.0° ± 7.5° (25°–62°)	40.5° ± 7.3° (23°–56°)	38.9° ± 7.5° (25°–62°)	36.7° ± 9.3° (14°–63°)	39.6° ± 7.9° (14°–63°)
Thoracic kyphosis	48.4° ± 9.3° (16°–74°)	49.7° ± 10.4° (22°–74°)	49.5° ± 10.7° (19°–72°)	52.7° ± 9.9° (28°–79°)	56.5° ± 12.0° (21°–81°)	50.1° ± 10.4° (16°–81°)
Lumbar lordosis	54.5° ± 9.9° (20°–84°)	55.1° ± 10.4° (33°–84°)	56.7° ± 11.2° (31°–79°)	54.3° ± 10.3° (33°–83°)	53.4° ± 12.1° (29°–84°)	54.8° ± 10.5° (20°–84°)
Spinosacral angle	130.7° ± 8.0° (102°–153°)	131.1° ± 7.4° (115°–148°)	131.7° ± 8.1° (112°–149°)	128.9° ± 7.9° (113°–151°)	126.7° ± 3.9° (106°–150°)	130.4° ± 8.1° (102°–153°)
Spinal tilt	90.9° ± 3.1° (80°–101°)	91.0° ± 3.3° (82°–100°)	91.3° ± 3.4° (82°–101°)	90.0° ± 3.9° (80°–98°)	90.0° ± 3.9° (77°–97°)	90.8° ± 3.4° (77°–101°)

Table 7.5 Distribution of global balance types reported for the normal adult population

Age group	Type 1	Type 2	Type 3	Type 4	Type 5	Type 6
<30 years	55.7%	29.1%	12.5%	2.0%	0%	0.7%
30–39 years	56.7%	26.2%	14.0%	2.4%	0.6%	0%
40–49 years	58.3%	27.2%	12.6%	0%	0%	1.9%
50–59 years	46.2%	35.9%	17.9%	0%	0%	0%
>60 years	47.1%	35.3%	16.2%	1.5%	0%	0%
All	54.6%	29.5%	13.7%	1.6%	0.1%	0.6%

Table 7.6 Racial differences in parameters of sagittal balance in the normal adult populations

	African-American	Caucasian	Asian	p Value	African-American vs. Caucasian p value	African-American vs. Asian p value	Caucasian vs. Asian p value
Lumbar lordosis (°)	57.3 ± 13.2	54.8 ± 10.5	48.6 ± 9.9	<0.001	0.489	<0.001	<0.001
Pelvic incidence (°)	57.2 ± 11.9	52.6 ± 10.4	48.8 ± 9.7	<0.001	0.021	<0.001	<0.001
Pelvic tilt (°)	15.5 ± 7.5	13.0 ± 6.8	13.2 ± 7.6	0.115	—	—	—
Sacral slope (°)	41.2 ± 9.1	39.6 ± 7.9	35.2 ± 7.7	<0.001	0.265	<0.001	<0.001

Table 7.7 Comparison of parameters of sagittal balance between normal pediatric and adult populations

Population	Pediatric	Adult
Pelvic incidence	46.0° ± 10.9° (23°–87°)	52.6° ± 10.4° (22°–89°)
Pelvic tilt	7.2° ± 8.2° (-13°–40°)	13.0° ± 6.8° (-7°–33°)
Sacral slope	38.9° ± 7.6° (18°–65°)	39.6° ± 7.9° (14°–63°)
Thoracic kyphosis	44.8° ± 10.6° (8°–84°)	50.1° ± 10.4° (16°–81°)
Lumbar lordosis	56.7° ± 11.4° (16°–102°)	54.8° ± 10.5° (20°–84°)
Spinosacral angle	132.1° ± 8.4° (103°–159°)	130.4° ± 8.1° (102°–153°)
Spinal tilt	93.2° ± 4.6° (76°–107°)	90.8° ± 3.4° (77°–101°)

Regional and global parameters of sagittal balance in the normal adult population are shown in ▶ Table 7.4 for different age groups. A recent study has reported significant racial differences in regional parameters, suggesting that pelvic incidence, sacral slope, and lumbar lordosis are larger in African-Americans than in Caucasians, and larger in Caucasians than in Asians (▶ Table 7.6).[20] Pelvic parameters are similar between adult males and females.[18] Thoracic kyphosis is significantly increased in adult females, but the difference is small (<3°). Similarly, lumbar lordosis, spinosacral angle, and spinal tilt are decreased in females, but the differences are small (<2°) and not likely to be clinically relevant.

When compared to the normal pediatric population, normal adults present increased pelvic incidence, pelvic tilt, and thoracic kyphosis, and decreased lumbar lordosis, spinosacral angle, and spinal tilt (▶ Table 7.7). However, sacral slope is similar from juvenile to elderly individuals, suggesting its prime importance in maintaining adequate sagittal balance. As for the pediatric population, spinosacral angle and spinal tilt remain within a narrow range in normal adults. Accordingly, it is expected that 95% of the normal adult population will present a spinosacral angle between 114° and 147°, and a spinal tilt between 84° and 97°. Interestingly, the line from the center of C7 vertebral body to the center of the upper sacral endplate used to measure the spinal tilt stands even closer to the vertical line in normal adults.

While 27% of juvenile and 11% of adolescent individuals stand with a C7 plumb line in front of the sacrum and hip axis

(types 3 and 6 global balance; ▶ Table 7.3), this proportion remains close to 14% during adulthood until middle age, before reaching 18% in late middle age individuals. Similarly, Laouissat et al[21] observed that 13% of asymptomatic adult subjects stand with a C7 plumb line in front of the sacrum and hip axis. They also found that a greater proportion of males had a C7 plumb line in front of the sacrum and hip axis (22% in males vs. 7% in females).

When analyzing global balance types, there are three main differences between normal pediatric and adult individuals. First, a greater proportion of adults stand with a retroverted pelvis (types 1, 2, and 3) (97.8% vs. 81.9%). Second, the proportion of individuals with type 2 global balance is markedly increased in adults (29.5% vs. 11.1%). Finally, the proportion of normal adults with type 4 global balance becomes very low in normal adults (1.6% vs. 12.2%).

Correlations between anatomical segments of the spine and pelvis are similar between normal children and adults (▶ Fig. 7.3), where pelvic incidence determines pelvic tilt and sacral slope, while sacral slope is highly correlated with lumbar lordosis. Spinosacral angle strongly relates to pelvic incidence and sacral slope, and spinal tilt is associated with global balance type. The only difference is that the correlation between spinosacral angle and spinal tilt is small in adults (r between 0.2 and 0.3) while it is moderate in children ($r = 0.4$).

Global balance in adults also differs with respect to the specific type of sagittal sacropelvic balance described in Roussouly classification[21,22]: type 1, sacral slope < 35° with short lumbar hyperlordosis; type 2, sacral slope < 35° with flat lumbar lordosis; type 3, sacral slope between 35° and 45°; type 3 + anteverted pelvis (AP), sacral slope between 35° and 45° with low or negative pelvic tilt; and type 4, sacral slope > 45°. In type 1 patients, the C7 plumb line usually falls behind the posterosuperior corner of the upper sacral endplate. For type 3-AP patients, the C7 plumb line typically falls on the upper sacral endplate, while it typically lies slightly in front of the anterosuperior corner of the upper sacral endplate for type 2 patients. The C7 plumb line usually falls between the hip axis and upper sacral endplate in types 3 and 4 patients.

7.6 Conclusion

Knowledge of normal sagittal balance is key when evaluating and treating patients with spinal pathologies. This chapter described reference values and key concepts of sagittal balance in normal children and adults. Sagittal balance and sacropelvic morphology change during growth to acquire stable sagittal balance and bipedal gait, and to accommodate for physiological and morphological changes occurring in children and adolescents. When compared to the normal pediatric population, normal adults present a different sagittal balance that needs to be considered. However, correlations between anatomical segments of the spine and pelvis are similar between normal children and adults.

References

[1] Kuntz C, IV, Shaffrey CI, Ondra SL, et al. Spinal deformity: a new classification derived from neutral upright spinal alignment measurements in asymptomatic juvenile, adolescent, adult, and geriatric individuals. Neurosurgery. 2008; 63(3) Suppl:25–39

[2] Mac-Thiong JM, Labelle H, Berthonnaud E, Betz RR, Roussouly P. Sagittal spinopelvic balance in normal children and adolescents. Eur Spine J. 2007; 16 (2):227–234

[3] Berthonnaud E, Dimnet J, Roussouly P, Labelle H. Analysis of the sagittal balance of the spine and pelvis using shape and orientation parameters. J Spinal Disord Tech. 2005; 18(1):40–47

[4] Glassman SD, Bridwell K, Dimar JR, Horton W, Berven S, Schwab F. The impact of positive sagittal balance in adult spinal deformity. Spine. 2005; 30 (18):2024–2029

[5] Harroud A, Labelle H, Joncas J, Mac-Thiong JM. Global sagittal alignment and health-related quality of life in lumbosacral spondylolisthesis. Eur Spine J. 2013; 22(4):849–856

[6] Mac-Thiong JM, Transfeldt EE, Mehbod AA, et al. Can C7 plumbline and gravity line predict health related quality of life in adult scoliosis? Spine. 2009; 34 (15):E519–E527

[7] Mangione P, Gomez D, Senegas J. Study of the course of the incidence angle during growth. Eur Spine J. 1997; 6(3):163–167

[8] Marty C, Boisaubert B, Descamps H, et al. The sagittal anatomy of the sacrum among young adults, infants, and spondylolisthesis patients. Eur Spine J. 2002; 11(2):119–125

[9] Tardieu C, Bonneau N, Hecquet J, et al. How is sagittal balance acquired during bipedal gait acquisition? Comparison of neonatal and adult pelves in three dimensions. Evolutionary implications. J Hum Evol. 2013; 65(2):209–222

[10] Mac-Thiong JM, Berthonnaud E, Dimar JR, II, Betz RR, Labelle H. Sagittal alignment of the spine and pelvis during growth. Spine. 2004; 29(15):1642–1647

[11] Mac-Thiong J-M, Labelle H, Roussouly P. Pediatric sagittal alignment. Eur Spine J. 2011; 20 Suppl 5:586–590

[12] Cil A, Yazici M, Uzumcugil A, et al. The evolution of sagittal segmental alignment of the spine during childhood. Spine. 2005; 30(1):93–100

[13] Voutsinas SA, MacEwen GD. Sagittal profiles of the spine. Clin Orthop Relat Res. 1986; 210:235–242

[14] Gutman G, Labelle H, Barchi S, Roussouly P, Berthonnaud É, Mac-Thiong JM. Normal sagittal parameters of global spinal balance in children and adolescents: a prospective study of 646 asymptomatic subjects. Eur Spine J. 2016; 25(11):3650–3657

[15] Roussouly P, Gollogly S, Noseda O, Berthonnaud E, Dimnet J. The vertical projection of the sum of the ground reactive forces of a standing patient is not the same as the C7 plumb line: a radiographic study of the sagittal alignment of 153 asymptomatic volunteers. Spine. 2006; 31(11):E320–E325

[16] Mac-Thiong JM, Roussouly P, Berthonnaud E, Guigui P. Sagittal parameters of global spinal balance: normative values from a prospective cohort of seven hundred nine Caucasian asymptomatic adults. Spine. 2010; 35(22):E1193–E1198

[17] Mac-Thiong JM, Wang Z, de Guise JA, Labelle H. Postural model of sagittal spino-pelvic alignment and its relevance for lumbosacral developmental spondylolisthesis. Spine. 2008; 33(21):2316–2325

[18] Mac-Thiong J-M, Roussouly P, Berthonnaud E, Guigui P. Age- and sex-related variations in sagittal sacropelvic morphology and balance in asymptomatic adults. Eur Spine J. 2011; 20 Suppl 5:572–577

[19] Yokoyama K, Kawanishi M, Yamada M, et al. Age-related variations in global spinal alignment and sagittal balance in asymptomatic Japanese adults. Neurol Res. 2017; 39(5):414–418

[20] Arima H, Dimar II Jr, Glassman SD, et al. Differences in lumbar and pelvic parameters among African American, Caucasian and Asian Populations. AAOS 2018 Annual Meeting, March 6–10 2018; New Orleans, LA

[21] Laouissat F, Sebaaly A, Gehrchen M, Roussouly P. Classification of normal sagittal spine alignment: refounding the Roussouly classification. Eur Spine J. 2018; 27(8):2002–2011

[22] Roussouly P, Gollogly S, Berthonnaud E, Dimnet J. Classification of the normal variation in the sagittal alignment of the human lumbar. 2005; 30(3):346–3–53

8 Sagittal Balance in the Elderly

Martin Gehrchen

Abstract

The aging spine is a continuum of a degenerative process that affects the sagittal balance in different degrees. The evolution of Roussouly spine shapes in the aging spine and the resulting involvement of the sagittal spine shape is described for each of the Roussouly types.

Keywords: aging spine, compensatory mechanisms, Roussouly classification, Roussouly type, sagittal balance

8.1 Introduction

The aging spine is most often characterized by the degenerative changes of the spine and their extent.[1,2,3,4] The pelvic incidence (PI) tends to increase linearly in adolescence with growing age until adulthood, then becomes a constant anatomical parameter.[5,6,7,8] The global and local spinal parameters (spinal lordosis [SL] and thoracic kyphosis [TK]) are closely dependent on the PI.[9,10]

To consider sagittal balance and normative shapes of the aging spine, it is important to understand, or at least make assumptions, as the change from the non-aging spine to the aging spine is a continuum with the development and growth of degenerative changes.[11] Thus, there is a gray zone where it can be difficult to differentiate between the young spine and the aging spine; however, degenerative changes of the spine such as disk degeneration and facet joint degeneration are signs that must be considered aging or the onset of aging. We cannot consider the aging process as a pathology; this is the natural evolution of extended life that affects the whole population whatever the initial shape of the global spinopelvic set. This chapter aims to characterize the aging spine and the implications of aging on the balanced spine shape in patients not previously operated on.

8.2 Classical Patterns of Aging Spine: Pelvis Retroversion with High Pelvic Incidence

Many attempts have been made to classify the adult aging spine.[12,13,14] All of them, however, are based on positional parameters and do not take the shape of the spine and its pathological evolution into account.[2,15,16] Lafage et al[17] showed the forward displacement of the gravity line and C7 plumb line in the aging population. Literature describing sagittal balance in the aging population is generally based on one pattern: loss of lumbar lordosis (LL) and increase of TK compensated for by a highly retroverted pelvis. It is well known that with age we may potentially lose height and the head may displace forward in relation to the pelvis. Loss of balance in the aging spine has several causes and sometimes they exist in combination. The main factor is the degenerative diskopathies that may

determine increased kyphosis in the thoracic and the lumbar region (decreased lordosis), although osteoporosis with fractures also induces the same problem as do neuromuscular conditions with a decreased muscular strength.[2,18,19] Scheuermann's disease and ankylosing spondylitis in variating degrees may, with aging, also impact sagittal balance significantly.[20,21]

A classic description of sagittal balance in aging associates forward flexion of the spine, pelvic retroversion (with hip extension), and in more severe situations knee flexion and femoral external rotation.[22] Progressive balance impairment is described over time by increasing muscle tiredness during daily activities inducing fatigue, discomfort, or pain.[22] Compensation of forward unbalance by high pelvic retroversion is a biomechanical property of pelvis with high PI. The act of walking impairs forward balance, thereby forcing the use of helping devices and limiting the ability to walk because of the limitation of hip extension. This situation may be even worse when there is associated arthritis of the hip or knee that compromises the diagnosis.

8.2.1 Spine and Hips Relation in Aging People with Retroverted Pelvis

Relations between hip positioning and worsening spinal shape may explain impairment from hip diseases or late hip prosthesis loosening. The progressive pelvic retroversion changes the acetabulum orientation (vertical positioning: acetabulum anteversion) and reduces the contact surface between femoral heads and acetabulum reduction.[23] In a normal hip joint, pressure on the cartilage may increase and induce wear on the cartilage and, later, arthritis. By the same mechanism, a total hip prosthesis may be compromised by decreasing contact between the head and acetabulum component, inducing polyethylene wearing and secondary loosening.

On the other hand, hip arthritis may reduce hip extension and worsen spinal imbalance by pelvic retroversion limitation. In this case, a decision regarding hip prosthesis has to be made before spinal surgery.[24] Sometimes, imbrication of hip arthritis and lumbar stenosis may result in diagnosis error between thigh pain as a result of the hip and neurological femoral pain.[25,26,27]

8.3 Aging Spine Evolution in Relation with Pelvic Incidence

If the previous description generally fits well with the balance of the features of aging, it describes mainly patients with higher PI and an increased tendency for more retroversion of the pelvis. This classic evolution of an aging person with high PI has led some authors to consider high PI as a specific pattern of aging people and a change in the position of sacroiliac joints as a cause of increasing PI with age. The poor angle variation related in those studies (3° to 4°) was sufficient to induce balance changes but remained within the limits of measurement error.

Relating the aging spine shape to the normal spine shape and looking at the different spine types according to Roussouly's classic four types[28] applied to the aging process, we can analyze the effect of aging on the shape of the spine. The contact forces in the posterior elements such as the facet joints increase with increased SL. The less the SL (kyphosis or flat back), the more impact there is on the disks. The classification thus can be helpful in determining where the high local stress zone is located in the spine in different types. The classification was updated recently with anteverted types 3 and 4 characterized with high SS and low PI in the normal population[29] (▶ Fig. 8.1).

In general, three courses are in play regarding degenerative changes and aging of the spine depending on whether changes are occurring in the TK, SL, or a combination of both. If the occurrence is in the transition zone between TK and SL, both zones can potentially be affected.

- Increasing spinal kyphosis caused by aging will move the head anteriorly in relation to the pelvis. The first changes will most likely be mild, and it will be very difficult to confirm it clinically; only magnetic resonance imaging (MRI) may confirm it in the very early stages. With increasing spinal kyphosis, extension of the spine will happen above and/or below and/or may be accompanied by retroversion of the pelvis (decreasing the lower SL) and increase of the upper SL until a point where no compensation above and below exists, and the spinal kyphosis is increased in general.
- Decreasing lower SL caused by aging will also tend to move the head anteriorly; however, an extension of the adjacent

levels will happen first, if possible. Here too, in the earlier stages, it may also be impossible to confirm it clinically, and only an MRI may document the early degenerative changes.[2,30] An increase in upper SL will accompany these changes as well.
- Increasing spinal kyphosis and decreasing lower SL in combination naturally will affect the position of the head faster, as the combination of changes has the same effect as the above-mentioned consequences.

The smaller the PI, the lower the potential for balance compensation of the spine by pelvis retroversion (increasing PT) and vice versa for higher PI. As a general biomechanical behavior, when the spine is flexible around a kyphosing event, an increased extension of the flexible spine above and/or below the local kyphosis will be seen.[2] But we must consider that in aging persons, the lack of muscular strength forbids this mechanism or at least is rapidly overpassed with muscle weakness. On the contrary, the second compensation mechanism is not compromised by muscles weakness. With progressive kyphosis, if the spine is rigid, the gravity line moves forward, and the pelvis rotates backward (retroversion), inducing a decrease in sacral slope (SS).[2,31,32,33,34] It thus seems both logical and crucial to implement Roussouly's four classic types (i.e., shape of spine) when evaluating the aging spine and its evolution to improve decision-making when surgical treatment is indicated.[28] Thus, the evolution of the sagittal alignment of the degenerative spine can be described based on the different types as proposed.[35] (For a description of the types in the normal population, see Chapter 7). For the degenerative spine, several types were identified such as "classic" type 1–4,

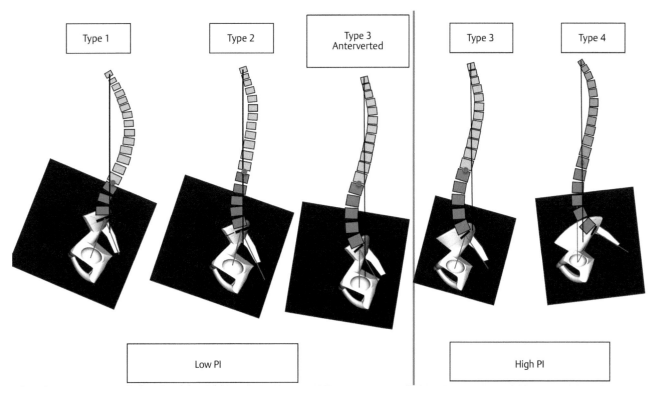

Fig. 8.1 The Roussouly classification integrating the anteverted pelvis shape. PI, Pelvic incidence.

anteverted types 3 and 4, false type 2, false type 2 + TK, false type 3, and the "kyphotic" group (lumbar and global).

The evolution of the aging spine based on the Roussouly classification of the normal spine can be described as follows depending on PI.[28,29]

8.3.1 Poorly Retroverted Pelvis (Low Pelvic Incidence < 50°)

Type 1

Compensation is developed low in the lumbar spine by increasing the LL if a kyphotic event occurs. If the spinal compensation mechanisms are consumed as a result of stiffness/degeneration, SL disappears, and if spine extension in the usually

kyphotic thoracolumbar area is insufficient, then there will be a "global kyphosis" with a small PI (▸ Fig. 8.2). Degenerative evolution of previous idiopathic thoracolumbar scoliosis may turn progressively the scoliosis deformity into a thoracolumbar kyphoscoliosis with small PI and sagittal patterns of type 1.

Type 2

There are small compensation abilities. Therefore, when a kyphotic event affects the thoracolumbar area, either an increase in LL will be seen on a small arch generating a type 1 (thoracolumbar kyphosis), or SL disappears generating a "lumbar kyphosis" type (if the thoracic spine can compensate with a hypokyphosis) or "global kyphosis" with a small PI (▸ Fig. 8.3). However, probably the most compromising

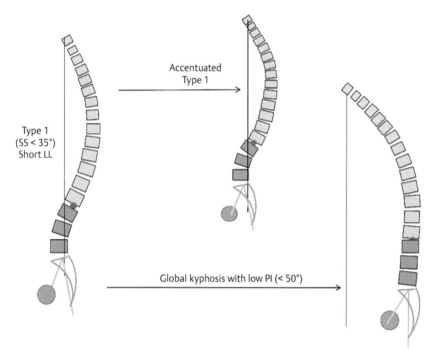

Fig. 8.2 Drawing showing the possible evolution of type 1 shape. PI, Pelvic incidence; LL, lumbar lordosis; SS, sacral slope.

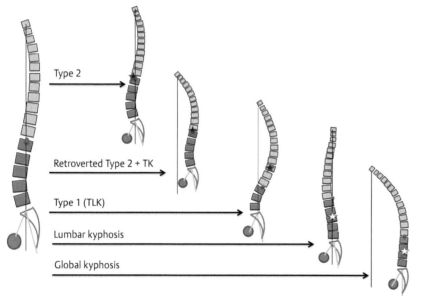

Fig. 8.3 Drawing showing the possible evolution of type 2 shape. TLK, thoracolumbar kyphosis.

situation is the combination of flat type 2 lordosis with a degenerative TK, which necessitates a global treatment in the case of surgical treatment. In the frontal plan, the occurrence of de novo lumbar scoliosis seems linked with small PI and type 2. The increasing disk pressure in the distal lumbar area explains the progressive loosening of the disks with lateral dislocations.

8.3.2 Strongly Retroverted Pelvis (High Pelvic Incidence > 50°)

Type 3

When SL decreases, compensation is seen in the mobile spine above and evolves to retroversion with a straight spine and a decrease in SS creating a false type 2. However, in aging people, the balance compensation by thoracic extension and hypokyphosis is probably limited by the muscle weakness. If the thoracic spine is too stiff, thoracic hypokyphosis does not occur, creating a false type 2 with TK with increased pelvic tilt (PT) (retroversion of the pelvis) as the only possible compensation mechanism. The ultimate evolution of type 3 is global kyphosis (with high PI) and maximally retroverted pelvis (▶ Fig. 8.4).

Type 4

The decreased SL induces a false type 3 with a retroverted pelvis. Subsequent evolution is as described for type 3 (▶ Fig. 8.5). It is with type 4 that we may encounter the higher retroverted pelvis with PT overpassing 35°.

This description of the evolution of the aging spine is the most reasonable that exists today. Clinical studies are emerging, and it seems that the classification (both classic and the above described one) can be advantageous in decision making: choosing and tailoring the right surgical strategy in individual patients. In a 2-year follow-up, a one-center study of 147 adolescent idiopathic scoliosis patients (non-aging population), the authors found that the incidence of proximal junctional kyphosis (PJK) was significantly higher in type 1 (50%) and type

4 (28%) at follow-up (overall incidence was 16%).[36] In a 2-year follow-up multicenter study of 314 ASD by Sebaaly et al,[37] it was found that ignoring restoration to the original shape according to the Roussouly classification of the degenerative spine showed a fivefold increased risk of mechanical complications.

When one assesses the sagittal shape in the elderly, thoracic or thoracolumbar kyphosis is a crucial point. First, control of the thoracic spine forces an extensive instrumentation up to the proximal thoracic spine that can be difficult to accept for an older patient. Maintaining the kyphosis involves compensating the balance by increasing lordosis below. This lordosis adaptation must consider the size of the PI. A small PI requires a short acute lordosis (type 1) or a small lordosis, and a high PI requires a longer lordosis but with a distal distribution (focused on L4, L5, S1). Sometimes, balance may be obtained by kyphosis reduction using kyphosis three-column osteotomy.[38,39,40] However, reduction must be slight according to LL reduction. If we reduce both kyphosis and lordosis too much, backward displacement of the upper thoracic spine with negative sagittal vertical axis induces a high risk of PJK.[41] It is easier to restore balance for a spine with a small PI because there is a small need of lordosis in type 2 spines. When a kyphosis is associated in a thoracic area with a small PI, the strategy of maintaining the kyphosis by transformation into type 1 is the most efficient and the less demanding strategy. With higher PI, the restoration of a big lordosis needs such a very strong technique such as pedicle subtraction osteotomy.

The frequent association of spinal stenosis and sagittal unbalance is generally difficult to treat. Simple local decompression may conduct to later destabilization of the spine, even with short local fusion, and recurrence of painful initial status may exist. On another hand, spinal reduction strategy could be excessive in older patients with poor general status. As expectancy of life in older patients may not display years or decades of life after surgery (relative limited follow-up time), one may assume that the study of sagittal balance in older patients after surgery may provide confusing conclusions.

Fig. 8.4 Drawing showing the possible evolution of type 3 shape. PI, Pelvic incidence; SS, sacral slope; TK, thoracic kyphosis.

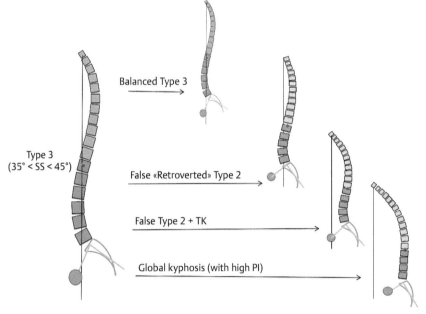

Type 3
(35° < SS < 45°)

Balanced Type 3

False «Retroverted» Type 2

False Type 2 + TK

Global kyphosis (with high PI)

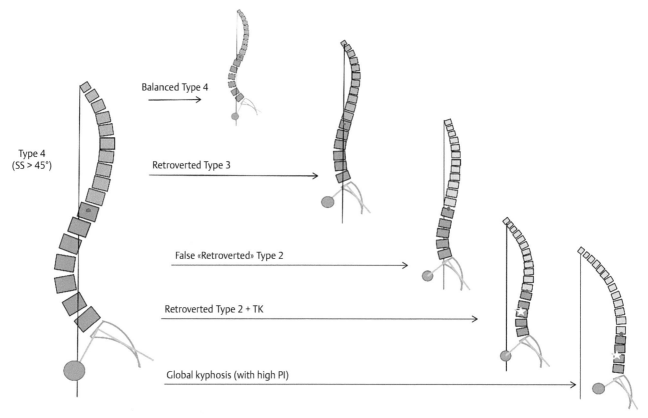

Fig. 8.5 Drawing showing the possible evolution of type 4 shape. PI, Pelvic incidence; SS, sacral slope; TK, thoracic kyphosis.

Longer fusions allowing reduction and stabilization have a high potential of pseudarthrosis and PJK mainly if the strategy of reduction tends to a perfect restoration. Hypercorrection with restoration of an ideal sagittal alignment, like Michelangelo's David, cannot be the aim of treatment in the elderly. Acceptance of maintaining kyphosis in the thoracic or thoracolumbar area is mandatory. A slight imbalance with a retroverted pelvis may be acceptable, and the use of a walking frame or stick could be integrated into the treatment.

8.4 Conclusion

Combining loosening of bony-disk support by degeneration and osteoporosis and muscle weakness, spinal unbalance in the elderly induces spinal kyphosis with or without compensation by pelvis retroversion depending on PI value. Association with knee or hip arthritis is frequent and must be taken into account in treatment strategy. Imbrication of spinal stenosis and deformity may be a big dilemma in treatment strategy when general clinical conditions are bad. Intermediate levels of reduction maintaining a part of kyphotic deformity may be more acceptable than "ideal" hypercorrection.

References

[1] Pollintine P, van Tunen MSLM, Luo J, Brown MD, Dolan P, Adams MA. Time-dependent compressive deformation of the ageing spine: relevance to spinal stenosis. Spine. 2010; 35(4):386–394

[2] Barrey C, Roussouly P, Perrin G, Le Huec J-C. Sagittal balance disorders in severe degenerative spine. Can we identify the compensatory mechanisms? Eur Spine J. 2011; 20 Suppl 5:626–633

[3] Ailon T, Smith JS, Shaffrey CI, et al. Degenerative spinal deformity. Neurosurgery. 2015; 77 Suppl 4:S75–S91

[4] Grubb SA, Lipscomb HJ, Coonrad RW. Degenerative adult onset scoliosis. Spine. 1988; 13(3):241–245

[5] Roussouly P, Pinheiro-Franco JL. Sagittal parameters of the spine: biomechanical approach. Eur Spine J. 2011; 20 Suppl 5:578–585

[6] Mac-Thiong JM, Roussouly P, Berthonnaud E, Guigui P. Age- and sex-related variations in sagittal sacropelvic morphology and balance in asymptomatic adults. Eur Spine J. 2011; 20 Suppl 5:572–577

[7] Mac-Thiong JM, Berthonnaud E, Dimar JR, II, Betz RR, Labelle H. Sagittal alignment of the spine and pelvis during growth. Spine. 2004; 29(15):1642–1647

[8] Mac-Thiong JM, Labelle H, Roussouly P. Pediatric sagittal alignment. Eur Spine J. 2011; 20 Suppl 5:586–590

[9] Vialle R, Levassor N, Rillardon L, Templier A, Skalli W, Guigui P. Radiographic analysis of the sagittal alignment and balance of the spine in asymptomatic subjects. J Bone Joint Surg Am. 2005; 87(2):260–267

[10] Boulay C, Tardieu C, Hecquet J, et al. Sagittal alignment of spine and pelvis regulated by pelvic incidence: standard values and prediction of lordosis. Eur Spine J. 2006; 15(4):415–422

[11] Brinjikji W, Luetmer PH, Comstock B, et al. Systematic literature review of imaging features of spinal degeneration in asymptomatic populations. AJNR Am J Neuroradiol. 2015; 36(4):811–816

[12] Kepler CK, Hilibrand AS, Sayadipour A, et al. Clinical and radiographic degenerative spondylolisthesis (CARDS) classification. Spine J. 2015; 15(8): 1804–1811

[13] Gille O, Challier V, Parent H, et al. Degenerative lumbar spondylolisthesis: cohort of 670 patients, and proposal of a new classification. Orthop Traumatol Surg Res. 2014; 100(6) Suppl:S311–S315

[14] Schwab F, Ungar B, Blondel B, et al. Scoliosis Research Society–Schwab adult spinal deformity classification: a validation study. Spine. 2012; 37(12): 1077–1082

[15] Obeid I, Boissière L, Yilgor C, et al. Global tilt: a single parameter incorporating spinal and pelvic sagittal parameters and least affected by patient positioning. Eur Spine J. 2016; 25(11):3644–3649

[16] Ryan DJ, Protopsaltis TS, Ames CP, et al. T1 pelvic angle (TPA) effectively evaluates sagittal deformity and assesses radiographical surgical outcomes longitudinally. Spine. 2014; 39(15):1203–1210

[17] Lafage V, Schwab F, Patel A, Hawkinson N, Farcy JP. Pelvic tilt and truncal inclination: two key radiographic parameters in the setting of adults with spinal deformity. Spine. 2009; 34(17):E599–E606

[18] Cortet B, Houvenagel E, Puisieux F, Roches E, Garnier P, Delcambre B. Spinal curvatures and quality of life in women with vertebral fractures secondary to osteoporosis. Spine. 1999; 24(18):1921–1925

[19] Vaccaro AR, Silber JS. Post-traumatic spinal deformity. Spine. 2001; 26(24) Suppl:S111–S118

[20] Wenger DR, Frick SL. Scheuermann kyphosis. Spine. 1999; 24(24):2630–2639

[21] Simmons EH. Kyphotic deformity of the spine in ankylosing spondylitis. Clin Orthop Relat Res. 1977; 128:65–77

[22] Roussouly P, Pinheiro-Franco JL. Biomechanical analysis of the spino-pelvic organization and adaptation in pathology. Eur Spine J. 2011; 20 Suppl 5: 609–618

[23] Siebenrock KA, Kalbermatten DF, Ganz R. Effect of pelvic tilt on acetabular retroversion: a study of pelves from cadavers. Clin Orthop Relat Res. 2003; 407:241–248

[24] Ben-Galim P, Ben-Galim T, Rand N, et al. Hip-spine syndrome: the effect of total hip replacement surgery on low back pain in severe osteoarthritis of the hip. Spine. 2007; 32(19):2099–2102

[25] Offierski CM, MacNab I. Hip-spine syndrome. Spine. 1983; 8(3):316–321

[26] Devin CJ, McCullough KA, Morris BJ, Yates AJ, Kang JD. Hip-spine syndrome. J Am Acad Orthop Surg. 2012; 20(7):434–442

[27] Fogel GR, Esses SI. Hip spine syndrome: management of coexisting radiculopathy and arthritis of the lower extremity. Spine J. 2003; 3(3):238–241

[28] Roussouly P, Gollogly S, Berthonnaud E, Dimnet J. Classification of the normal variation in the sagittal alignment of the human lumbar spine and pelvis in the standing position. Spine. 2005; 30(3):346–353

[29] Laouissat F, Sebaaly A, Gehrchen M, Roussouly P. Classification of normal sagittal spine alignment: refounding the Roussouly classification. Eur Spine J. 2018; 27(8):2002–2011

[30] Fujiwara A, Tamai K, Yamato M, et al. The relationship between facet joint osteoarthritis and disc degeneration of the lumbar spine: an MRI study. Eur Spine J. 1999; 8(5):396–401

[31] Barrey C, Jund J, Noseda O, Roussouly P. Sagittal balance of the pelvis-spine complex and lumbar degenerative diseases. A comparative study about 85 cases. Eur Spine J. 2007; 16(9):1459–1467

[32] Barrey C, Jund J, Perrin G, Roussouly P. Spinopelvic alignment of patients with degenerative spondylolisthesis. Neurosurgery. 2007; 61(5):981–986, discussion 986

[33] Jackson RP, McManus AC. Radiographic analysis of sagittal plane alignment and balance in standing volunteers and patients with low back pain matched for age, sex, and size. A prospective controlled clinical study. Spine. 1994; 19 (14):1611–1618

[34] Jackson RP, Kanemura T, Kawakami N, Hales C. Lumbopelvic lordosis and pelvic balance on repeated standing lateral radiographs of adult volunteers and untreated patients with constant low back pain. Spine. 2000; 25(5):575–586

[35] Sebaaly A, Grobost P, Mallam L, Roussouly P. Description of the sagittal alignment of the degenerative human spine. Eur Spine J. 2018; 27(2):489–496

[36] Ohrt-Nissen S, Bari T, Dahl B, Gehrchen M. Sagittal alignment after surgical treatment of adolescent idiopathic scoliosis-application of the Roussouly classification. Spine Deform. 2018; 6(5):537–544

[37] Sebaaly A, Gehrchen M, Silvestre C, Kharrat KE, Bari T, Kreichati G, et al. Restoring the spinal shape in adult spinal deformity according to the Roussouly classification and its effect on mechanical complications: a multicentric study (in preparation)

[38] Kiaer T, Gehrchen M. Transpedicular closed wedge osteotomy in ankylosing spondylitis: results of surgical treatment and prospective outcome analysis. Eur Spine J. 2010; 19(1):57–64

[39] Cho K-J, Kim K-T, Kim W-J, et al. Pedicle subtraction osteotomy in elderly patients with degenerative sagittal imbalance. Spine. 2013; 38(24): E1561–E1566

[40] Lenke LG, Sides BA, Koester LA, Hensley M, Blanke KM. Vertebral column resection for the treatment of severe spinal deformity. Clin Orthop Relat Res. 2010; 468(3):687–699

[41] Kim HJ, Bridwell KH, Lenke LG, et al. Patients with proximal junctional kyphosis requiring revision surgery have higher postoperative lumbar lordosis and larger sagittal balance corrections. Spine. 2014; 39(9):E576–E580

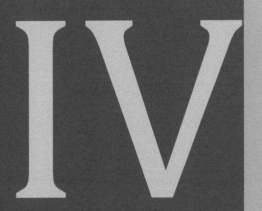

Part IV

The Sagittal Balance of the Spine in Pathology

IV

9 Local Stresses: Segmental Mechanism of Low Back Pain and Degeneration, and Stresses According to Spinal Orientation—Contact Forces Theory

Amer Sebaaly, João Luiz Pinheiro-Franco, and Pierre Roussouly

Abstract

The human spine assumes the body verticality compared with quadrupeds. This global vertical orientation of the spine and pelvis induces a permanent stronger action of the gravity on the spinal structures. The normal spine physiology can be compared to the function of a crane that is governed by a tripod of mechanical forces: the anterior downward force of the gravity (weight of the patient), the posterior forces of the muscles to erect the spine that allow walking, and the effect of the belly shape in this system, but only two main forces act in pathology: the weight gravity and posterior muscle force (MF). The total contact force on the spinal unit is the sum of these two acting forces. On the other hand, the distribution of the same vertical force is different depending on the sagittal orientation of the vertebrae. This induces different contact forces orientation is the various spinal shapes. Thus, the identification of various spinopelvic morphotypes allows understanding the physical distribution of forces induced by body weight and muscle counterbalance, regarding spinal unit orientation and range of motion. An abnormal overstress may explain the mechanical origin of pain and spine degeneration.

Keywords: Contact forces, Spinal shapes, spinal degeneration, Roussouly classification

9.1 Introduction

The spinal column forms the axial skeleton and is a complex multiarticular system that supports the head and the trunk with economical transfer of the loads to the lower limbs. This system is under the control of the central nervous system and the local muscles and allows smooth force transfer without any increase of degenerative changes. While assuring this biomechanical role, the spinal column protects the neural elements (spinal cord, cauda equina, and nerve roots) and vascular elements (vertebral artery). While all vertebrates have a common spinal structure by vertebral unit alignment, the human spine must assume the body verticality compared with quadrupeds in which the spine behaves like a bridge between anterior and posterior legs. In quadrupeds, the thoracic and lumbar spine has almost nothing to support regarding the gravity because of its horizontal position. Their intervertebral disks aligned with their horizontal spine do not suffer direct vertical compression forces from gravity (▶ Fig. 9.1). The only pressure is produced by horizontal forces during acceleration by the posterior legs. This propulsion force from the posterior legs is transmitted by a very anteverted pelvis through a vertical sacral plateau positioned forward the femoral heads. In opposition to other bipeds like dinosaurs or birds, human

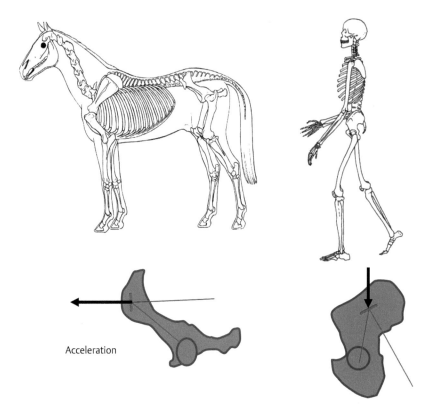

Acceleration

Fig. 9.1 Comparison of pelvis orientation: quadruped versus human. In quadrupeds, the pelvis is tilted forward with a vertical sacral plateau to provide a horizontal force and acceleration. In human, the pelvis is tilted backward to support the vertical body weight.

bipedalism is characterized by the verticality. The global vertical orientation of the spine and pelvis induces a permanent stronger action of the gravity on the spinal structures. It is of paramount importance to maintain the standing position in the most physically economical and stable system.

Spinal stability was defined by the American Academy of Orthopedic Surgeons as "The capacity of the vertebrae to remain cohesive and to preserve the normal displacements in all physiological body movements."[1] The spinal stability implies the transfer of power forces between the upper and lower limbs with active generation of forces in the trunk. This allows prevention of early biomechanical deterioration of spine components by reduction of the energy expenditure during muscle action.[2] Another factor of stability is provided by the limited segmental mobility, but a global harmonious spinal flexibility linked to the association of the whole segmental unit. The segmental mobility has been extensively studied for each level of the spine[3,4] and is characterized by a small range of motion rarely exceeding 5° to 6°.

This chapter reviews the mechanisms of low back pain generation focusing on contact forces and forces transmission while applying novel findings of spinal alignment on the generation of these forces. Mechanisms of segmental motion overpassing are also analyzed with its possible painful action.

9.2 Historical Review

Even though anatomy of the spine has been quite well described by Hippocrates and then Galen, and very precisely by Vesalius during the 16th Century, it was Giovanni Alfonso Borelli who approached its mechanical function in the book *De Motu Animalium*. He described the muscles–joint interactions and the forces acting on the spine in various situations (see Chapter 1). Later, Jean Cruveilhier used Euler's law to demonstrate how successive spinal curvatures favor the spinal resistance. During the 19th century, numerous authors, mainly in Germany, tried to determine the position of the center of gravity and more precisely to define the position of the center

of mass at each level of the human body. In 1987, Duval-Beaupère published a technique using a gamma-ray scanner to identify the mass of successive body scans and the position of their respective body mass centers. Based on the notion of spinal unit, many authors (Panjabi, Dimnet) described the intervertebral motion. Recently, using the crane concept, Dimnet defined the combination of different gravity and muscles forces that induce a global contact force on each level.

9.3 Functional Spinal Unit and Normal Range of Motion

The spinal biomechanical unit is the functional spinal unit (FSU). An FSU is formed by two adjacent vertebrae with one intervertebral disk and corresponding ligaments (▶ Fig. 9.2).[5] The FSU's main function is to provide spinal movement while protecting the neural elements. Another function of the FSU is to transmit the weight of the body to the lower limbs via the pelvis and the femoral heads.[5] The FSU function relies greatly on the anatomy of its components as well as on the interactions between the bony structures, the surrounding muscles and ligaments, and the control of the central nervous system.[2]

In everyday activity, the vertical loads on the spine are thought to be around 500–1000 N, nearly twice the body weight. These compressive forces increase to nearly 5000 N with lifting, achieving nearly half the failure load.[6] The transmission of these loads is assured by the anatomy of the vertebral bodies, the intervertebral disk, and the facets and the sagittal curvatures of the spine.[2]

The vertebral body anatomy and architecture plays an important role in the load transmission. The load-bearing ability increases from 200 N in cervical vertebra to around 8000 N in the lower lumbar vertebrae. This is caused by the increasing size of the vertebral body going from the cervical spine to the lumbar spine (C1 has no vertebral body and S1 has the largest vertebral body). This increase of size of the vertebral bodies abides by Wolff's law: "bones adapt their mass and

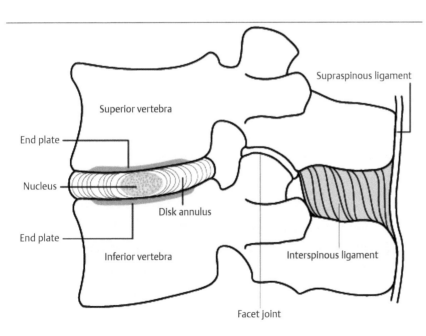

Fig. 9.2 A functional spinal unit is formed by the two adjacent vertebrae, the facet joints, the intervertebral disk, and the surrounding ligaments.

Superior vertebra

End plate

Nucleus

Disk annulus

End plate

Inferior vertebra

Supraspinous ligament

Interspinous ligament

Facet joint

architecture in response to the magnitude and direction of forces applied to them." Bony microarchitecture also plays an important role in the load transmission. In normal vertebrae, the trabecular bone is arranged with vertical and horizontal trabeculae. While the vertical trabecular system transmits the compressive forces, the horizontal system decreases the bending forces on the vertical system by transmitting the bending forces to the outer cortical shell.[7] With osteoporosis, there is a rarefaction of the horizontal system with elongation of the vertical system. This phenomenon is more marked in the anterior body, thus the prevalence of anterior wedge osteoporotic fractures.[8]

The intervertebral disk is another actor in the load transmission. It has the proprieties of both a ligament (tension resisting) and a synovial joint (compression resisting). The orientation of the fibers of the annulus fibrosus limits the movements of the FSU in axial (limits rotation), sagittal (limiting flexion, extension), and coronal planes (limiting side bending). On the other hand, the nucleus pulposus acts as a spacer between the two endplates and as a shock absorber and load transmitter. It is interesting to note that the same unit has very different functions in quadrupeds compared to humans. In quadrupeds, intervertebral disks are used for motion stabilization and for propulsion forces transmission but no gravity support, whereas in humans, gravity loads are the main constraints the FSU has to sustain. This may explain the apparent disk fragility in humans who develop more diskopathies than quadrupeds.

The final load-transmitting components are the articular facets. The articular facets contribute to the posterior column (in the Denis model) and acts primarily counteracting shear forces. Similar to vertebral bodies, the shape, size, and orientation of the facets change from C1 to S1 to accommodate the increasing load transmission requirements. Classically, it has been stated that for a normal spine, the intervertebral disk receives more than 90% of the loads. There is concern on the definition of a normal spine. Contemporary studies have shown that there are various spine shapes from more straight (or less curved) to more curved and that the stress/load bearing is divided between disk forward and facets backward, depending on the sagittal orientation of the FSU. With increasing disk degeneration, causing loss of disk height, the loads are transmitted via the posterior facets that receive more than half of the compressive loads. This induces facet joints hypertrophy and osteoarthritis.

As the disk acts as a synovial articulation, it could be compared to another osteoarticular articulation as, for example, the knee or the elbow. Every joint has a normal range of motion that, when beyond it, movement is painful (hyperextension and hyperflexion). This principle is applied to an FSU albeit with a lesser range of motion (5°) compared to the elbow. With the degenerative cascade, the range of motion is ultimately decreased by degenerative changes. Disk degeneration limits flexion and brings the hyperflexion threshold closer to the average position, whereas facet joints arthritis limits hyperextension and brings the hyperextension threshold close to the average position (▶ Fig. 9.3). When the FSU is in a hyper lordosis state, the remaining possibility of increasing extension is limited. In this kind of structure (i.e., type 1 lordosis), an increasing thoracolumbar kyphosis induces a painful caudal compensation by increasing the distal lordosis in an already much-extended area. As the painful caudal position in extension is very close to the neutral posture, an excessive postural lordosis such as supine with knees extended may be quickly intolerable. If hyperextension is needed (like in osteoporotic fracture in the thoracolumbar area in type 1 lordosis), the hyperextension is painful and generates low back pain and there is increased risk of facet hypertrophy (▶ Fig. 9.4). Therefore, the back pain of these patients is relieved by lying on the side and rounding the back. On the other hand, an FSU in hypolordosis has the average positioning closer to a hyperflexion threshold. This phenomenon is seen is type 2 spines where the patient may adopt a lumbar kyphosis alignment as a result of multilevel diskopathies. Back pain is generated by the inability to escape the hyperflexion zone and the patients are relieved by lying in a hyperextended position (▶ Fig. 9.5). In addition, different degenerative mechanisms would also modify this range of motion of the FSU (▶ Fig. 9.6).

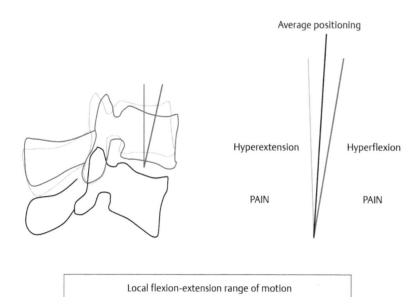

Average positioning

Hyperextension

PAIN

Hyperflexion

PAIN

Local flexion-extension range of motion

Fig. 9.3 Normal range of motion of the functional spinal unit (FSU). The average position is around the bisector of the angle between maximum flexion and maximum extension. Note that the average range of motion of the FSU is ~ 5°.

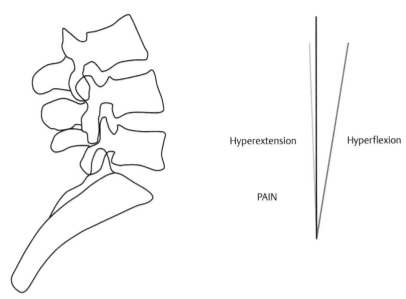

Fig. 9.4 Functional spinal unit in hyperextension. The average positioning is near the extension threshold. Further extension would induce pain.

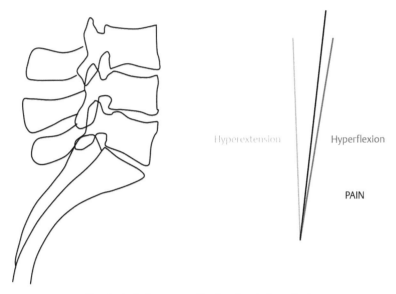

Fig. 9.5 Functional spinal unit in hyperflexion. The average positioning is near the flexion threshold. Further flexion would induce pain.

9.4 The Crane Principle and Contact Forces

The normal spine physiology can be compared to the function of a crane that is governed by a tripod of mechanical forces: the anterior downward force of the gravity (weight of the patient), the posterior forces of the muscles to erect the spine that allow walking, and the effect of the belly shape in this system. The belly shape is different between men and women and changes with age. In younger patients, contraction of abdominal muscles increases the rigidity of the abdomen and helps the spine in supporting forward forces. In older patients, abdominal muscles weaken and the belly size increases. Women's fatty depositions are concentrated around the hips and buttock areas before menopause (gynoid disposition), whereas the fat is concentrated around the belly in men and postmenopausal women (android deposition). In addition, the belly shape is somewhat different in men and postmenopausal women. Men's bellies are round and puffy (with more musculature) allowing it to function as a shock absorber by maintaining higher intra-abdominal pressure and helps in fighting the anterior angulation of the spine and kyphosis. On the other hand, the postmenopausal woman's belly shape is fluffy and, in ptosis, acting as an increasing force to the anterior angulation of the spine (▶ Fig. 9.7). In pathology, the belly action is poor and, to simplify the crane system, the belly shape function will be removed from the equation and we will only discuss the two

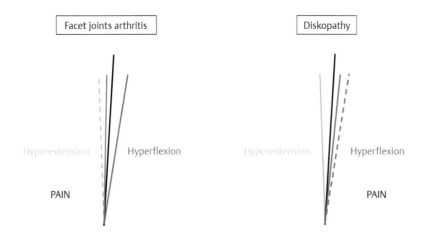

Fig. 9.6 Effect of degenerative changes on the range of motion of the functional spinal unit. Facet joint arthritis would decrease the extension limit, whereas diskopathy will decrease the flexion limit.

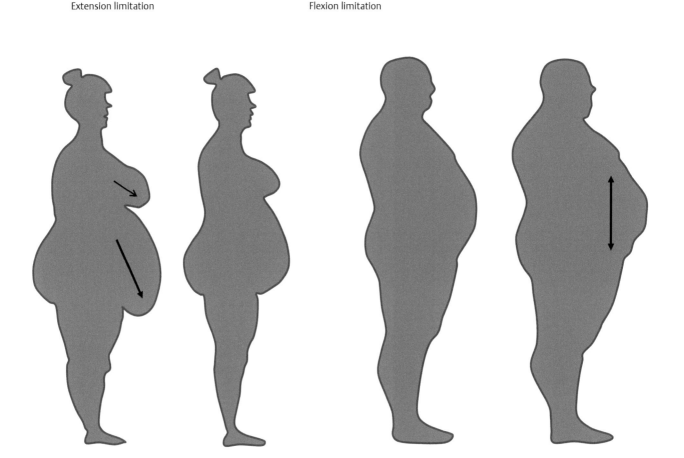

Fig. 9.7 Difference in the form of the belly between men and women. Men have a puffy round belly allowing anterior support, whereas the anterior forces of the belly and the breast in women tend to displace anteriorly the gravity line.

main acting forces: the weight gravity and posterior muscle force (MF).

Weight gravity is not caused by the total weight that applies on the ground but at each spinal level if we consider the vertical force linked to the mass over the level of the spine where this force acts. The more caudal is the level (like in lumbosacral area), the higher the force. This was the center of the barycentrometry theory of Duval-Beaupère. Using a gamma-ray scan, the authors were able to determine the body mass and the corresponding center of mass of each spinal segment above the pelvis. With the Duval-Beaupère technique, each functional segment unit has its own evaluation and the gravity acting on it is calculated by the sum of gravity of the different segments above. When using the force plate technique, the gravity on the whole body is calculated.

It is not sure that both gravity on one vertebral unit and global gravity are equivalent. But as they are close, the idea of approximation is acceptable. Nonetheless, this study was experimental and difficult to use in clinical routines. To define more easily the global gravity line, some authors combined a force plate and standing X-rays to position the vertical projection of the center of mass on the ground and report it on the X-rays.

Center of mass falls always down on the foot surface and passes close to the center of femoral heads. Even if it is not totally accurate, we may consider that the centers of mass of each anatomical segment over the pelvis are, by approximation, close to the global gravity line.

Posterior muscles action is a result of paraspinal, posterior abdominal muscles that go against the body mass forces (BMFs). This mechanical system may be assimilated as a crane with the spine corresponding to the pylon. On one side of the pylon, body mass forces are acting forward, and on the other side, posterior muscles are counteracting backward. Contact force acting on the pylon is the sum of BMFs and MFs. To balance the system, if "A" is the distance from BMF to the pylon and "B" from MF to the pylon, the equation would be $A \times BMF = B \times MF$. When BMF is closer to the spine, only a small MF is necessary. If BMF displaces forward, MF cannot compensate by a backward displacement and MF must increase, increasing the contact force applied on the spine, because the contact force is an addition of BMF + MF (BMF is constant and MF increases) (▶ Fig. 9.8).

The main objective of this system is to have the gravity force line behind the femoral heads to maintain an economical balance and the ability of the humans to walk in a vertical stance. In fact, as shown in ▶ Fig. 9.8, the moment of the force is equal to the force times the level arm of this force. Because the erector muscle level arm is constant, and to maintain a balanced spine, the increase of the moment of the gravity force will induce a higher workload from the posterior erector muscles, generating increased potentials and the fatigability of this muscular group. The result of this system is a contact force on the lower disks that increases with the imbalance of this system (▶ Fig. 9.8).

9.5 Pressure and Shear Forces in Normal Spine

When the Euler law is applied to spinal curvatures, the resistance for compression is proportional to the squared number of curvatures plus one (R=[(Number of curves)^2 + 1] × K) with a minimum of 1 when there is no curve as in a straight spine. In fact, within an FSU, the normally vertical compressive forces will be divided into two forces: one force is parallel to the intervertebral disk and tries to displace the vertebra anteriorly or posteriorly (the shear force), and the other is perpendicular to the disk that tends to stabilize the FSU with the drawback of higher intradiskal pressures (▶ Fig. 9.9).

The distribution of the same vertical force is different depending on the sagittal orientation of the vertebrae. In fact, vertebrae that are located in the apex of a curve (apex of the spinal lordosis or the apex of spinal kyphosis) are practically horizontal. The vertical force of weight transmission is divided into a small shear component and a much higher compressive component. On the other hand, vertebrae located at the ends of the curves tend to be more inclined with a higher shear component and a lesser compression component (▶ Fig. 9.9).

This biomechanical concept may explain several findings in normal and pathological conditions. First, it is well documented

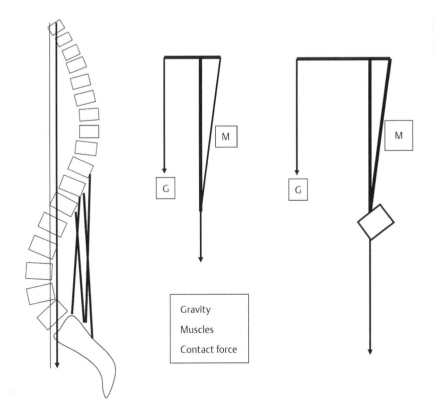

Fig. 9.8 Contact forces definition and compensation of the muscle forces to decrease the effect of forward displacement of the gravity line.

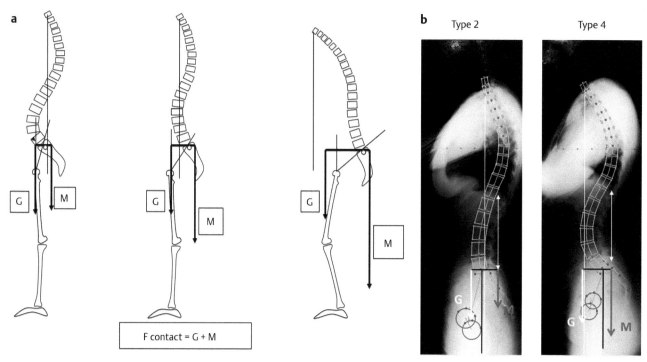

Fig. 9.9 Drawing showing the increase of the difference of the contact forces between types 2 and 4 and in pathological conditions (**a**). Contact forces are shown on full spine sagittal X-ray (**b**).

that the most common location of lumbar diskopathies is at L4-L5.[9] This could be explained by the fact that the L4-L5 disk is horizontally oriented in the majority of the cases and is subject to higher compressive loads and, thus, higher intradiskal pressures. Second, the degeneration profile is different depending on the spinal shape as defined by Roussouly et al[10] (Chapter 6). As a matter of fact, Roussouly et al stated that type 2 spines have a higher prevalence of multilevel disk degeneration while type 4 spines had higher prevalence of spondylolisthesis.[11] The degeneration in type 2 spines is mainly caused by the higher compressive component in a relatively straight spine. Degeneration of the disk is the primum movens of the degenerative cascade in this spinopelvic type. On the other hand, the inclination of the L4 and L5 vertebrae induces high contact forces on the posterior facets, determining facet joints hypertrophy and osteoarthritis as well as high shear forces favoring vertebral slippage and spondylolisthesis.

One spinal type is less explored in the literature: type 1 or thoracolumbar kyphosis. This spinal type is associated with low PI, low SS, lower number of vertebrae comprised in the lordosis, and a lordosis apex located in the L5 vertebra. In this type, there are practically no shear forces on the L5-S1 articulation with higher pressures on the posterior facets and thus higher L5-S1 facet joint degeneration.[12] There are low rates of L5-S1 degeneration as most of the compressive forces are focused on the facets. Even more, there are higher rates of L2-L3 retro spondylolisthesis, mainly because of the great inclination of the L2-L3 FSU, rendering it more susceptible to the increased shear forces and then to retrolisthesis.

9.6 Application of Biomechanical Principles in Pathology

The combination of FSU orientation and positioning with the global shape of the spine may be used for explaining mechanical spinal disorders. An observation of spinal mechanics shows that an overstress in flexion or in extension may explain local pain by hypermotion and hyperpressure because of a local spinal orientation. For example, in type 4, back where spinal lordosis is overcurved in extension, pressure on the facets is favored by a double effect: localization of the contact forces on the posterior elements and FSU hyperextension. This mechanism may generate low back pain even before evidence of degeneration. As explained in Chapter 10, mechanisms and localization of degeneration are strongly linked with specific mechanical stress according to each spinopelvic morphotype.

It is evident that proximal junction kyphosis (PJK) has an important mechanical component and the theory of stress distribution according to the spinal architecture allows possible new explanations. Based on two different situations, we constructed the local junctional contact force (▶ Fig. 9.10). In case 1, the insufficient lumbar reduction is compensated by pelvic retroversion. The posterior displacement of the spine positions the junctional area far backward from the gravity projection. This fact combined with a vertical straight thoracic spine may explain the junctional overstress and the PJF (proximal junctional failure). In case 2, a too-long spinal lordosis inflicts on the

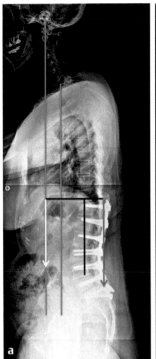 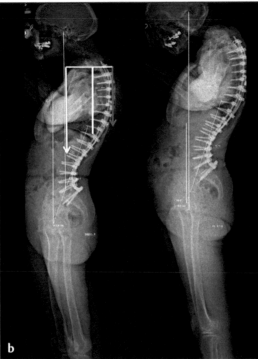

Fig. 9.10 (a) Case 1 showing insufficient balance restoration, causing thoracic hyperextension. This increases muscles activity and induces dramatic increase in contact forces. The result is a proximal junctional failure. **(b)** Case 2 shows a forward displacement of the gravity line with insufficient muscle compensation inducting the proximal junction kyphosis.

thoracic spine a backward position compared to the head. The head gravity has a very strong force moment that cannot be compensated by posterior muscles inducing a PJF.

9.7 Conclusion

Verticality of the human body has imposed specific mechanical stresses on the set spine and pelvis to counteract the gravity. The aim of an ideal balance is to minimize these stresses on the different spinal structures: vertebral bodies, disks, and facet joints. The identification of various spinopelvic morphotypes allows understanding the physical distribution of forces induced by body weight and muscle counterbalance, regarding spinal unit orientation and range of motion. An abnormal over-stress may explain the mechanical origin of pain and spine degeneration. After surgical treatment, position induced by an arthrodesis may disturb the mechanical forces distribution and induce unexpected complications such as PJK.

References

[1] Kirkaldy-Willis W. Presidential Symposium on Instability of the Lumbar Spine: Introduction. Spine. 1985;10(3):254

[2] Izzo R, Guarnieri G, Guglielmi G, Muto M. Biomechanics of the spine. Part I: spinal stability. Eur J Radiol. 2013; 82(1):118–126

[3] Oxland TR. Fundamental biomechanics of the spine—what we have learned in the past 25 years and future directions. J Biomech. 2016; 49(6):817–832

[4] Stagnara P, De Mauroy JC, Dran G, et al. Reciprocal angulation of vertebral bodies in a sagittal plane: approach to references for the evaluation of kyphosis and lordosis. Spine. 1982; 7(4):335–342

[5] Kowalski RJ, Ferrara LA, Benzel EC. Biomechanics of the spine. Neurosurg Q. 2005; 15(1):42–59

[6] Wilke HJ, Neef P, Caimi M, Hoogland T, Claes LE. New in vivo measurements of pressures in the intervertebral disc in daily life. Spine. 1999; 24(8): 755–762

[7] Pollintine P, Dolan P, Tobias JH, Adams MA. Intervertebral disc degeneration can lead to "stress-shielding" of the anterior vertebral body: a cause of osteoporotic vertebral fracture? Spine. 2004; 29(7):774–782

[8] Sebaaly A, Rizkallah M, Bachour F, Atallah F, Moreau PE, Maalouf G. Percutaneous cement augmentation for osteoporotic vertebral fractures. EFORT Open Rev. 2017; 2(6):293–299

[9] Weinstein JN, Lurie JD, Tosteson TD, et al. Surgical vs nonoperative treatment for lumbar disk herniation: the Spine Patient Outcomes Research Trial (SPORT) observational cohort. JAMA. 2006; 296(20):2451–2459

[10] Roussouly P, Gollogly S, Berthonnaud E, Dimnet J. Classification of the normal variation in the sagittal alignment of the human lumbar spine and pelvis in the standing position. Spine. 2005; 30(3):346–353

[11] Roussouly P, Pinheiro-Franco JL. Biomechanical analysis of the spino-pelvic organization and adaptation in pathology. Eur Spine J. 2011; 20 Suppl 5: 609–618

[12] Scemama C, Laouissat F, Abelin-Genevois K, Roussouly P. Surgical treatment of thoraco-lumbar kyphosis (TLK) associated with low pelvic incidence. Eur Spine J. 2017; 26(8):2146–2152

10 Mechanisms of Spinal Degeneration According to Spinopelvic Morphotypes

João Luiz Pinheiro-Franco and Pierre Roussouly

Abstract:
The sagittal balance of the spine has been recognized as one of the new pillars in spine surgery. The analyses of pelvic parameters, spinal parameters and the assessment of the global balance of the spine are providing new perspectives on the surgical treatment of spinal pathologies. Spinal curvatures are characterized by their length and angle, where among the humans there are shorter lordoses and longer lordoses with higher and lower angles. The distribution of angles throughout the lordotic curve is however, not always homogeneous and has led to the classification of four spinopelvic morphotypes.

By employing the sacral slope (SS) and the pelvic incidence (PI) on lateral radiographs, Roussouly et al have classified four spinopelvic morphotypes according to four lordosis types. These authors observed a trend in patterns of spinal degeneration according to the type of presenting lordosis. It has been suggested that differences in spinal degeneration are also dependent on different patterns of spinal architecture, as exerted gravitational and muscle forces apply different patterns of mechanical stresses on spinal articulations. The classification of these degeneration patterns detailed in this chapter provides the specialist a better understanding of the natural history of spinal degeneration for each specific spinopelvic morphotype and therefore, serves as an impetus to promote more appropriate treatments.

Keywords: spinopelvic, spinopelvic types, types of lordosis, sagittal balance, Roussouly classification, sagittal balance classification, natural history of degenerative disc disease, natural history of spinopelvic types, spinopelvic morphotypes, effect of sagittal balance in spine degeneration, disc degeneration, posterior facet degeneration, pathological spinal shapes, spinal stenosis, pelvis retroversion

10.1 Introduction

The sagittal balance of the spine has been recognized as one of the new pillars in spine surgery. The analyses of pelvic parameters, spinal parameters, and the assessment of the global balance of the spine are providing new perspectives on the surgical treatment of spinal pathologies. Recognized since Hippocrates, the sagittal spinal segmentation has limited the lumbar lordosis (LL) between T12 and S1. More recently, Stagnara et al[1] and Berthonnaud et al[2] have redefined the functional borders of human distal lordosis with respect to an inflection point where lordosis transitions into kyphosis. Spinal curvatures are thereafter characterized by their length and angle, where among the humans there are shorter lordoses and longer lordoses with higher and lower angles. The distribution of angles throughout the lordotic curve is, however, not always homogeneous and has led to the classification of four spinopelvic morphotypes.

By employing the sacral slope (SS) and the pelvic incidence (PI) on lateral radiographs, Roussouly et al have classified four spinopelvic morphotypes according to four lordosis types.[3] These authors observed a trend in patterns of spinal degeneration according to the type of presenting lordosis. It has been suggested that differences in spinal degeneration are also dependent on different patterns of spinal architecture, as exerted gravitational and muscle forces apply different patterns of mechanical stresses on spinal articulations. The classification of these degeneration patterns detailed in this chapter provides the specialist a better understanding of the natural history of spinal degeneration for each specific spinopelvic morphotype and, therefore, serves as an impetus to promote more appropriate treatments.

10.2 Distal Spinal Lordosis and Pelvic Incidence as Sagittal Balance Modifiers

As described in Chapter 6, the authors emphasize herein differences in nomenclature: LL and distal spinal lordosis (DSL). Based on functional segmentation (Berthonnaud et al[2]), the new term DSL is defined as the part of the spine in extension between the S1 endplate and the inflection point where lordosis transitions into kyphosis (▶ Fig. 10.1). The classic usage of LL remains, that being, lordosis between T12-L1 and the S1 plateau.

LL and SS are integrally related to pelvic orientation ($r = 0.85$), which is strongly influenced by the PI ($r = 0.83$).[4] Stagnara found a strong correlation between LL and SS.[1] Likewise, an important correlation was found between LL and PI[1,5] in asymptomatic lower back pain (LBP) individuals.[6] Usually, the presence of a small PI equates to a smaller SS. The wide variability of SS in accordance with PI values was demonstrated by Roussouly, which led to his classification of four types of spinopelvic morphologies.[7]

10.3 Distal Spinal Lordosis Geometrical Analysis[8]

The radiological quantification of lordosis has been studied and demonstrated through a variety of ways. The arc of circle system of Berthonnaud et al[2] demonstrated that lordosis could be mathematically expressed as having two contiguous arcs of circle tangents in the horizontal line drawn from the apex of the lordosis (apex level is determined by the vertical line drawn tangentiating the anterior-most part of the convex side of lordosis).[2] The horizontal line crossing the apex of lordosis creates two arcs of a circle: the upper arc of the lordosis (from the apex horizontal line to the inflection point where lordosis bends into kyphosis) and the lower arc of the lordosis (from the

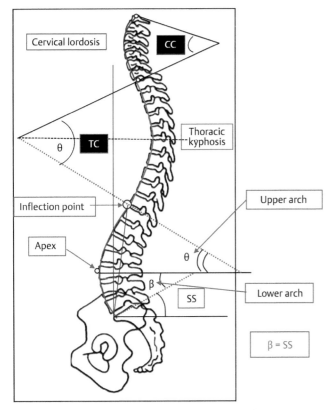

Fig. 10.1 Functional spinal sagittal segmentation based on the inflection point (Berthonnaud et al[2]). CC, Cervical curve; SS, sacral slope; TC, thoracic curve.

apex horizontal line to the sacral endplate). The angle of the lower arc and the SS are the same angle.[3]

Based on spinal lordosis/kyphosis segmentation, Roussouly et al developed a classification of four lordosis types, according to the concordances of the SS and the PI (Chapter 6). The main distinction among lordotic curves is the magnitude of the lower arc of lordosis. From geometric constructions, the lower arc of DSL is equal to SS. In agreement with the same geometric principle, the upper arc of DSL is equal to the lower arc of spinal kyphosis. DSL analysis thus consisted of the analyses of both the lower arc (equal to SS) and the upper arc. To segment it, SS was divided into three categories: low (<35°), average (35° < SS < 45°), and high (>45°) SS.

10.3.1 Low SS (<35°)

Type 1 Lordosis (Thoracolumbar Kyphosis)

There is a small SS (<35°) with a corresponding very small lower arc. The apex of lordosis is very low. The lordosis is very short and there is an acute angle concentrated in the lower arc with a significant backward displacement of the top of the lordosis. The weighbridge angle is acutely positive. As lordosis is very small, the maximal thoracic kyphosis (TK) is large and extends caudally beyond L2. The number of vertebrae comprised in this distal spinal lordosis (DSL) is reduced (≤3).

Type 2 Lordosis (Flat Back)

This lordosis is flat, and the angle of weighbridge is from positive to zero. The lordosis is also small. The inflection point is higher than that for type 1, as is the apex of the lordosis and the number of vertebrae included in the lordosis. TK is flat thereby corresponding with the flat lordosis.

10.3.2 Average SS (35° < SS < 45°)

Type 3 Lordosis (Harmonious)

Theoretically, this is the harmonious spine; the inflection point resides at the thoracolumbar junction. Lordosis is divided between two similar arcs. The apex is at the center of L4. There are usually four to five vertebrae in the lordosis. The angle of weighbridge is from positive to zero.

10.3.3 High SS (45°)

Type 4 Lordosis (Hypercurved)

Also known as the greater lordosis, SS is high, with the lower arc also being large (>45°). The distal spinal lordosis is long composed of more than five vertebrae included in the curve. The apex of lordosis is high (above L4) and the inflection point is also high, beyond the classic T12-L1 limits. The toggle angle is generally from zero to negative. The TK is generally much curved in correspondence with higher lordosis.

Roussouly et al observed that types 1 and 2 lordoses usually have lower PI values, while types 3 and 4 generally have higher PI values.[9] The authors have also noticed subjects with a very small or even negative pelvic tilt (PT) of < 10° in very anteverted pelvises. This situation may allow for SS > 40° even with a small PI, recognized as an anteverted type 3 with a small PI.[10] The PI value suggests a tendency for LL morphotypes; however, to extract an LL value from PI is an inexact extrapolation (▶ Fig. 10.2).

10.4 Lumbar Lordosis and Thoracic Kyphosis Angle

Spinal parameters LL and TK are interdependent. Jackson and McManus[11] observed a significant correlation between LL and TK.[6] The method of tangent arcs of circle segmentation applies to the thoracic spine. There is a direct relation between the upper arc of LL and the lower arc of TK. A change in one induces a change in the reciprocal segment of the other depending on the flexibility of the spine. This is more relevant in type 1 (too-small lower LL arc) where the total LL depends mostly on the upper arc of LL, which is forced to compensate for the higher, lower arc of TK in the thoracolumbar area.

TK may extend beyond the thoracolumbar area. Sometimes, both LL and TK curves are separated by a straight segment composed of a variable number of vertebrae. The importance of this disposition has not been well validated and requires further study.

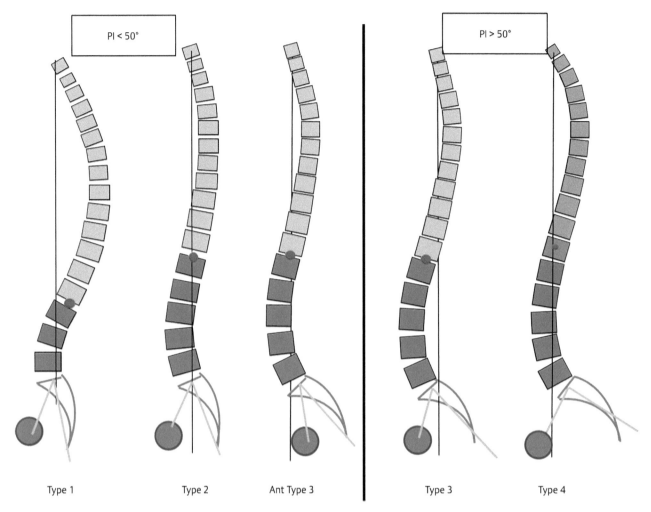

PI < 50°

PI > 50°

Type 1   Type 2   Ant Type 3   Type 3   Type 4

Fig. 10.2 Roussouly's classification according to the pelvic incidence.

10.5 Contact Forces: Resultant from Gravity and Muscular Action

We postulate a correlation between the spinopelvic morphotypes and the degenerative patterns found in computed tomography (CT) scans and magnetic resonance imaging (MRI). In the nonbalanced spine, there is a mechanical trend for forward gravitational forces to prevail over counteracting back muscle forces. These contact forces, the sum of both gravitational and muscular action, may load more strongly on the anterior parts of the spine (i.e., vertebrae and disks or the posterior elements of the spine, that is, zygapophyseal facet joints), depending on the morphology of one's spinopelvic structure. Individuals with flat spine or very poor lordosis curvature tend to present contact force loading predominantly in the anterior elements: disks and vertebrae. Inversely, a prominently curved lordosis produces higher loading in the posterior facet joints. Futhermore, the greater the tilt of the sacral plate, the greater are the resultant shear-slipping forces.

In Chapter 4, a spinal model using finite elements confirms this variation of loading action in agreement with the spinopelvic types.

In the "flat back," that is, type 2, the resultant forces are located forward in the lumbar spine, promoting high disk pressures. In type 1, combining both short hypercurved DSL and thoracolumbar kyphosis (TLK), load stress acts predominantly posteriorly on facet joints in the distal spinal lordosis area, but acts more anteriorly in TLK, creating a forward hyperpressure on disks in the TLK area.

In cases of greater lordosis, as in type 4, the resultant forces are displaced posteriorly over the posterior facet joints. This sagittal orientation contributes to bone remodeling in the facet arthrosis, lumbar narrow canal, and olisthesis (degenerative spondylolisthesis) in the distal end of the curve where the disks are more tilted. It becomes clear that the sagittal spinopelvic structure defines which specific alterations will occur through aging and natural degenerative processes. Each of the four spinopelvic morphotypes have a trend to produce specific outcomes in CT scans and MRIs[7,8] (▶ Fig. 10.3)

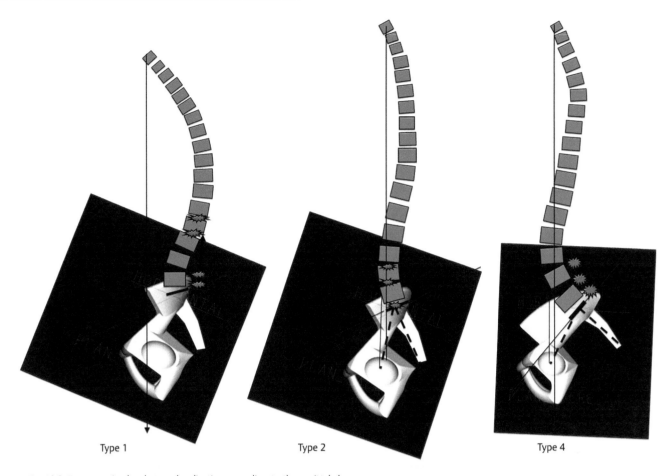

Type 1   Type 2   Type 4

Fig. 10.3 Degenerative local stress localization according to the sagittal shape.

10.6 Effect of Sagittal Balance Alignment on Local Intervertebral Degeneration

According to the sagittal balance classification in asymptomatic individuals, we postulate that there are different patterns of degenerative evolution depending on each type.

10.6.1 Type 1 Lordosis

These individuals present a small SS (< 35) and a small PI (< 45). The DSL is composed of very few vertebrae, and the top of the maximal lordosis is markedly displaced posteriorly. This short distal hyperlordosis combines with a thoracolumbar kyphosis (TLK). There is a succession of two strongly curved segments that induces forward hyperpressure on the disks in thoracolumbar area and a backward hyperextension in the lumbar area that produces greater stresses on the posterior facet joints. With aging, the thoracolumbar kyphotic zone suffers disk overloading and there is often disk degeneration in this area associated with retrolisthesis in the junctional zone (L2-L3), indicating an attempt to recover lordosis and balance. The spine constantly seeks for a better global balance. The small distal lordosis, under hyperextension, usually spares disks L4-L5 and L5-S1, but there is interspinous processes conflict and facet

arthrosis. The distal hyperextension could explain radicular pain while standing, as neuroforamens are decreased. This hyperextension might cause L5 isthmic lyses through the nutcracker phenomenon. The possibilities of pelvic retroversion as a compensatory mechanism for sagittal imbalance are minimal as the PI is small. The global final architecture of type 1 remains type 1 with curvature acutization. A type 1 cannot turn into another type by natural degenerative evolution (▶ Fig. 10.4).

10.6.2 Type 2 Lordosis

Type 2 lordosis is described as a spine with a small SS (< 35°) and a usually small PI (< 45°). The DSL is not high and the change of orientation of the curve from lordosis to kyphosis is smooth. This is a quite vertical structure. As the disks in the lumbar spine have minimal tilting near to the horizontal line, the disks suffer the main loads in the lumbar spine. Individuals with type 2 lordosis are supposed to undergo early lumbar disk degeneration during their lifetime, as well as precocious central disk herniation. Several authors have shown that a smooth straight lordosis is associated with disk herniation, low LL, and SL.[12,13]

Barrey,[14] in his doctoral thesis, showed that disk herniations that occur in patients under 45 years old tend to be present in type 2 lordosis. Inversely, patients older than 45 years old with lumbar disk herniation present all four types of spinopelvic structure. In a recent study (unpublished data), authors found a prevalence of

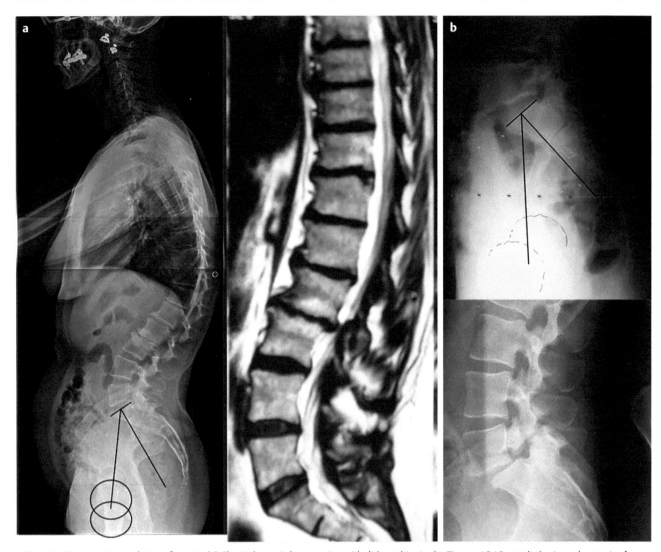

Fig. 10.4 Degenerative evolution of type 1. **(a)** Classical type 1 degeneration with diskopathies in the TL area, L2-L3 retrolisthesis, and posterior facet joints arthritis L4, L5, S1. **(b)** L5 isthmic lysis by the nutcracker mechanism as a result of distal hyperextension stress.

type 2 lordosis in patients with de novo lumbar degenerative scoliosis. In the final degenerative evolution, a type 2 spine generally loses few LL with few increasing PT, thus remaining type 2. As PI is small, retroversion possibilities are poor (▶ Fig. 10.5).

10.6.3 Type 3 Lordosis

Type 3 is well-balanced spine, theoretically less prone to a specific pattern of spinal degeneration. There may exist diskopathies, facet arthritis, or both, with, at the beginning, a slight increase of PT to compensate for a small decrease of lordosis remaining a type 3 because SS does not reach less than 35°.

10.6.4 Type 4 Lordosis

Type 4 is a large and long lordosis. The forces act especially on the posterior elements of the lumbar spine. The sacral inclination is great; there is a morphological predisposition to facet arthritis. In younger individuals, the disks are protected from early degeneration as the loading is more posterior. Because of higher SS, there is a predisposition of type 4 for L5-S1

spondylolisthesis by increasing shearing forces (approximately 80% of L5 isthmic lyses present PI greater than 60°). Highly curved type 4 may develop early facets degeneration because of the constant facet hyperpressure. These patients initially present a painful lower back without any signs of degeneration. Facet joints degeneration occurs progressively: foramen stenosis, articular cyst, and facet loosening mainly in L4-L5 with degenerative spondylolisthesis. Until this occurs, LL remains or is poorly altered maintaining the type 4 or turning into a type 3 with a slight retroversion (▶ Fig. 10.6).

10.7 Morphology of Posterior Elements

Roussouly postulated that the sagittal alignment would be correlated to the morphology of posterior elements (i.e., facet joints and interspinous processes). The mathematical representation of lordosis, according to the arc of a circle model, defines two arcs of a circle. Both have telltale signatures in their radii. In type 4 lordosis, the arcs have smaller radii, which means there is less

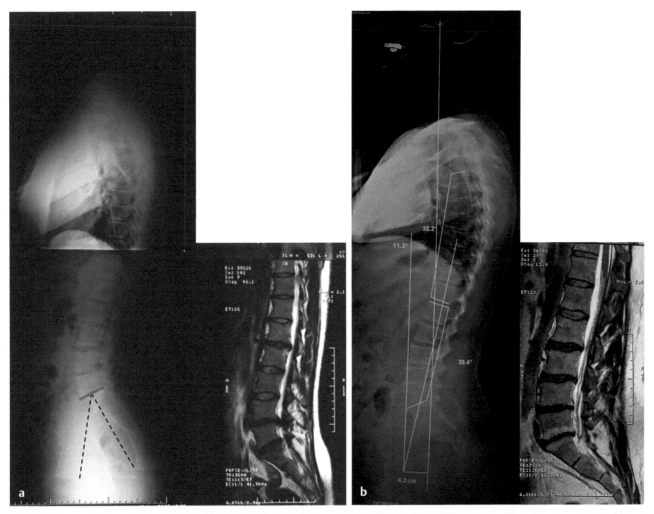

Fig. 10.5 Degenerative evolution of type 2. **(a)** Central disk herniation in a 30-year-old man. **(b)** Multilevel lumbar diskopathies in a 45-year-old woman.

space for posterior elements of vertebrae (i.e., facet joints and interspinous processes). Facets are supposed to be smaller explaining for their "weakness" and possible loosening that induces degenerative spondylolisthesis. However, interspinous process conflict could be an associated process. In type 2 lordosis, there are two arcs of a circle with higher radii, with probable more space for posterior vertebral elements. Roussouly hypothesizes that zygapophyseal joints are probably larger in type 2 than in type 4 lordosis. In addition, with a small size in certain women, this may explain the frailty of posterior facets and the production of degenerative spondylolisthesis. Anatomical or radiological studies on the size of spinal elements for each type of lordosis should be performed to confirm this (▶ Fig. 10.7).

10.8 How Degeneration Induced by Specific Sagittal Balance Patterns May Produce Neurological Compression

Neurological damage by canal stenosis (central or foraminal) is the main feature of spinal degeneration. Although the main

concepts of the sagittal balance effects have just recently been recognized, the neurological troubles associated with spinal degeneration are well known for a much longer time. The main aim of neurosurgical treatment for the degenerative spine is nerve decompression. The association between lumbar canal stenosis and sagittal balance has been studied recently but no real correlations were found between PI values and neurologic compression. Barrey showed that in subjects with degenerative L4-L5 spondylolisthesis, the PI was higher than in a referent asymptomatic population. Likewise, this author affirmed that early disk herniation is predominant in low PI individuals. Thus, there are different ways on how the local spinal degeneration induced by the spinal shape may induce stenosis:

• Type 1: In the thoracolumbar area, the increasing kyphosis has a poor effect on the central canal diameter. The only risk to the nervous system is the common L2L3 retrolisthesis as a result of the severe slope of L3. In the lumbar area, the increasing short distal hyperlordosis may induce a distal foraminal stenosis. The foraminal closure increases in standing position when the lordosis compensation is maximal. This may explain the occurrence of radicular pain only in the standing position and the lack stenosis on the MRI because of the lying position during this exam.

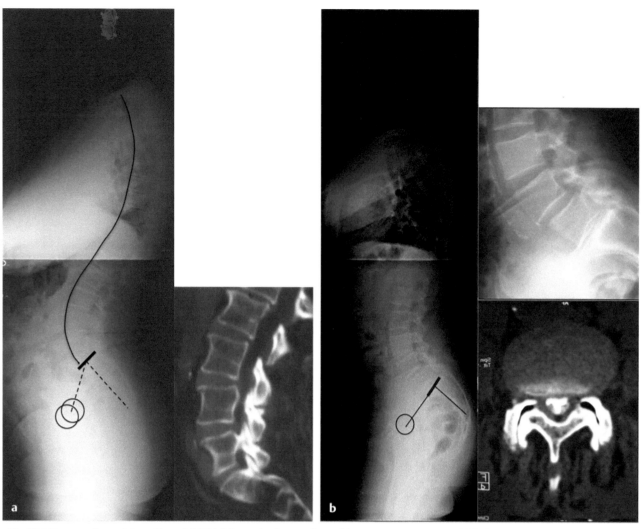

Fig. 10.6 Degenerative evolution of type 4. **(a)** Painful posterior facets arthritis. **(b)** Degenerative L4-L5 spondylolisthesis by posterior facets loosening.

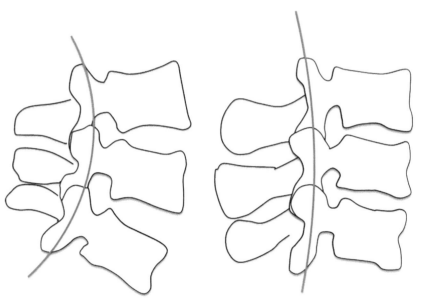

Fig. 10.7 On the left, the posterior intervertebral distance is shorter as a result of a smaller radius in a very curved lordosis like in type 4. Articular facet joints and spinous processes are smaller. On the right, in a flatter lordosis, the radius is longer with longer intervertebral posterior distance. Facet joints and spinous processes are bigger, preventing increasing extension.

- Type 2: The hyperpressure on the disks explains the predominance of diskopathies with early disk herniation and the possibility of central stenosis by central disk protrusion. A combination of multilevel diskopathies with marked facets arthritis may lead to central stenosis. The natural large size of facet joints may reduce the canal diameter.
- Type 4: Hyperlordosis conducts to facet joints hyperpressure and initially to foraminal stenosis as in type 1. Later, facet joints arthritis may produce compressive cysts until facet joint alteration and loosening, inducing degenerative spondylolisthesis with corresponding stenosis.

10.9 Distribution of Morphotypes in the Population

Barrey studied the distribution of spinopelvic morphotypes in a series of 160 subjects without symptoms and obtained the following distribution: 21.2%, 11.2%, 37.5%, and 30.0% in lordosis types 1, 2, 3, and 4, respectively. Morphotypes 1 and 2 corresponded to less than 35% of the asymptomatic population.[14] Types 3 and 4 were present in more than 65% of asymptomatic subjects. However, these morphotypes were responsible for more than 85% of degenerative olisthesis and were also found in the disk herniations subgroups. In types 1 and 2, spondylolisthesis occurred in a very limited number of cases. These results demonstrate that every spinopelvic morphotype can produce distinct degenerative events, but there is a clear tendancy for straighter lordosis types to cause early disk problems and for higher lordosis types to result in more facet joint processes, as well as olisthesis and lumbar narrow canal. These findings remain to be replicated.

10.10 How Degeneration May Affect the Spinal Structure

Degeneration occurs in a functional segmental unit of the spine or in multiple units. In the spine, degeneration may affect the anteriorly placed intervertebral disks or the posteriorly placed facet joints. Degeneration is a progressive process related to aging and is influenced by local mechanical stresses as a result of different anatomical architectures. In the end, degeneration may destroy the articulations and induce dislocation and instability as a local effect and change the global spinal architecture, generally by increasing segmental flexion through segmental kyphosis.

In Chapter 11, it was shown how compensatory mechanisms of the spine build up with increasing kyphosis: extension of the flexible spine above and below the kyphotic segment. In the thoracic area, the kyphosis may be
- Normal, poorly affected.
- Decreased by compensation mechanism.
- Increased either because of structural shape or by local degeneration and muscle weakness (mainly in the elderly).

Kyphosis may affect also thoracolumbar or lumbar area. Elsewhere in this book, it has been also demonstrated that pelvic retroversion is the main compensatory mechanism

favored by high PI. It is primarily the most important compensatory mechanism for those subjects who lose lordosis. Inversely, for individuals with low PI, this mechanism of pelvic retroversion is poor and limited.

With aging, the sagittal balance of normal asymptomatic individuals may change. The identification in the elderly population of the original spinopelvic morphotype is of paramount importance. Thus, regarding these degenerative evolutions (of the spinopelvic morphotypes), the authors propose a classification of the different pathological shapes initiating from normal shapes based on a combination of structural deformities and compensation:
- No-change shape: Types 1, 2, 3, and 4 may remain a type 1, 2, 3, and 4, respectively. Sagittal balance is poorly or nonaffected with aging.
- Sagittal balance is affected (there is forward displacement of C7 plumb line or increasing sagittal vertical axis [SVA]):
  - Nonpelvic retroversion or poor pelvic retroversion as a result of a small PI that forbids this mechanism (sagittal unbalance because of increasing thoracic or TLK).
  - Retroverted shapes: degeneration creates a loss of lordosis and/or an increasing kyphosis inducing compensation by pelvic retroversion (PT > 25°). This situation is a characteristic of higher PI individuals (PI > 55°) (compensation by decreasing TK, no compensation: normal TK, degenerative TLK).
- Global kyphotic shapes: the corresponding lumbar spine is in hypolordosis or in kyphosis where the spine is generally globally in kyphosis with a severe global imbalance. C7 plumb line is widely forward the femoral heads, and SVA is very high. Retroverted pelvic compensation overpasses but still depends on the PI value. In some cases, the thoracic spine widely compensates by using lordosis shape to maintain the global balance over the pelvis.

In summary:
- Type 1 stays in type 1 or turns into global kyphosis without retroversion.
- Type 2 may
  - Stay in type 2.
  - Turn into type 2 + TK.
  - Turn into type 1.
  - Turn into lumbar kyphosis with compensated thoracic lordosis.
  - Turn into global kyphosis without retroversion.
- Types 3 and 4 may
  - Stay in types 3 or 4 slightly retroverted.
  - Turn into retroverted false type 1.
  - Turn into retroverted false type 2 + TK.
  - Turn into retoverted false type 2 (compensated hypokyphosis).
  - Turn into global kyphosis with retroverted pelvis.

10.10.1 How to Identify Spinopelvic Morphotypes during Aging

With aging, in older patients, diskopathies and a decrease in disk height may lead to a loss of lordosis and to changes in the global architecture with sagittal compensation through pelvic retroversion. Furthermore, kyphosis may occur. The analysis of spinopelvic types can be deceptive in older patients. Pelvic retroversion and segmental kyphosis must be analyzed, particularly in these older patients. Herein, the retroverted and the kyphotic shapes related to aging and spine degeneration are presented:

10.10.2 Retroverted Shapes

Retroverted shapes are possible evolutions of morphotypes 3 and 4. Loss of lordosis with aging may be compensated for by pelvic retroversion to obtain a better sagittal balance. Higher abilities of pelvic retroversion are the privilege of individuals with higher PI values (types 3 and 4). The retroverted shapes usually occur in patients with high PI, essentially types 3 and 4 spinopelvic morphologies. The loss of lordosis decreases SS, which may reach values inferior to 35°. Together, low lordosis and low SS may produce an aspect of a type 2 spinopelvic morphotype, but the astute clinician will notice that the pelvis is retroverted and the PI is high. Therefore, regarding the compensatory mechanisms in the thoracic area, there is the possibility of two evolutive situations from types 3 and 4 to retroverted shapes:
- Retroverted type 2 with TK.
- Retroverted type 2 with thoracic compensation and hypokyphosis.

In some cases, degenerative kyphosis occurs at a thoracic-lumbar level, giving a type 1 shape with a retroverted pelvis. It is important to note that the loss of lordosis is mainly dependent on the distal diskopathies L4-L5, L5-S1, affecting mainly the inferior arc of lordosis. Restoration of physiological lordosis by surgery should correct this lower arc in curvature and angle.

10.10.3 Kyphotic Shapes

An uncommon extreme degenerative evolution may present, through disk degeneration, the transformation of an LL into a kyphosis. This situation may occur, whatever the PI value.

In low PI (<50°) spines, depending on the thoracic compensation, some other situations may exist:
- Lumbar kyphosis with compensation in thoracic lordosis.
- Lumbar kyphosis without compensation producing a global kyphosis with a poorly retroverted pelvis.
- A specific case possible is the association of type 2 with a pronounced TK.

With high PI (PI > 50°), it is possible to find
- The disappearance of LL that creates a global kyphosis with a retroverted pelvis.

In summary, each initial spinopelvic morphotype has its own pattern of sagittal shape transformation under degenerative evolution:
- Type 1 cannot change into another shape; it remains type 1 with increasing curvatures. A loss of lordosis could induce a global kyphosis (▶ Fig. 10.8).
- Type 2 generally remains as a type 2. Regarding the level in the spine where kyphosis occurs, type 2 may turn into (▶ Fig. 10.9, ▶ Fig. 10.10)
  ○ Type 2 with TK.
  ○ Type 1 in the case of thoracolumbar localization.
  ○ Lumbar kyphosis with thoracic compensation in lordosis.
  ○ Global kyphosis with poor pelvic retroversion.
- Types 3 and 4 may stay as types 3 and 4, maybe displaying a slight retroversion. In the case of kyphotic evolution, as there is a higher probability for pelvic retroversion as a result of the higher PI, such cases may change into (▶ Fig. 10.11, ▶ Fig. 10.12)

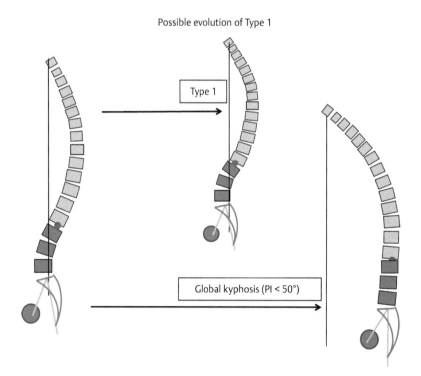

Possible evolution of Type 1

Type 1

Global kyphosis (PI < 50°)

Fig. 10.8 Illustration depicts possible outcomes of a type 1 spinopelvic morphotype. On the right, note that global kyphosis and PI are less than 50.

Possible evolution of Type 2

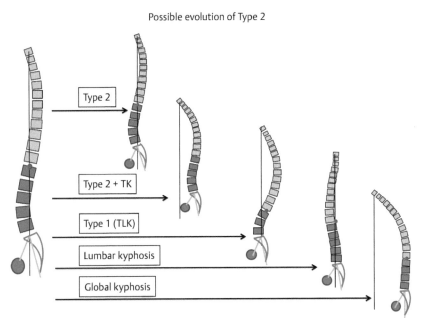

Fig. 10.9 Illustration depicting possible outcomes of a type 2 spinopelvic morphotype. Note that degeneration in a type 2 may mimic a type 1, with pelvic retroversion and even lower sacral slope.

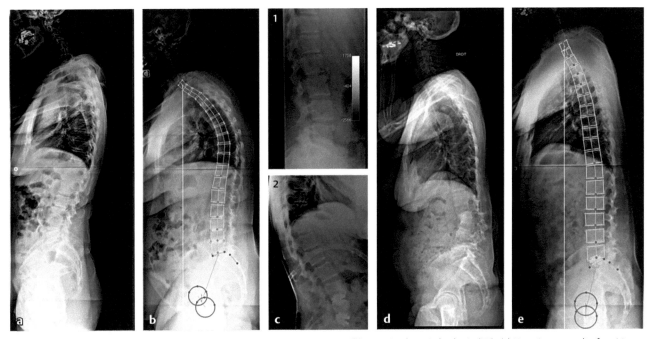

Fig. 10.10 Radiological examples of type 2 evolution. **(a)** Type 2 stays type 2. **(b)** Type 2 + thoracic kyphosis (TK). **(c)** Type 1 as a result of an L1 fracture. **(d)** Lumbar kyphosis with thoracic lordosis. **(e)** Global kyphosis without retroverted pelvis.

○ False retroverted type 1.
○ False retroverted type 2 with TK.
○ False retroverted type 2 with a flat thoracic spine.
○ Global kyphosis with a retroverted pelvis.

Ferrero et al[15] identified a subgroup of patients with low PT that presented global anterior sagittal misalignment. The authors have suggested that this may be because of insufficient pelvic compensation in this cohort. This situation seems to correspond with an anteverted type 3. Because of the limited number of such cases, this anteverted type 3 has not been well

identified. The evolution of anteverted type 3 cannot be commented on with certainty, but anteverted type 4 with back pain and irreducible lordosis may suggest a similar evolution of such cases (▶ Fig. 10.13).

10.11 Conclusion

LL is not the same for every individual. The arc of a circle mathematical model by Berthonnaud et al provides a quintessential perspective for understanding the geometry of the lumbar spine.

Possible evolution of Type 3, 4

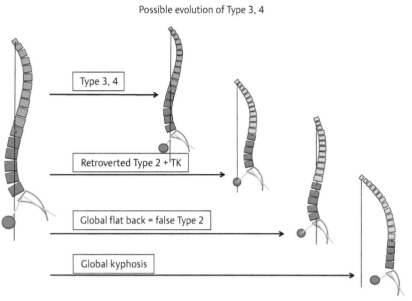

Fig. 10.11 Illustration depicts possible outcomes of types 3 and 4 spines.

Type 3, 4

Retroverted Type 2 + TK

Global flat back = false Type 2

Global kyphosis

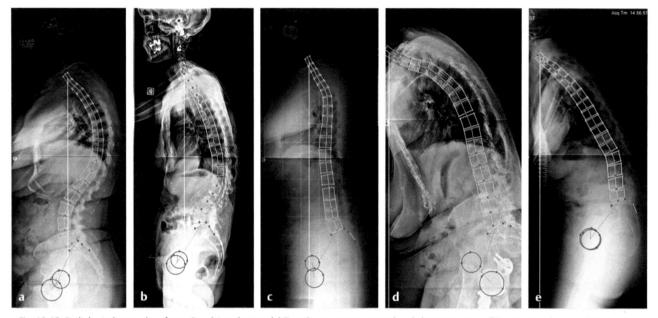

Fig. 10.12 Radiological examples of type 3 and 4 evolutions. **(a)** Type 3 or 4 sometimes with a slight retroversion. **(b)** Retroverted type 1. **(c)** False type 2 with double compensation (retroverted pelvis and thoracic hypokyphosis). **(d)** False type 2 + thoracic kyphosis (severe global unbalance because of insufficient compensation by pelvic retroversion). **(e)** Global kyphosis with retroverted pelvis.

Until recently, the concept of spinopelvic morphotypes was not recognized. The sum of gravitational forces and counteracting muscular action, combined with the spinopelvic morphotype have demonstrated that, with aging, there is a tendency to certain patterns of spinal degeneration to occur according to specific morphotypes. DSL is a new term that defines the distal curve of human spine in extension. More studies are requested to illuminate this rich area of research. Treatment options should consider the spinopelvic morphotype analysis as they should aim to restore sagittal balance according to the PI.

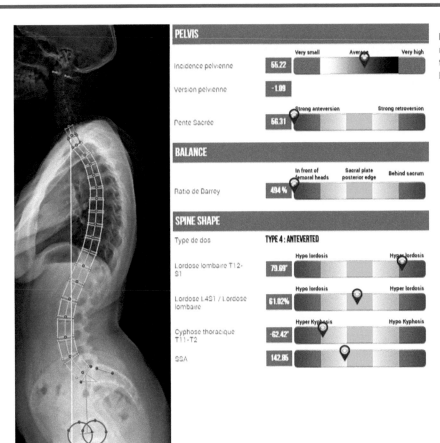

Fig. 10.13 Anteverted type 4 induced by abnormal lumbar hyperlordosis giving an inadequate type 4 lordosis with a pelvic incidence of 50°. Possible evolution of a previous type 3?

References

[1] Stagnara P, De Mauroy JC, Dran G, et al. Reciprocal angulation of vertebral bodies in a sagittal plane: approach to references for the evaluation of kyphosis and lordosis. Spine. 1982; 7(4):335–342

[2] Berthonnaud E, Dimnet J, Roussouly P, Labelle H. Analysis of the sagittal balance of the spine and pelvis using shape and orientation parameters. J Spinal Disord Tech. 2005; 18(1):40–47

[3] Roussouly P, Berthonnaud E, Dimnet J. Geometrical and mechanical analysis of lumbar lordosis in an asymptomatic population: proposed classification (in French). Rev Chir Orthop Reparatrice Appar Mot. 2003; 89(7):632–639

[4] Legaye J, Duval-Beaupère G, Hecquet J, Marty C. Pelvic incidence: a fundamental pelvic parameter for three-dimensional regulation of spinal sagittal curves. Eur Spine J. 1998; 7(2):99–103

[5] During J, Goudfrooij H, Keessen W, Beeker TW, Crowe A. Toward standards for posture. Postural characteristics of the lower back system in normal and pathologic conditions. Spine. 1985; 10(1):83–87

[6] Vialle R, Levassor N, Rillardon L, Templier A, Skalli W, Guigui P. Radiographic analysis of the sagittal alignment and balance of the spine in asymptomatic subjects. J Bone Joint Surg Am. 2005; 87(2):260–267

[7] Roussouly P, Pinheiro-Franco JL. Biomechanical analysis of the spino-pelvic organization and adaptation in pathology. Eur Spine J. 2011; 20 Suppl 5:609–618

[8] Roussouly P, Pinheiro-Franco JL. Sagittal parameters of the spine: biomechanical approach. Eur Spine J. 2011; 20 Suppl 5:578–585

[9] Roussouly P, Gollogly S, Berthonnaud E, Dimnet J. Classification of the normal variation in the sagittal alignment of the human lumbar spine and pelvis in the standing position. Spine. 2005; 30(3):346–353

[10] Laouissat F, Sebaaly A, Gehrchen M, Roussouly P. Classification of normal sagittal spine alignment: refounding the Roussouly classification. Eur Spine J. 2018; 27(8):2002–2011

[11] Jackson RP, McManus AC. Radiographic analysis of sagittal plane alignment and balance in standing volunteers and patients with low back pain matched for age, sex, and size. A prospective controlled clinical study. Spine. 1994; 19 (14):1611–1618

[12] Barrey C, Jund J, Noseda O, Roussouly P. Sagittal balance of the pelvis-spine complex and lumbar degenerative diseases. A comparative study about 85 cases. Eur Spine J. 2007; 16(9):1459–1467

[13] Rajnics P, Templier A, Skalli W, Lavaste F, Illes T. The importance of spinopelvic parameters in patients with lumbar disc lesions. Int Orthop. 2002; 26 (2):104–108

[14] Barrey C. Equilibre Sagittal Pelvi-Rachidien et Pathologies Lombaires Degeneratives [these doctorat], Université Claude-Bernard, Lyon, France; 2004

[15] Ferrero E, Vira S, Ames CP, et al. International Spine Study Group. Analysis of an unexplored group of sagittal deformity patients: low pelvic tilt despite positive sagittal malalignment. Eur Spine J. 2016; 25(11):3568–3576

11 Sagittal Imbalance Compensatory Mechanisms

Martin Gehrchen

Abstract

The compensatory mechanisms are described for both flexible and stiff spines and in relation to Roussouly types with examples, including illustrative figures. Examples of decision making where the surgeon can easily make the wrong decision are included in this chapter.

Keywords: balance, compensation, compensatory, imbalance incompensation

11.1 Introduction

This chapter will focus mainly on the compensatory mechanisms of keeping an upright position and a horizontal gaze when balance is affected. This natural adaptation to any kyphosing event is the body's effort at self-preservation. So, whatever the pathologies involved in the kyphosing event, the body composition's self-preservation, to keep upright gait and horizontal gaze, is the driver in these compensatory mechanisms.[1,2,3,4] A description of this is partly found in Chapter 9, but a more systematic description will be given in this chapter (with examples) of the causal pathology.

The kyphosing event can occur in any part of the spine, but this chapter focuses on the thoracolumbar (TL) spine. In general, kyphosing events may occur over many segments as in multilevel degenerative processes or, for example, in Scheuermann's disease or, more acutely, osteoporosis, fractures, or short segmental degeneration.[5,6,7,8] In addition, there is a significant number of iatrogenic causes for kyphosing events such as postlaminectomy syndrome (flat back) or a lumbar spine fusion in relative kyphosis.[9,10] Less known, hyperlordosis may bring specific compensations to counteract paradox imbalance. We shall not treat specific situations of hyperlordosis in neuromuscular diseases here. Natural hyperlordosis may accompany a pelvis with very high pelvic incidence (PI). A less recognized but worse situation is iatrogenic hyperlordosis caused by surgical overcorrection of lumbar lordosis.

11.2 Compensatory Mechanism of a Kyphosing Event

11.2.1 Pelvic Retroversion

The first well-known and described compensatory mechanism for a sagittal imbalance is pelvic retroversion.[11] First described in severe kyphosis of ankylosing spondylitis (AS), pelvic posterior rotation around the femoral head axis was constant with a decreasing sacral slope (SS) frequently calculated as close to 0° (close to horizontal). Later, using the Duval-Beaupère parameters—PI, pelvic tilt (PT), and SS—a relation was established between PT and SS.[12] At that time, the reciprocal positioning of the hips and knees was not clear, and the hip position was frequently considered in flexion but, in reality, they were in extension. The last frequent feature of severe kyphosis in AS was the knee position in flexion.

What Is the Mechanical Effect of the Pelvic Retroversion?

The posterior pelvis rotation around the femoral heads induces a physical effect and a shape transformation.

- Physical effect: A kyphosing event wherever the place in the spine displaces forward the gravity of the body above. To counteract this gravity force displacement, the pelvis acts like a reverse pendulum around the femoral heads and moves the body back to ensure the gravity line position is inside the feet area.
- Shape transformation: We have seen previously that the lumbar lordosis is closely linked with SS and that a small lordosis accompanies a small SS. This is the same in pathology in the case of decreasing lordosis, by degeneration, for example, SS decreases. If SS decreases, PT increases. There is a coupling mechanism between pelvic retroversion, decreasing SS, and decreasing lordosis.

How the Pelvic Shape Influences the Mechanism of Retroversion

To know the different pathways of compensation, it is necessary to fully understand the limitations and implications of the PI and the implications of the magnitude of the PI.[13] A patient with a high PI may have more pelvic retroversion for compensation than a patient with low PI. This is geometrically explained by the angular relation: $PI = PT + SS$, where PT indicates the magnitude of rotation of the pelvis around the femoral heads and the SS, the slope of the sacral plateau.[14] If we consider that, in the standing position, the lower virtual value of SS that the system can reach is zero in low PI, there is a lesser ability of pelvic retroversion than with a high PI. In other words, to reach a high PT (strong retroversion), a patient must have a high PI. For the same quantity of kyphosis, in AS, the global balance (C7 plumb line) appears in a better position in a higher PI where the compensatory mechanism of retroversion is stronger than in a patient with a lower PI (▶ Fig. 11.1). A high level of retroversion is always a specificity of a pelvis with high PI. Following Roussouly's classification, a highly retroverted pelvis (PT > 25°) characterizes the degenerative evolution of types 3 and 4. Types 1 and 2 have a poor ability for retroversion.

What Are the Limitations of Pelvic Retroversion Mechanism?

We have seen that the maximal compensation of SS would be 0°, which means a horizontal position of the sacral plateau. Virtually, for a PI of 60°, PT could reach 60°. This mechanism is limited by the ability of the hip extension (HE),[15] maintaining the femoral shafts strictly vertical, then 60° probably overpasses this possibility. When the maximum HE is reached, the mechanism of pelvis retroversion must use a new and lower axis of rotation. This is why knee flexion occurs inducing a tilt of the femoral shaft. Mangione and Sénégas described an angle between the femoral shaft and vertical axis called the pelvic femoral angle (PFA).[16] We write the relation: PT = HE + PFA (▶ Fig. 11.2). As PT considers both HE and PFA, PFA does not have to be taken into account in surgical strategy. PT correction is sufficient to correct both knee flexion and HE. For example, a patient with a severe kyphosis has a PT = 35°, the HE limit is 20°, and the patient needs to tilt the femoral shaft to 15° to reach a PT value of 35°. If simulating the correction, the surgeon tries to obtain PT = 15°; in this situation, hips turn in their normal range of rotation (< 20°). Knees are no longer in flexion; the femoral shaft may be vertical without a tilt.

What Are the Main Clinical Issues of High Pelvic Retroversion?

Muscle action is important for maintaining pelvis retroversion, mainly gluteus and posterior thigh muscle action. This may be misinterpreted as sciatica. However, the most important effect is the alteration of walking.[17] During gait, when one leg is in the posterior position, the HE must be free to maintain a balanced pelvis. If the hips are locked in extension, the forward femoral

tilt induces an anteverted pelvis positioning and a global forward tilt of the spine above. If the retroverted pelvis mechanism seems efficient to correct the sagittal body balance in the standing position, during walking, this mechanism loses its positive effect and strongly impairs the balance (▶ Fig. 11.3).

Different classifications of sagittal balance were based on the retroversion level. Hresko classified the balance of high-grade spondylolisthesis by the level of retroversion; the most retroverted was considered the most unbalanced. The more PT increases, the more sacral plateau positioning moves backward. This may explain the close relation between PT and C7PL forward displacement translated by increasing SVA or Barrey ratio (BR). Based on this, Barrey proposed a sagittal spinal balance classification in degeneration divided into three categories (▶ Fig. 11.4)[17,18,19]:

- Type A or normal spinal balance: Characterized by global balance of the trunk measured BR < 100% (C7PL behind femoral heads and posterior edge of the sacral plateau) and 10° < PT < 25°; lower limbs are completely extended in the standing position.

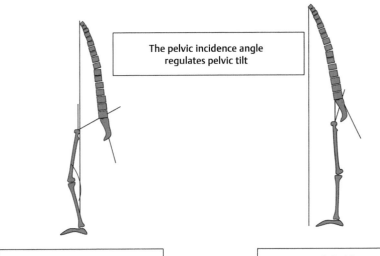

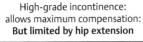

Fig. 11.1 Pelvic tilt compensation according to pelvic incidence (PI). On the left, with high PI, there is a better ability of pelvis retroversion but with the possibility of reaching the limits of hip extension. On the right, note low PI, with less possibility of pelvis retroversion and less compensation of global imbalance, but no effect on hip limitation.

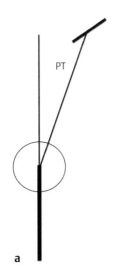

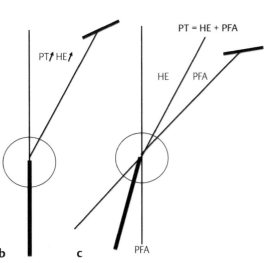

Fig. 11.2 (a) In normal standing position, pelvis rotation is in a neutral position. Femurs are vertical. (b) When pelvic tilt (PT) increases, hip extension (HE) increases until its own limit. Femurs stay in a vertical position. (c) When hip extension is overpassed, femurs must tilt by knee flexion to increase PT over HE limits. PFA, Pelvic femoral angle.

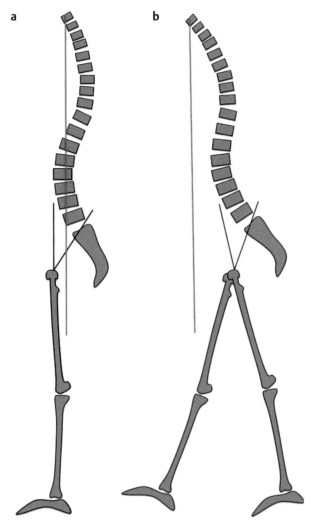

Fig. 11.3 (a) When the pelvis is retroverted in a standing position, the patient seems balanced. (b) When walking, the pelvis tilts forward driving by the femoral forward tilt during gait, impairing balance.

- Type B or compensated balance: Global balance of the trunk is still normal BR (< 100%) but the pelvis is retroverted (PT > 25°). The lower limbs show extension of the hips (femur straight) and the knees are in full extension. This means that the HE can reach up to 25°.
- Type C or uncompensated balance: Global balance of the trunk shows a positive C7 value that generally falls in front of the femoral heads, and the pelvis shows a PT in retroversion. In the lower limbs, extension of the hips (pelvic retroversion) and flexion of the knees are evident. HE is overpassed.

This classification is dependent on the hips' range of motion. If the hips are poorly mobile (inflammation, arthritis), the knees' flexion compensation may occur with a lower value of PT.

11.2.2 Spinal Extension Compensation

Barrey's classification emphasizes only the pelvic retroversion as a compensatory mechanism. A second method of compensation is the active extension of the spine above and below a kyphosing event.[5] This mechanism exists only when the spine is flexible and when muscles are strong enough to erect it. This mechanism may be painful either by muscle overactivity and/or by posterior facets constraints. This mechanism may be located at any level of the spine.

- In lordotic areas, cervical or lumbar spine, the compensation appears as an increasing extension and angle of lordosis. This effect is limited by the intervertebral extension ability. The local stressed spine may be fully extended, very curved, in hyperlordosis in a very flexible cervical or lumbar spine. This is the case of spinal shape with a high ability of extension such as type 1 or type 4 in Roussouly's classification. In the case of a rigid or poorly extended spine—either because of the structure such as in the flat type 2 or a degenerative spine (▶ Fig. 11.5)—when local extension is overpassed, an abnormal local hyperextension may occur with a listhesis effect at its maximum.[5] This mechanism may explain the origin of L5 lysis nutcracker mechanism in type 1 lordosis because of the distal lumbar hyperlordosis.
- In thoracic kyphotic areas, the expression of active extension of the spine is a decreasing kyphosis and sometimes, at its maximum, an inversion of the curve orientation with lordosis in place of kyphosis. The hypokyphotic thoracic compensation may not be identified clearly. In degenerative pathology, this compensation is a specificity of types 3 and 4. Initially, a curved or hypercurved lordosis as a result of a high PI has a curved thoracic kyphosis (TK) in correspondence. The degenerative loss of lordosis may induce both mechanisms, decreasing SS and increasing PT, on the one hand and, on the other hand, decreasing TK. This global flattening of the spine with a low SS gives a type 2 aspect but with a retroverted pelvis and a high PI. It is a trap in surgical sagittal balance restoration. When restoring an adequate lumbar lordosis by surgical correction, there is a risk of losing the thoracic hypokyphosis compensation and of turning a flat thoracic spine into kyphosis. In the case of fusion until T10, the kyphosis evolution of the spine above because of the loss of compensation is constant and explains a kind of proximal junctional kyphosis (PJK). In the case of extended instrumentation to the proximal thoracic spine maintaining the hypokyphosis, there is a risk of spine flexion below the top of instrumentation with loosening, or above with PJK development. Even if the fusion and instrumentation are stable, an inadequate reduction of the compensatory thoracic spine is always uncomfortable for the patient and may lead to complaints the physician may be unable to explain (▶ Fig. 11.6).

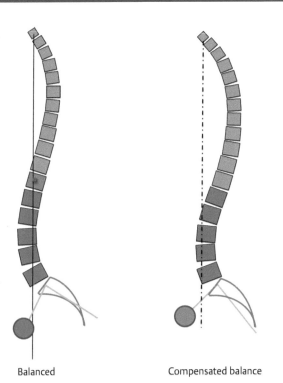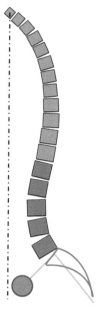

Fig. 11.4 Barrey types: balanced, compensated balance, and unbalanced.

Balanced   Compensated balance   Unbalanced

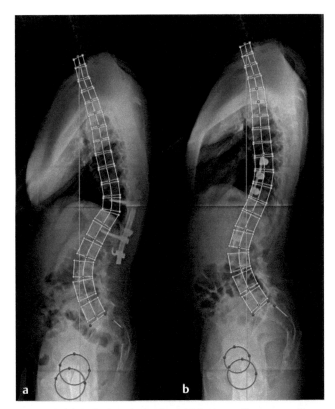

Fig. 11.5 **(a)** Kyphotic malunion in an L1 fracture with compensation above (hypokyphosis) and below (hyperlordosis). **(b)** After surgical reduction, improvement of both compensations.

11.3 Compensatory Mechanisms of Lordosing Event

If the compensatory mechanism for a kyphosing event is well identified, the hyperlordosis effect is less well known. In children, until the end of their growth, a situation with pelvic anteversion (low, even negative PT) and C7PL forward of the femoral heads was first described by Mac-Thiong et al.[20] A lower PI at that time of life could be a partial explanation. Recently, Laouissat added a new type in Roussouly's classification combining a type 3 lordosis with a small PI, characterized by a pelvis anteversion to reach a value of SS in correspondence with a higher lordosis named anteverted type 3.[21] This situation was found in an asymptomatic population, and we have no proof of a particular imbalance or a specific worse evolution of anteverted type 3.

In pathology, a natural situation of hyperlordosis is type 4 with high PI (> 45°). In some cases, hyperlordosis is so severe that PT may reach a value < 10°. This situation is very painful because of facet hyperload. When the patient is able to decrease the lordosis, the pain disappears. If rehabilitation with active pelvis retroversion seams evident, the patient is generally unable to maintain the pelvis in a better, more retroverted position, as if the hyperlordosis was the "primum movens" and forbids pelvis retroversion. In very painful low back pain, we propose a lumbosacral fusion with a small decrease of lordosis allowing better pelvis positioning (▶ Fig. 11.7).

Pathology is very different in iatrogenic situations. The new techniques of reduction combining osteotomies and

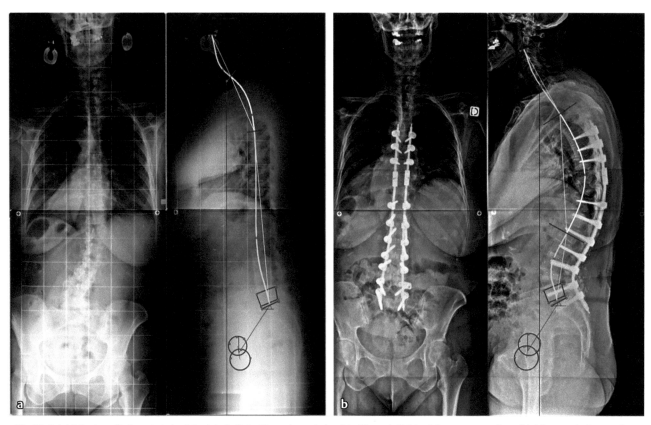

Fig. 11.6 **(a)** False type 2, the whole back is globally flat with a retroverted pelvis. Thoracic flat back is a compensation. **(b)** After surgical correction, lordosis restoration contributes to a kyphosation of the thoracic spine.

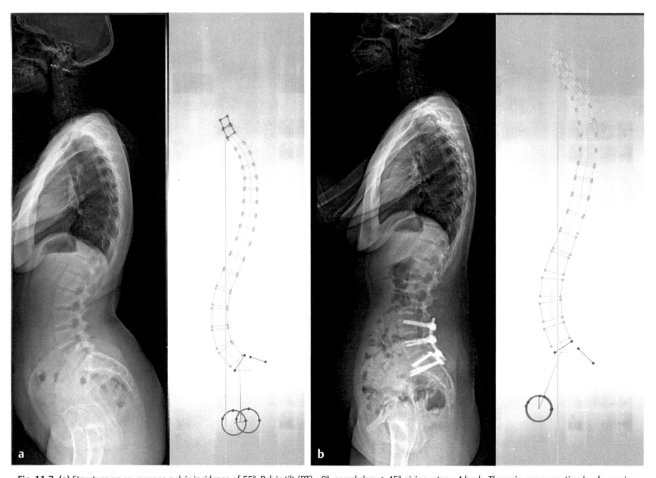

Fig. 11.7 **(a)** Structure on an average pelvic incidence of 55°. Pelvic tilt (PT) = 0°, sacral slope > 45° giving a type 4 back. Thoracic compensation by decreasing kyphosis. **(b)** Arthrodesis with slight reduction of lordosis restoring a positive PT, a better positioning of C7PL, even with an increasing thoracic kyphosis.

instrumentation has contributed to some overcorrection of lordosis, mainly in cases with low PI, transforming types 1 and 2 into anteverted type 3. This new situation is never well balanced if the anterior PT—due to the inadequate lordosis—displaces the center of mass forward and is playing as a forward imbalance inducing thoracic compensation by reducing the kyphosis. This is a paradoxal situation in which an increasing lordosis induces a forward imbalance. The frequent big mistake is to increase the lordosis by various osteotomies. The only option is to reduce the lordosis by "reverse" osteotomies (posterior opening instead of closing). This technique allows a better pelvis position and restores a better thoracic curvature. (▸ Fig. 11.8)

There are different examples of compensatory mechanisms as follows:

- General kyphosation of several adjacent segments like multilevel disk degeneration or Scheuermann's disease:
  ○ Thoracic region: Increased kyphosis in the thoracic spine induces extension (increased lordosis) below the kyphosation (and above in the cervical region). This will increase the lordosis below if the spine is flexible and can lead to severe muscle fatigue and increased load on the facet joints, inducing further discomfort and pain. The same can be seen in the cervical region. The compensatory mechanism is dependent on the magnitude of the PI and, thus, on the quantity of pelvis anteversion that can be reached. When the anteversion compensatory mechanism of the pelvis is consumed and if the kyphosation increases, a retroversion of the pelvis can be seen trying to maintain horizontal gaze. In the cervical spine, hyperlordosis is sometimes seen with a so-called swan neck. ▸ Fig. 11.9 shows the evolution of a Scheuermann patient at 8, 15, and 21 years where the lordosis is still significant. Any degeneration in the lumbar

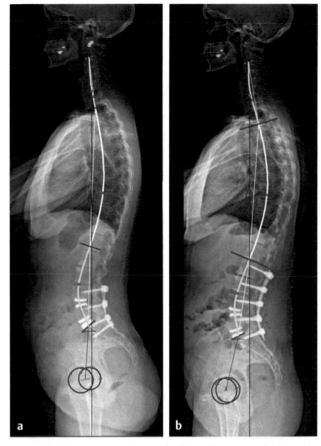

Fig. 11.8 (a) Iatrogenic inadequate lordosis with anteverted pelvis and hypo-thoracic kyphosis (TK) compensation. **(b)** Paradoxical effect of decreasing lordosis restoring a better global balance and relaxing TK.

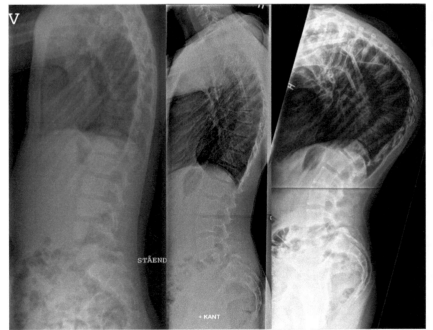

Fig. 11.9 Evolution of spine shape in a single male patient with Scheuermann's disease at age 8, 15, and 21 years.

region from that point will result in retroversion of the pelvis in this specific case. The same will happen in extended degeneration in the thoracic spine, and when the compensation is consumed, spinal lordosis (SL) will disappear producing a global kyphosis.

○ TL region: Again, the increase of kyphosis induces extension (lordosis) below and above the kyphosation area and, thus, extension of TK and SL in the flexible spine. If the spine is rigid, retroversion of the pelvis is seen. This situation can also be seen in the TL Scheuermann or extended degeneration in the TL area (▶ Fig. 11.10).

○ Lumbar region: This is a classic degenerative event, and loss of SL will induce extension of the segments above if the spine is flexible. If the spine is rigid, the only compensatory possibility is the retroversion of the pelvis.

- Local kyphosation of segments such as postfracture or osteoporotic fracture: The process is the same as for general kyphosation, but compensatory mechanisms are more extended as a result of the local process involving only a few segments.

- Iatrogenic kyphosation are most likely the most frequent kyphotic spine mechanism type after the kyphosing degenerative disk process. In this chapter, only lumbar iatrogenic kyphosation will be presented. In principle, there is no difference in whether the kyphosation results from a postlaminectomy (flat back) syndrome or a postfusion situation except that there might be some mobility left in the former. The most common compensation mechanism is extension of the TK (hypokyphosation) as a result of the lumbar kyphosis and later retroversion of the pelvis. If the thoracic spine is rigid, the only possible compensatory mechanism is pelvic retroversion. Often, a fixation of a retroverted pelvis can be seen if the balance has not been addressed at the index operation (▶ Fig. 11.11). Furthermore, the same radiological situation can be present no matter what spine shape was present. In ▶ Fig. 11.12, two cases of fixation of the lumbar spine in relative kyphosis are shown, one being a type 1 spine and the other being type 4. The same radiologic presentation is observed. However, the pelvic parameters are quite different, indicating a different treatment solution (▶ Fig. 11.13a, b). This well illustrates the importance of the parameters and the foundation of the interpretation of the radiographs.

- High-grade L5S1 spondylolisthesis: The position of L5 relative to the sacrum may be approximate to a severe lumbosacral kyphosis. Both compensatory mechanisms express pelvis retroversion and extension of the whole spine and lordosis reaching the whole thoracic spine. After surgical correction of lumbosacral kyphosis, the compensatory mechanisms disappear spontaneously (▶ Fig. 11.14).

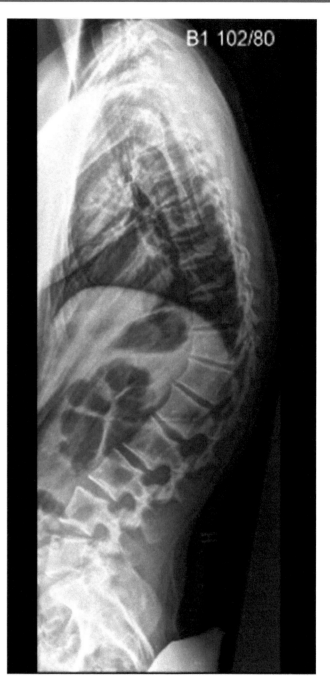

Fig. 11.10 Thoracolumbar Scheuermann demonstrating compensatory mechanisms above and below the thoracolumbar region.

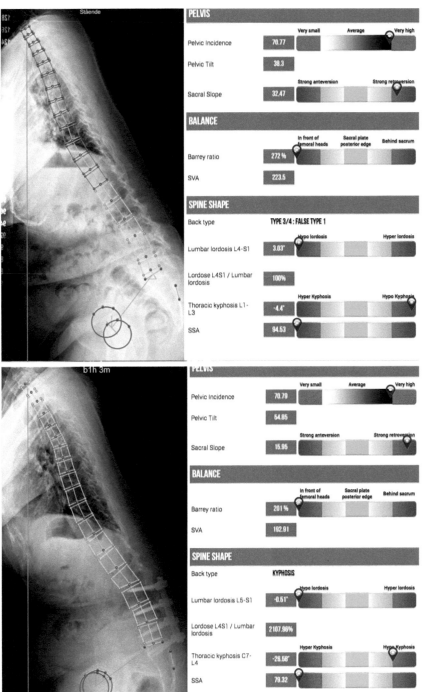

Fig. 11.11 Type 4 spine fixed in relative kyphosis. Preop at the top and 4 months postop at the bottom.

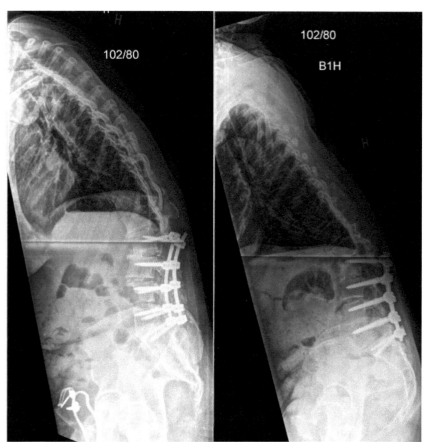

Fig. 11.12 Induced hypokyphosation in a type 1 and a type 4 spine with iatrogenic fixated lumbar kyphosis.

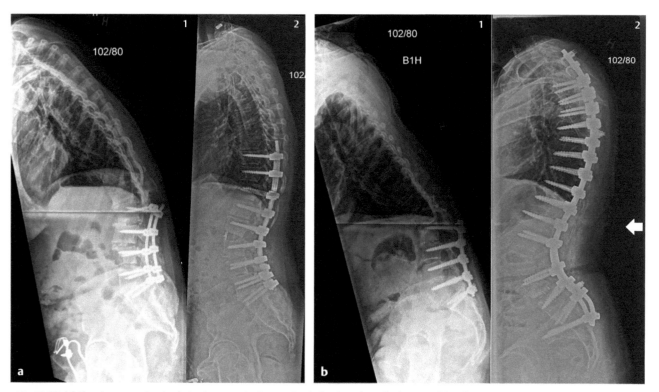

Fig. 11.13 **(a)** Showing correctional solution in a type 1 spine previously fixed in relative kyphosis, and **(1)** after correction using the posterior lumbar interbody fusion (PLIF) technique at the failed mobile segment L2-L3 **(2)**. **(b)** Showing correctional solution in a type 4 spine previously fixed in relative kyphosis **(1)** and after correction with restoration of kyphosis and lordosis **(2)**.

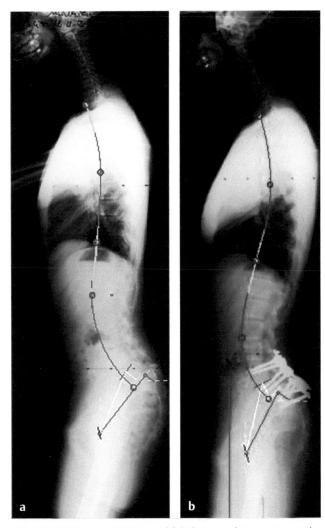

Fig. 11.14 (a) Grade IV L5S1 spondylolisthesis combining retroverted pelvis and long hyperlordosis to compensate the lumbosacral kyphosis (LSK). **(b)** After reduction strategy (LSK reduction), both compensations disappear restoring a good balance.

As illustrated above, the compensatory mechanisms are logical, however complex, and one must try different approaches to comprehending these mechanisms to understand fully the compensatory mechanisms.

References

[1] Roussouly P, Nnadi C. Sagittal plane deformity: an overview of interpretation and management. Eur Spine J. 2010; 19(11):1824–1836

[2] Dubousset J. Three-dimensional analysis of the scoliotic deformity. In: Weinstein SL, ed. The Pediatric Spine: Principles and Practice. New York, NY: Raven; 1994:479–496

[3] Vidal J, Marnay T. Sagittal deviations of the spine, and trial of classification as a function of the pelvic balance (in French). Rev Chir Orthop Repar Appar Mot. 1984; 70 Suppl 2:124–126

[4] Vidal J, Marnay T. Morphology and anteroposterior body equilibrium in spondylolisthesis L5-S1. Rev Chir Orthop Repar Appar Mot. 1983; 69(1): 17–28

[5] Barrey C, Roussouly P, Perrin G, Le Huec J-C. Sagittal balance disorders in severe degenerative spine. Can we identify the compensatory mechanisms? Eur Spine J. 2011; 20 Suppl 5:626–633

[6] Wenger DR, Frick SL. Scheuermann kyphosis. Spine. 1999; 24(24):2630–2639

[7] Cortet B, Houvenagel E, Puisieux F, Roches E, Garnier P, Delcambre B. Spinal curvatures and quality of life in women with vertebral fractures secondary to osteoporosis. Spine. 1999; 24(18):1921–1925

[8] Vaccaro AR, Silber JS. Post-traumatic spinal deformity. Spine. 2001; 26(24) Suppl:S111–S118

[9] Lu DC, Chou D. Flatback syndrome. Neurosurg Clin N Am. 2007; 18(2): 289–294

[10] Potter BK, Lenke LG, Kuklo TR. Prevention and management of iatrogenic flat-back deformity. J Bone Joint Surg Am. 2004; 86-A(8):1793–1808

[11] Lafage V, Schwab F, Patel A, Hawkinson N, Farcy JP. Pelvic tilt and truncal inclination: two key radiographic parameters in the setting of adults with spinal deformity. Spine. 2009; 34(17):E599–E606

[12] Debarge R, Demey G, Roussouly P. Sagittal balance analysis after pedicle sub-traction osteotomy in ankylosing spondylitis. Eur Spine J. 2011; 20 Suppl 5:619–625

[13] Legaye J, Duval-Beaupère G, Hecquet J, Marty C. Pelvic incidence: a funda-mental pelvic parameter for three-dimensional regulation of spinal sagittal curves. Eur Spine J. 1998; 7(2):99–103

[14] Vaz G, Roussouly P, Berthonnaud E, Dimnet J. Sagittal morphology and equili-brium of pelvis and spine. Eur Spine J. 2002; 11(1):80–87

[15] Lazennec J-Y, Brusson A, Rousseau M-A. Hip-spine relations and sagittal bal-ance clinical consequences. Eur Spine J. 2011; 20 Suppl 5:686–698

[16] Mangione P, Sénégas J. Sagittal balance of the spine. Rev Chir Orthop Repar Appar Mot. 1997; 83(1):22–32

[17] Roussouly P, Pinheiro-Franco JL. Biomechanical analysis of the spino-pelvic organization and adaptation in pathology. Eur Spine J. 2011; 20 Suppl 5: 609–618

[18] Le Huec JC, Charosky S, Barrey C, Rigal J, Aunoble S. Sagittal imbalance cas-cade for simple degenerative spine and consequences: algorithm of decision for appropriate treatment. Eur Spine J. 2011; 20 Suppl 5:699–703

[19] Barrey C, Jund J, Noseda O, Roussouly P. Sagittal balance of the pelvis-spine complex and lumbar degenerative diseases. A comparative study about 85 cases. Eur Spine J. 2007; 16(9):1459–1467

[20] Mac-Thiong JM, Labelle H, Roussouly P. Pediatric sagittal alignment. Eur Spine J. 2011; 20 Suppl 5:586–590

[21] Laouissat F, Sebaaly A, Gehrchen M, Roussouly P. Classification of normal sag-ittal spine alignment: refounding the Roussouly classification. Eur Spine J. 2018; 27(8):2002–2011

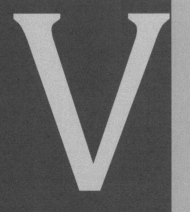

Part V

The Non Scoliotic Spine

12 Isthmic Lytic Spondylolisthesis—The Physiopathology, Classification, and Treatment Better Explained by the Sagittal Balance

Hubert Labelle, Jean-Marc Mac-Thiong, Stefan Parent, and Pierre Roussouly

Abstract

Global sagittal plane alignment is important to consider in both adult and pediatric patients with L5-S1 spondylolisthesis. Clinicians treating this disorder need to be aware that normal sagittal balance of the hip-spinopelvic axis is frequently disrupted and that it is insufficient to limit their evaluation and base their treatment plan strictly on the local L5-S1 area. The proposed classification based on sagittal alignment emphasizes that subjects with L5-S1 spondylolisthesis are a heterogeneous group with various adaptations of their posture and that clinicians need to keep this fact in mind for evaluation and treatment. Abnormal spinopelvic alignment alters the biomechanical stresses at the lumbosacral junction and the compensation mechanisms used to maintain an adequate posture. Patients with high-grade spondylolisthesis (HGS) associated with a postural abnormality has provided a compelling rationale to reduce and realign the spondylolisthesis deformity, thus restoring global spinal alignment and improving the biomechanical environment for fusion. Recent evidence supports the contention that reduction of HGS improves overall global hip-spinopelvic balance by correcting the local kyphotic deformity and partly reducing vertebral slippage, and that reduction is not associated with a greater risk of developing neurologic deficits compared with arthrodesis in situ.

Keywords: classification, spinopelvic balance, spondylolisthesis, surgical reduction

12.1 Why Is Sagittal Balance So Important in Spondylolisthesis?

Spondylolysis is a defect in the pars articularis of a vertebra. It can occur independently or in association with spondylolisthesis, most frequently at the level of L5-S1. Spondylolisthesis is the forward displacement of one vertebra with respect to the adjacent caudal vertebra. Spondyloptosis is a 100% translation of one vertebra on the next caudal vertebra.

This chapter focuses on developmental spondylolisthesis and on the less frequently encountered stress fracture, the two most frequent types seen in children, adolescents, and young adults. It is not meant to be a comprehensive review of spondylolisthesis but to focus on sagittal balance as it applies to this disorder and show how it can help to better understand physiopathology, classification, and treatment. It is assumed that the reader has the basic understanding of the disease.

In the past two decades, there has been much development in the understanding of the disorder, as significant new knowledge on sagittal spinopelvic balance has been acquired. In 2005, the Spine/Scoliosis Research Society summary statement in the *Spine* focus issue devoted to spondylolisthesis[1] stressed the point that "…global sagittal plane alignment is important in both adult and pediatric patients with spondylolisthesis. In patients with high-grade developmental spondylolisthesis, this has provided a compelling rationale to reduce and realign the spondylolisthesis deformity, thus restoring global spinal balance and improving the biomechanical environment for fusion." Improved understanding of the complex relationship between spondylolisthesis and human standing posture was gained by stopping to concentrate on the local L5-S1 junction and rather focus on the global sagittal picture using long-standing lateral sagittal X-rays of the spine and pelvis and, more recently, with full-body sagittal radiological images using EOS low-radiation technology[2] (▶ Fig. 12.1).

From the evolutionary standpoint, two important observations indicate the importance of sagittal balance in the development of this disorder. First, although many authors have searched for a spondylolytic lesion at birth, a pars defect has

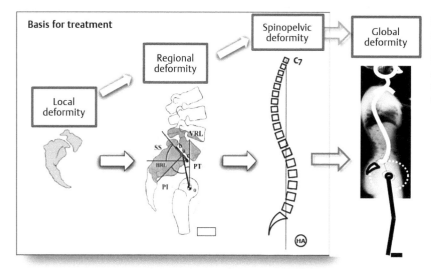

Fig. 12.1 Improved understanding in spondylolisthesis over the past two decades has been gained by studying pathological changes not only in the local L5-S1 area, but also the regional deformity using spinopelvic measures, the spinopelvic balance, and, more recently, the global changes occurring at the lower extremities.

never been reported in a newborn. The earliest cases of spondylolysis have been found in children between the ages of 6 weeks and 10 months.

In a prospective study of 500 first-grade children, Fredrickson et al[3] found a prevalence of spondylolysis of 4.4% at 6 years old, 5.2% at 12 years old, 5.6% at 14 years old, and 6% in adulthood. Thus, spondylolysis/listhesis is intimately linked to the standing posture. Tardieu et al[4] have studied how sagittal balance is acquired during bipedal gait acquisition by comparing neonatal and adult pelvises in 3D (▶ Fig. 12.2). During gait acquisition, the relationship between the sacrum and acetabula are modified through the mobility and malleability of the S-I joints, as indicated by very significant changes in pelvic incidence (PI) values. Before walking, hip flexion and anterior vertebral flexion induce an anterior location of the trunk center of gravity. After walking, femoral extension and lumbar lordosis induced by muscular actions increase sacral slope (SS) and PI, creating a backward displacement of the center of gravity behind the femoral heads, a basic characteristic of human standing posture, which will set and control all spinopelvic relationships from childhood to adulthood.

Second, spondylolysis has not been reported in quadrupeds, only in bipeds. Furthermore, there are no known cases reported in nonambulatory humans. Evolution from the quadrupedal to the bipedal posture in primates and humans has been allowed by progressive and very significant changes in the shape and position of the pelvis and spine and of their supporting ligaments and muscles (▶ Fig. 12.3). A quadruped has no lumbar lordosis and a more longitudinal and narrow-shaped pelvis. In sharp contrast, a human has a well-developed lumbar lordosis and a much "rounder" pelvic shape, a situation that has gradually evolved in primates along with the transition to the bipedal posture. These changes in shape and morphology of the pelvis are crucial to the understanding and management of spondylolisthesis, a disorder that is closely linked to the bipedal posture and associated with activities involving a lordotic effect on the lumbar spine, such as gymnastics.

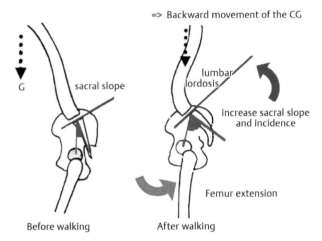

Fig. 12.2 Important changes in sagittal posture before and after walking age are brought about by changes in pelvic morphology with a significant increase in pelvic incidence, and corresponding changes in hip-spinopelvic posture with a backward displacement of the center of gravity behind the femoral heads increase in sacral slope and lumbar lordosis, combined with loss of hip flexion position.

12.2 Why Standard Spondylolisthesis Classification Systems, although Useful, Are Insufficient to Understanding Physiopathology and Help Guide Treatment

The most commonly used classification systems are the Meyerding,[5] the Wiltse,[6] and the Marchetti and Bartolozzi[7] classifications.

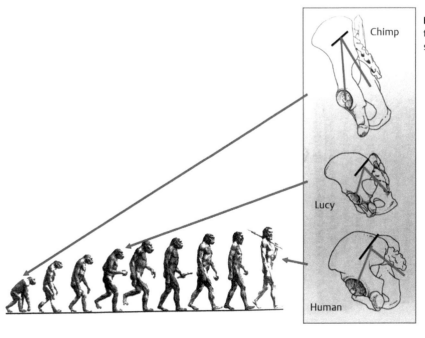

Fig. 12.3 Evolution of pelvic morphology through time: pelvic incidence (PI) increases with transition to the upright posture.

Meyerding described the simplest system of grading, and the least comprehensive classification, which is based only on the severity of the forward displacement of the cranial vertebra with respect to the caudal vertebra, with no consideration for the very important lordotic or kyphotic relation between the two. The caudal vertebra is divided into four parts. Grade I means a translation of the cranial vertebra of 0% to 25%, grade II of 25% to 50%, grade III of 50% to 75%, and grade IV of 75% to 100%. Grade V was added later, describing the ptosis of the cranial vertebra. Unfortunately, he did not specify the landmarks to use on the cranial vertebra. Bourassa-Moreau et al[8] have demonstrated that various landmarks have been used by many authors, creating significant variations on the interpretation of slip severity caused by the various lordotic and kyphotic relationship of L5-S1. Consequently, they proposed a standardized method, shown in ▸ Fig. 12.4, which is recommended when using the Meyerding classification.

Wiltse divided spondylolisthesis into five types, based on radiological findings. It is useful to differentiate between the various etiologies of this pathology:

- Type I (dysplastic) involves a congenital defect of the lumbosacral facet joints.
- Type II (isthmic), where the lumbosacral facets are normal but the listhesis is caused by a defect in the pars. The subtypes are IIA with a stress fracture, IIB with a pars elongation, and IIC with an acute pars fracture.
- Type III (degenerative) is secondary to degenerative osteoarthritis of the facet joints and intervertebral disk.
- Type IV (traumatic) results from an acute fracture of posterior elements other than the pars interarticularis.
- Type V (pathologic) is associated with destruction of posterior elements as result of a systemic or local bone disease.

Marchetti and Bartolozzi developed a classification system based on the developmental origin versus the acquired forms of spondylolisthesis, thereby providing some insight into the etiology and prognosis of spondylolisthesis:

- Developmental spondylolisthesis is divided into two major types (high and low dysplastic), depending on the severity of

bony dysplastic changes present in the L5 and S1 vertebrae and on the risk of further slippage. Dysplastic facet joints and spina bifida of L5 and/or S1 are frequent in both types, but, in addition, the high dysplastic type is associated with significant lumbosacral kyphosis (LSK), trapezoidal L5 vertebra, hypoplastic transverse processes, and sacral doming with verticalization of the sacrum, while the low dysplastic type is associated with a relatively normal lumbosacral profile, a rectangular L5 vertebra, preservation of a flat upper endplate of S1, and no significant verticalization of the sacrum.

- Acquired spondylolisthesis is secondary to trauma, surgery, a pathologic disease, or a degenerative process: the traumatic form can be a result of either an acute or stress fracture. Typically, a stress fracture occurs in young athletes and is distinct from the isthmic dysplastic type of spondylolisthesis.

Thus, the Meyerding classification is useful, but insufficient, for grading severity of the displacement. The other two classifications are useful to identify the underlying pathology, but they are of little help in understanding physiopathology or guiding surgical treatment. As stated earlier, this chapter focuses on developmental spondylolisthesis (Marchetti and Bartolozzi) and on the less frequently encountered Wiltse type II stress fracture, the two most frequent types seen in children, adolescents, and young adults.

12.3 Etiology and Physiopathology Are Better Explained Using Sagittal Balance

The exact etiology of spondylolysis/listhesis remains unknown but it is most likely multifactorial, as various hereditary, traumatic, biomechanical, growth, and morphological factors have been reported to play a role.[9] They are shown in ▸ Fig. 12.5. Among many of these factors, sagittal balance plays a crucial and central role, which will be discussed further.

12.3.1 Trauma

Spondylolysis/listhesis occurs only in bipeds and predominantly at L5-S1 (87%), but also at L4-L5 (10%) and L3-L4 (3%). Several authors suggest that spondylolysis is caused by a stress fracture secondary to repetitive microtrauma at the pars level. In the case of spondylolisthesis without an isthmic defect, elongation of the posterior elements can be a result of repeated microfractures and subsequent healing, as the L5-S1 disk bond slowly fails, allowing anterior translation of L5. In the upright posture, the pars articularis is submitted to high shear, compressive, and tensile loads during flexion and extension movements. Accordingly, there is an increased prevalence of spondylolysis and spondylolisthesis among athletes in certain sports involving repetitive alternate flexion–extension loading such as gymnastics, weight lifting, and football.

12.3.2 Biomechanics

The body weight transmitted to the lumbosacral junction is supported by the L5-S1 disk, the L5-S1 facet joints, the posterior

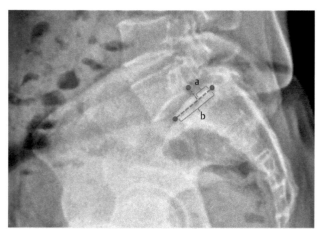

Fig. 12.4 Modified Meyerding technique for grading spondylolisthesis: a perpendicular to the sacral plate is drawn from the posteroinferior corner of the L5 vertebral body. Degree of slip is length "a" over length "b," expressed in percentage. A low-grade slip is between 0% and 49%, a high-grade slip is 50% and higher.

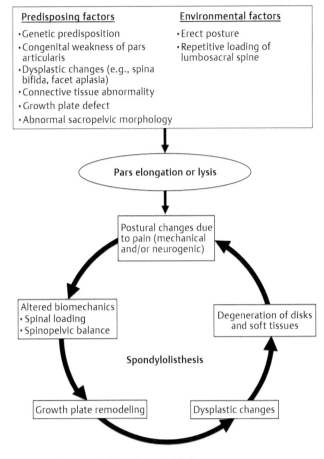

Predisposing factors	Environmental factors
•Genetic predisposition	•Erect posture
•Congenital weakness of pars articularis	•Repetitive loading of lumbosacral spine
•Dysplastic changes (e.g., spina bifida, facet aplasia)	
•Connective tissue abnormality	
•Growth plate defect	
•Abnormal sacropelvic morphology	

Fig. 12.5 Physiopathology of spondylolisthesis.

ligaments, and the sacrospinalis and multifidus muscles. Under normal upright conditions, the facet joints support the majority of the shear force, while the L5-S1 disk supports most of the compression at the lumbosacral junction. In spondylolysis, the facet joints are not functional and most of the shear stresses at L5-S1 are transferred to the disk, which predisposes to degeneration of the disk and subsequent spondylolisthesis. With progression of spondylolisthesis, there is a further decrease in disk stiffness and an increase in stresses across the lumbosacral junction. A variable amount of dysplasia, such as with spina bifida occulta, facet, or laminar aplasia, is also common and can further disturb the normal posterior bony hook/catch at the lumbosacral junction. Connective tissue disorders with associated lax ligaments or abnormal bone can also predispose to spondylolisthesis, such as in Marfan, Ehlers–Danlos syndrome, and osteogenesis imperfecta.

12.3.3 Growth Plate Disturbance

Progression of spondylolisthesis mainly occurs during skeletal growth and is less likely after skeletal maturity. The risk of slip progression is generally low (4% to 5%). Factors associated with an increased risk of slip progression include female gender, presentation at a young age, severity of slip at presentation, developmental type, increased slip angle, and a high degree of bony

dysplasia. If slip severity is less than 30% at presentation, then further slipping is unlikely.

Remaining growth is also an important predictor of progression. Previous studies support the role of a biomechanical weakness in the vertebral growth plate as an important mechanism in slip progression. In the growing child, increased stress in the L5-S1 disk can be associated with bony remodeling through the growth plates, particularly the upper and anterior endplate of S1. Involvement of the upper S1 endplate can further contribute to the progression of the spondylolisthesis in a process similar to the progression of Blount's disease where progressive tibia vara develops as a result of asymmetric pressures on the growth plate in the upright position (▶ Fig. 12.6). This process explains the frequent development of sacral doming and the trapezoidal shape of L5 frequently encountered in high-grade spondylolisthesis (HGS). Once again, the standing posture is crucial to explain how these changes occur and how asymmetrical pressures on the anterior part of the growth plates create secondary doming of the sacrum in HGS.[10]

12.4 Hip-Spinopelvic Balance and Morphology

Sagittal sacropelvic morphology and orientation modulates the geometry of the lumbar spine and, consequently, the mechanical stresses at the lumbosacral junction. In L5-S1 spondylolisthesis, it has been clearly demonstrated over the past decade that sacropelvic morphology is frequently abnormal and that, combined with the presence of a local lumbosacral deformity and dysplasia, can result in an abnormal sacropelvic orientation as well as in a disturbed global sagittal balance of the spine.[1] These findings have important implications for the evaluation and treatment of patients with spondylolisthesis, especially for those with a high-grade slip.

When compared with normal populations, pelvic morphology is clearly abnormal, as indicated by PI, which is significantly higher[11,12,13] in spondylolisthesis, and the difference in PI tends to increase in a direct linear fashion as severity of the spondylolisthesis increases.[11] The cause–effect relationship between pelvic morphology and spondylolisthesis remains to be clarified. By virtue of the relationship between morphology (PI) and spinopelvic balance (pelvic tilt [PT], SS, L5I, LSK, C7 plumb line, etc.) described in previous chapters, all other measures of spinopelvic balance are also significantly different in control populations compared to subjects with L5-S1 spondylolisthesis,[11,13] especially in HGS where the relationship between the spine and the pelvis is distorted (▶ Table 12.1). Strong correlations are found between PI, L5I, PT, SS, and LSK and lumbar lordosis.[14] In high-grade slips with sacral doming, the measurement of PI, SS, and LSK is not as reliable, as they depend on the sacral plate, which is then irregular and domed. Contrarily, L5I (▶ Fig. 12.7) is not affected by sacral doming as it is measured with the superior L5 endplate, which offers a better inter- and intrarater reproducibility over the superior S1 endplate.[15] It is thus the preferred measurement to assess the disturbed relation between the spine and pelvis, particularly in HGS. Similarly, PT is a more reliable measure in HGS, as it does not depend on the sacral plate.

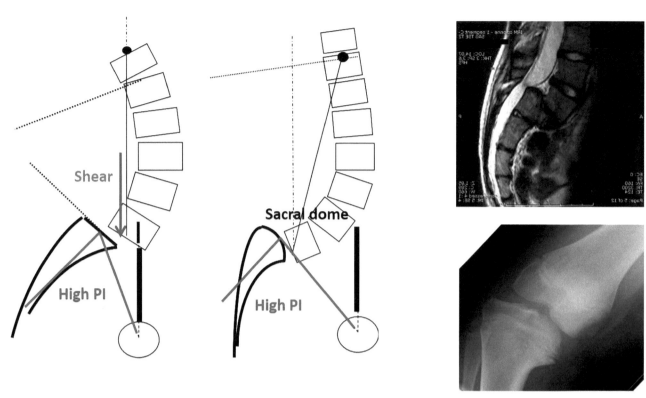

Fig. 12.6 How shear forces on the anterior growth plate of S1 can create a sacral dome in a process similar to Blount's deformity. PI, Pelvic incidence.

Table 12.1 Mean values (and standard deviation) of pertinent sagittal sacropelvic measurements in subjects with spondylolisthesis compared to a control population

	Normal children and adolescents[a] (n = 341)	Normal adults[b] (n = 160)	Developmental spondylolisthesis[c]				
			Grade 1 (n = 21)	Grade 2 (n = 91)	Grade 3 (n = 74)	Grade 4 (n = 17)	Grade 5 (n = 11)
Pelvic incidence	49.1 (11.0)	51.8 (5.3)	57.7 (6.3)	66.0 (6.9)	78.8 (5.6)	82.3 (7.2)	79.4 (10.2)
Sacral slope	41.4 (8.2)	39.7 (4.1)	43.9 (4.8)	49.8 (4.2)	51.2 (5.7)	48.5 (7.6)	45.9 (13.5)
Pelvic tilt	7.7 (8.0)	12.1 (3.2)	13.8 (3.9)	16.2 (5.4)	27.6 (5.7)	33.9 (5.2)	33.5 (5.4)

[a]Values from Mac-Thiong et al.[34]
[b]Values from Berthonnaud et al.[35]
[c]Values from Labelle et al.[12]

In a static standing position, the way SS and PT balance refers to the concept of sacropelvic balance. Members of the Spinal Deformity Study Group (SDSG) have specifically investigated sacropelvic balance in low-grade spondylolisthesis (LGS) and HGS. Roussouly et al[16] proposed two different subgroups of sacropelvic balance observed in subjects with LGS, which could be related to the etiology. In their opinion, patients with high PI and SS have increased shear stresses at the lumbosacral junction, causing more tension on the pars interarticularis at L5, and ultimately a pars defect (▶ Fig. 12.8). Conversely, patients with a low PI and a smaller SS have impingement of the posterior elements of L5 between L4 and S1 during extension, thereby leading to repetitive impingement of the pars interarticularis of L5 by the posterior facets of L4 and S1 during extension movements, a "nutcracker" effect on the L5-S1 pars (▶ Fig. 12.6). The clinical relevance of these findings is that because PI is always much greater than normal in HGS,[12] it is assumed that the risk of progression in the low-grade subgroup with a normal PI is much lower than in the subgroup with an abnormally high PI value. It is hypothesized that the subgroup with normal PI corresponds to acquired traumatic cases with an acute or stress fracture (Marchetti and Bartolozzi[7] classification) in subjects with a normal sacropelvic morphology, whereas the other subgroup with high PI is associated

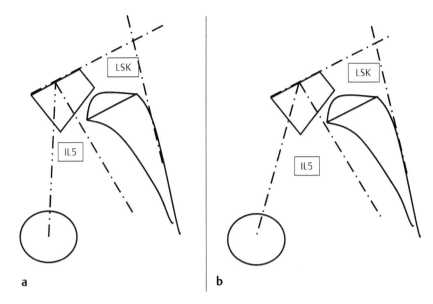

Fig. 12.7 In the presence of sacral doming, L5 incidence angle (IL5) and lumbosacral kyphosis (LSK) are more reliable than pelvic incidence (PI) and sacral slope (SS) as they are not dependent on the sacral plate for their measurement. In this example, when comparing situations **(a)** and **(b)**, Il5 is clearly different in both cases, and not influenced by the sacral doming at L5S1. The measurement of lumbosacral kyphosis (LSK) using the Dubousset technique (DUB LSK) is illustrated in both **(a)** and **(b)**.

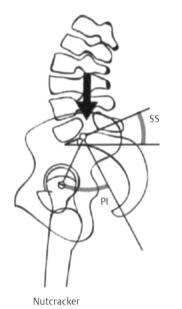

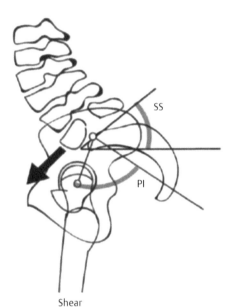

Nutcracker　　　　　　Shear

Fig. 12.8 The two sacropelvic balances observed in subjects with low-grade spondylolisthesis. SS, Sacral slope; PI, pelvic incidence.

with more dysplastic developmental cases. As for HGS, Hresko et al[17] have identified two subgroups of patients: balanced versus unbalanced pelvis (▸ Fig. 12.9). The "balanced" group includes patients standing with a high SS and a low PT, a posture similar to the subgroup of normal individuals with high PI, whereas the "unbalanced" group includes patients standing with a retroverted pelvis and a vertical sacrum, corresponding to a low SS and a high PT. Each new subject with HGS can be classified by using the raw SS and PT values or, in borderline cases, by using the nomogram (▸ Fig. 12.10) provided by Hresko et al.[17] Recently, Sebaaly et al[15] have demonstrated that

L5I and /or PT values can be used reliably and more easily to identify these two basic pelvic postures. Subjects with PT values ≤ 25° and/or L5I values ≤ 60° are in the balanced pelvis group. Subjects with PT values > 25° and/or L5I values > 60° belong to the unbalanced group.

In a static standing position, the way the spine and the pelvis balance themselves refers to the concept of spinopelvic balance. By using a postural model of spinopelvic balance showing the relationships between parameters of each successive anatomical segment from the thoracic spine to the sacropelvis, Mac-Thiong et al[18] have observed that a relatively normal

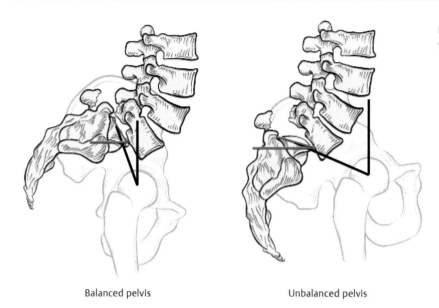

Fig. 12.9 The two pelvic postures found in high-grade spondylolithesis.

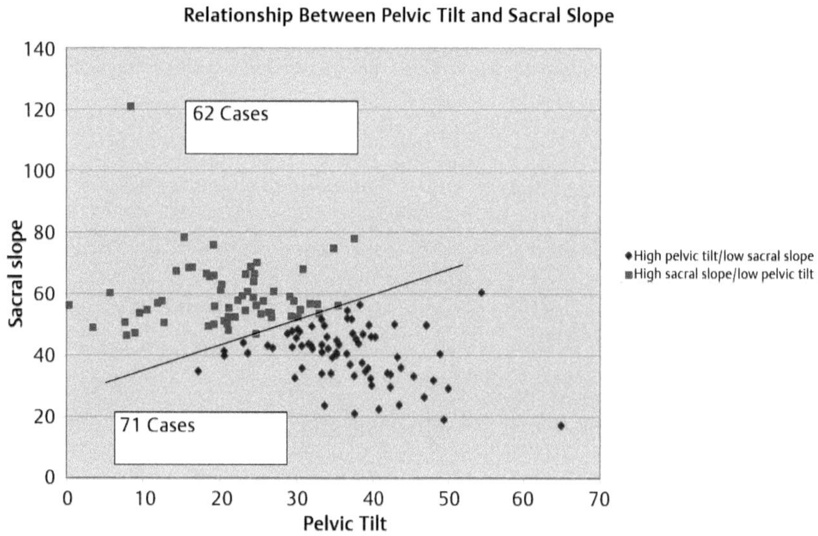

Balanced pelvis   Unbalanced pelvis

Fig. 12.10 Nomogram from Hresko et al[17]: in pink, the balanced pelvis; in blue, the unbalanced pelvis.

posture is maintained in LGS, whereas posture is clearly abnormal in HGS. In HGS, the spinopelvic balance is particularly disturbed in the subgroup with an unbalanced sacropelvis, as described by Hresko et al.[17] They also reported that for most patients with spondylolisthesis (low grades and balanced high grades), the global spinopelvic balance (position of C7 vertebral body over the femoral heads) was relatively constant with the C7 plumb line projecting behind the femoral heads, regardless of the local lumbosacral deformity and particularly with the alignment of the C7 plumb line with respect to S1, indicating the predominant influence of the sacropelvis in the achievement of a normal global spinopelvic balance.

A few studies have correlated spinopelvic and sacropelvic balance with health-related quality of life (HRQoL) measures. Tanguay et al[19] have demonstrated that increased LSK has a significant association with a decrease in the physical aspect of the quality of life for patients with adolescent L5-S1 spondylolisthesis. The effect of LSK is particularly important for patients with HGS, independent of the slip percentage. Therefore, LSK

values should be included in the routine evaluation of patients with spondylolisthesis, to fully appreciate the severity of the deformity and its clinical impact on the quality of life of patients. Glavas et al[20] studied techniques of LSK measurement used in the literature and found that the technique described by Dubousset (DUB LSK; ▸ Fig. 12.7) was the only measurement of LSK that showed a gradation along the spectrum from normal to HGS. They also found that DUB LSK was the most correlated to slip percentage. Moreover, they proved that it had the best inter- and intrarater reliability, and the upper sacral endplate doming does not interfere with its measurement. Correlation between DUB LSK and L5I is strong both in the normal population[15] and in the HGS population. Harroud et al,[21] in a cohort of subjects with HGS, have noted that an increasing positive sagittal alignment was related to a poorer SRS-22 total score, especially when the C7 plumb line (C7PL) is in front of the hip axis. Global sagittal alignment using C7PL should therefore always be assessed in patients with HGS.

Recently, Mac-Thiong et al[22] reported on the importance of evaluating the presence of hip flexum in the standing position using the proximal femoral flexion angle ([PFA]; ▶ Fig. 12.11). PFA is significantly higher in HGS subjects compared to normals. A PFA ≥ 10° is proposed as a criterion to define abnormal PFA. PFA was increased in HGS and increased along with deteriorating sagittal balance and HRQoL.

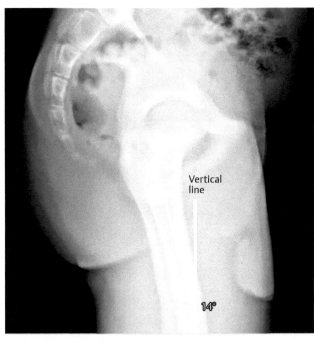

Fig. 12.11 Proximal femoral flexion angle measurement.

12.5 Postural Compensation Mechanisms in Spondylolisthesis

In the presence of abnormal sacropelvic balance and progressive spondylolisthesis, the lumbosacral alignment and the global sagittal alignment can be altered (▶ Fig. 12.12). In addition to the translational slip of L5 on top of S1, an angular deformity appearing as LSK can occur. Forward global spinal balance, as measured by a plumb line from C7 to the sacrum and forward spinal–pelvic balance, as measured by a plumb line from C7 to the hip axis and/or hip flexum can also be observed, especially in HGS. In response to the progressively abnormal sacral–pelvic, lumbosacral, and global balance, the center of gravity of the torso tends to be displaced anteriorly, therefore inducing forward displacement of the anterior part of L5, while the posterior part of L5 remains attached to the posterior soft tissues. In subjects with spondylolisthesis and a high PI (the majority of subjects), there is a high SS and PT with an increased lumbar lordosis to keep the center of gravity and C7 plumb line behind the hips to maintain a balanced posture. This first compensation mechanism occurs by increasing the intervertebral segmental lordosis and/or by including more vertebrae in the lordotic segment. For each patient, there is a maximal attainable lumbar lordosis beyond which the patient will then attempt to maintain a balanced posture by progressive retroversion of the pelvis. This second compensation mechanism induces a progressive retroversion of the pelvis and a progressive verticalization of the sacrum. Because each subject has a fixed PI, SS decreases along with the retroversion of the pelvis and PT increases as the sacrum becomes vertical. When the limit of these two compensation mechanisms is reached, the patient develops sagittal trunk imbalance, most

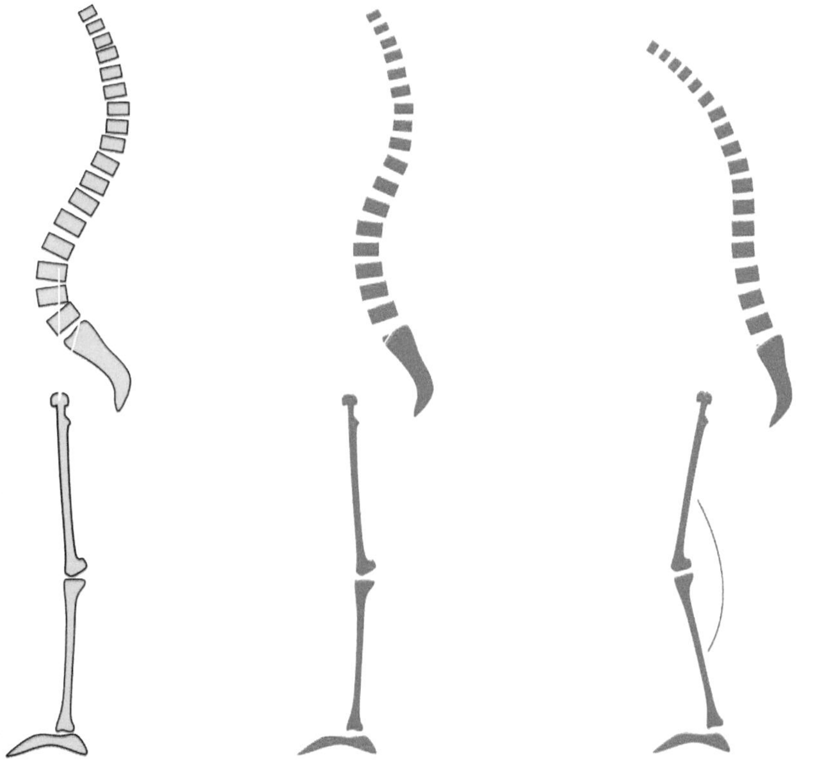

Fig. 12.12 Compensation mechanisms in spondylolisthesis: pelvic tilt increases as the pelvis becomes more vertical (retroversion). As maximal retroversion is achieved, knee and hip flexion increase to maintain spinal balance. Finally, the spine becomes unbalanced with displacement of the C7 plumb line in front of the femoral heads.

often characterized either by compensatory hip flexion, by forward leaning of the trunk with positive sagittal imbalance of the spine, or a combination of both. In addition, in immature subjects, increased LSK and L5I, combined with the anterior slipping of L5, induce higher pressure on the anterior part of the S1 growth plate, which itself leads to decreased growth of the anterior sacrum according to the Hueter–Volkmann Law, inducing progressive rounding of the sacrum and the so-called sacral dome deformity often seen in HGS (▶ Fig. 12.6). This doming combined with progressive L5-S1 disk deterioration creates further LSK and increase of L5I, further disrupting the global hip-spinopelvic balance, up to a spondyloptosis.

12.6 How Can Global Sagittal Balance Be Incorporated into a Classification System?

The findings described in the previous section have stimulated a renewed interest for the radiological evaluation and classification of spinopelvic alignment in L5-S1 spondylolisthesis. The SDSG reported a classification system[23] in six different sagittal spinopelvic postures, based on the radiographic measurement of slip grade and spinopelvic alignment (PI, sacropelvic, and spinal balance). Refinements to this classification have been added more recently based on the new findings reported in the previous section on the contribution of L5I[15] and hip flexum deformity,[22] resulting in an updated classification presented in ▶ Fig. 12.13 that is still based on the initial six sagittal postures. The rationale of the classification was derived from the analysis of a multicenter radiological database of patients with L5-S1 developmental or acquired stress fracture spondylolisthesis, containing standing lateral radiographs of the spine and pelvis of 816 subjects with grades 1 to 5 spondylolisthesis, aged between 10 and 40 years, and collected from 43 spine surgeons in North America and Europe. The classification is based on five important sagittal characteristics that can be assessed on standing sagittal radiographs of the spine, pelvis, and proximal

femurs: (1) the grade of slip (low or high), (2) the PI (low, normal, or high), (3) the spinopelvic balance (balanced or unbalanced), (4) the LSK and L5I, and (5) hip flexum (PFA). Accordingly, six different postures can be identified with two subtypes of type 5.

To classify a patient, the degree of slip is quantified first from the lateral standing radiograph, using the modified Meyerding technique[5] (▶ Fig. 12.4) to determine whether it is low grade (grades 0, 1, and 2, or < 50% slip) or high grade (grades 3, 4, and spondyloptosis, or ≥ 50% slip). Next, the sagittal balance is measured by determining sacropelvic and hip-spinopelvic alignment, using measurements of PI, SS, PT, IL5, LSK, PFA, and the C7 plumb line.

For LGS, three types of sacropelvic balance can be found (▶ Fig. 12.14): type 1, the nutcracker type, a subgroup with low PI (< 45°); type 2, a subgroup with normal PI (between 45° and 60°); and type 3, the shear type, a subgroup with high PI (> 60°).

For HGS, three types are also found (▶ Fig. 12.15). Each subject is first classified as having a balanced or an unbalanced sacropelvis using the nomogram of SS and PT provided by Hresko et al[17] (▶ Fig. 12.10); if not available, PT can also reliably be used with a cut-off value of 26°, subjects with a PT < 26° being classified as balanced, and subjects with a PT value ≥ 26° classified as an unbalanced sacropelvis.[15] Next, hip–spine balance is determined using the C7 plumb line for the spine and proximal PFA to evaluate hip flexum. If the C7 plumb line falls over or behind the femoral heads, the spine is balanced, whereas if it lies in front of the femoral heads, the spine is unbalanced. A hip flexum is present if the PFA ≥ 10° (▶ Fig. 12.11). In this case, it is important to obtain sagittal X-rays of the hip, proximal femurs, and spine with the patient standing with the knees in maximal extension, as a hip flexum can cause improper classification into a type 5 while the classification should in fact be a type 6, becoming apparent with the lateral radiographs with the knees in extension (▶ Fig. 12.16). In our experience, the hip–spine complex is almost always balanced in LGS and in HGS with a balanced sacropelvis and, therefore, hip–spinal balance needs to be measured mainly in high-grade deformities with an unbalanced pelvis (types 5 and 6). Therefore, the three types in

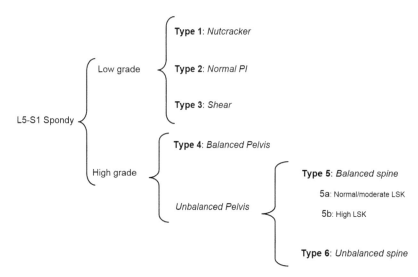

Spondylolisthesis Sagittal Balance Classification

Fig. 12.13 Spondylolisthesis sagittal balance classification. LSK, Lumbosacral kyphosis.

L5-S1 Spondy

Low grade
- **Type 1**: *Nutcracker*
- **Type 2**: *Normal PI*
- **Type 3**: *Shear*

High grade
- **Type 4**: *Balanced Pelvis*
- *Unbalanced Pelvis*
  - **Type 5**: *Balanced spine*
    - 5a: Normal/moderate LSK
    - 5b: High LSK
  - **Type 6**: *Unbalanced spine*

HGS are type 4, balanced pelvis, type 5, unbalanced pelvis with balanced spine, and type 6, unbalanced pelvis with an unbalanced spine. ▶ Fig. 12.14 and ▶ Fig. 12.15 illustrate clinical examples of these six basic postures. In addition, following the demonstration that increased LSK is associated with a decrease in HRQoL in HGS,[19] two subtypes of type 5 posture have been

Low grade types

1- Low PI < 45°   2- PI = 45° to 60°   3- High PI > 60°

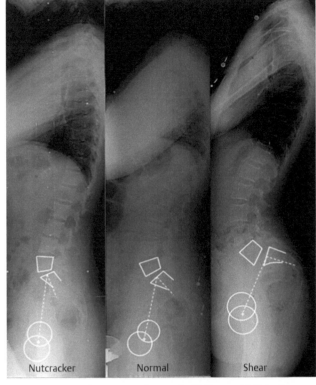

Nutcracker   Normal   Shear

Fig. 12.14 Sagittal postures in low-grade L5-S1 spondylolisthesis.

recognized: type 5a, associated with a normal or low LSK (as measured by Dubousset's lumbosacral angle ≥ 80°), and type 5b, associated with high LSK (as measured by Dubousset's lumbosacral angle < 80°). ▶ Fig. 12.17 shows the two type 5 subtypes. In a clinical assessment of this refined version of the classification system, Mac-Thiong et al.[24] found improved and substantial intra- and interobserver reliability similar to other currently used classifications for spinal deformity, with overall intra- and interobserver agreements of 80% (kappa: 0.74) and 71% (kappa: 0.65), respectively.

The proposed classification emphasizes that subjects with L5-S1 spondylolisthesis are a heterogeneous group with various adaptations of their posture and that clinicians need to keep this fact in mind for evaluation and treatment. Abnormal spinopelvic balance alters the biomechanical stresses at the lumbosacral junction and the compensation mechanisms used to maintain an adequate posture. The clinical relevance of this classification is shown in ▶ Fig. 12.18 and will be discussed in the following section.

12.7 How Can Sagittal Balance Help Guide Treatment?

12.7.1 Clinical Relevance for Low-Grade Spondylolisthesis

Subjects with L5-S1 spondylolisthesis are a heterogeneous group with various adaptations of their posture that clinicians need to keep in mind for evaluation and treatment. Low grades with normal or low PI tend to be Wiltse's type II or Bartolozzi's acquired type, while low grades with high PI and all high grades are Wiltse's type I or Bartolozzi's developmental type. Thus, it is important to follow closely low grades with high PI as they are the ones most at risk of further progression. Because PI is always much greater than normal in HGS, this suggests that the risk of progression in skeletally immature subjects with types 1

Type 4   Type 5A   Type 5B   Type 6

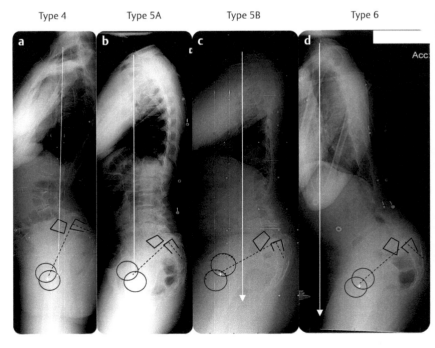

Fig. 12.15 Sagittal postures in high-grade spondylolisthesis. **(a)** Type 4 posture with a balanced and horizontal sacrum, and a balanced spine with the C7 plumb line falling behind the femoral heads (yellow line). **(b)** Type 5A posture with an unbalanced/vertical sacrum, a balanced spine, and a lumbosacral angle more than 80°. **(c)** Type 5B posture, with an unbalanced/vertical sacrum, a balanced spine, and a lumbosacral angle less than 80°. **(d)** Type 6 posture with both an unbalanced sacrum/pelvis and spine.

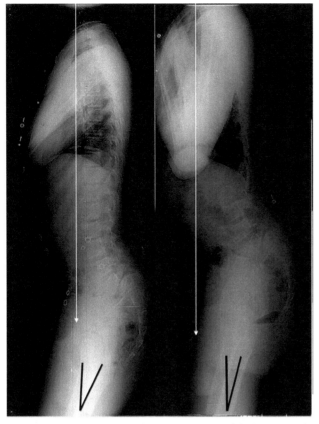

Fig. 12.16 It is important to obtain sagittal X-rays of the hip, proximal femurs, and spine with the patient standing with the knees in maximal extension, because a hip flexum can cause improper classification into a type 5 while the classification should in fact be a type 6, becoming apparent on the lateral radiographs with the knees in extension.

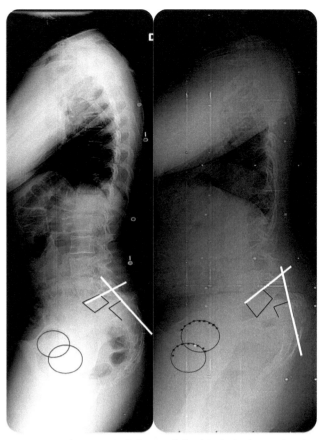

Fig. 12.17 Subtypes 5a and 5b: in 5a (left side), the lumbosacral angle ([LSA], in white) is ≥ 80°. In 5b, LSA is < 80°.

L5-S1 Spondylolisthesis Classification

Fig. 12.18 Clinical relevance.

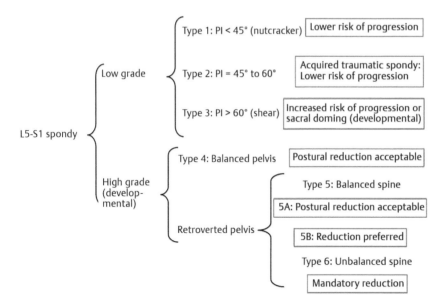

L5-S1 spondy
- Low grade
  - Type 1: PI < 45° (nutcracker) — Lower risk of progression
  - Type 2: PI = 45° to 60° — Acquired traumatic spondy: Lower risk of progression
  - Type 3: PI > 60° (shear) — Increased risk of progression or sacral doming (developmental)
- High grade (developmental)
  - Type 4: Balanced pelvis — Postural reduction acceptable
  - Retroverted pelvis
    - Type 5: Balanced spine
      - 5A: Postural reduction acceptable
      - 5B: Reduction preferred
    - Type 6: Unbalanced spine
      - Mandatory reduction

and 2 with lower or normal PI may be lower than in the shear type 3 with abnormally high PI and SS values, imposing higher shear stresses at the L5-S1 junction. In these subjects as well as those with type 4 alignment, there is an increased lumbar lordosis to keep the center of gravity and C7 plumb line behind the hips to maintain a balanced posture.

Asymptomatic individuals with an incidental finding of spondylolysis or low-grade, low-dysplastic developmental spondylolisthesis require no treatment or activity restrictions. However, high dysplastic patients are at greater risk for progression and should be seen at regular intervals (6 months) with radiographs until skeletal maturity.

12.7.2 Clinical Relevance for HGS: Reduction versus Fusion in Situ?

The traditional treatment for HGS has been in situ posterolateral L5-S1 fusion with no attempt at reduction of the slip, and several publications over the past decades have shown good long-term results with this approach. In previous decades, in situ L5-S1 fusion techniques have been associated with fewer neurological complications than reduction, instrumentation, and circumferential fusion techniques, but at the expense of less improvement in sagittal alignment and a higher risk of pseudarthrosis. In an evidence-based literature review done up until 2007 on the subject of reduction versus in situ fusion, Transfeldt and Mehbod[25] were unable to identify any level I or II evidence on this subject, the best evidence being provided by five retrospective comparative studies (level III). They were thus unable to formulate clear guidelines for treatment of HGS based on the best evidence available in the published literature.

Has anything changed over the past decade? While the need for reduction in the surgical treatment of HGS is still debated, there has been a clear shift of choice of surgical technique by spinal surgeons away from the traditional in situ posterolateral L5-S1 fusion toward reduction, instrumentation, and circumferential fusion. This is supported by the fact that almost all articles on HGS published in the past decade report on instrumentation ± reduction of HGS. The only reports discussing in situ fusion without instrumentation are long-term results of cases done prior to this decade. This evolution in technique can be explained by two factors: first, an improved understanding of sagittal spinopelvic alignment, which is the subject of this chapter and, second, improved methods of reduction, fusion, and spinopelvic fixation with the use of pedicle screws and improved sacropelvic methods of fixation.

In HGS, sacropelvic morphology is clearly abnormal and creates an abnormal sacropelvic orientation as well as a disturbed global sagittal balance of the hip–spine axis. These findings have important implications for the evaluation and treatment of patients with spondylolisthesis, and especially for those with a high-grade slip. Although more outcome studies are needed before a definitive treatment algorithm can be established for each type of spondylolisthesis in the classification presented previously, it is suggested that for subjects with a type 4 spinopelvic posture, forceful attempts at reduction of the deformity may not be required and that instrumentation and fusion after simple postural reduction by prone positioning of patients under anesthesia on the operating table may be all that is necessary to maintain adequate

sagittal alignment, as adequate sagittal spinopelvic alignment is already present in these subjects. For subjects with a type 5 posture, in which the pelvis is unbalanced, reduction and realignment procedures should preferably be attempted; but in subtype 5a, instrumentation and fusion after postural reduction may also be sufficient to achieve adequate sagittal alignment, as spinal alignment is maintained and LSK is within normal limits. Reduction and realignment procedures would appear to be necessary in type 5b and 6 deformities where sagittal alignment is severely disturbed. While the need for reduction in the surgical treatment of L5-S1 spondylolisthesis is still debated, a recent therapeutic level III evidence-based review[26] supports the contention that reduction of HGS improves overall spine biomechanics by correcting the local kyphotic deformity and reducing vertebral slippage, and that reduction is not associated with a greater risk of developing neurologic deficits compared with arthrodesis in situ.

In the recent largest multicenter study of the results of reduction in HGS, Mac-Thiong et al[27] compared the HRQoL using the SRS-22 questionnaire before and after surgery in young patients with low- and high-grade lumbosacral spondylolisthesis, and demonstrated that HRQoL was significantly improved by surgery, especially for high-grade patients. Thus, while the need for reduction in the surgical treatment of L5-S1 spondylolisthesis is still debated, many studies published in the last decade support the value of this classification for the decision-making process.[26,27,28,29,30]

12.7.3 How and What to Reduce?

The goals of surgery in high-grade developmental L5-S1 spondylolisthesis are to prevent progression, to restore global spinal alignment and normal biomechanics, and to relieve symptoms. The decision to proceed with surgical treatment may include the following:

- The degree of slip (greater than 50% in the growing child or greater than 75% in a skeletally mature adolescent).
- The documentation of progression beyond 30% slippage.
- The persistence of functional impairment, pain, or neurological symptoms despite appropriate nonsurgical treatment.
- Progressive postural deformity (cosmetic dissatisfaction) or gait abnormality.

A variety of techniques and methods of fixation for achieving reduction and/or fusion have been proposed, with posterior spinopelvic fixation coupled with L5-S1 interbody support by posterior lumbar interbody fusion/transforaminal lumbar interbody fusion now performed by most authors. Significant improvement of sagittal balance is noted after surgical reduction of HGS.[31,32] Whatever the surgeon's preferred technique, Agabegi and Fischgrund[30] concluded, in a recent literature review, that circumferential (360°) fusion is superior to posterolateral fusion in HGS, resulting in a decreased incidence of pseudarthrosis, and that achieving a solid fusion improves outcome. This is also supported by the study of Mac-Thiong et al,[27] the largest series to demonstrate improved HRQoL after reduction in HGS.

Whatever the technique used during surgery, the first goal should be to reduce as completely as possible the L5-S1 LSK,[32] as this is the primary abnormality causing pelvic retroversion and progressive imbalance of the hip-pelvis-spine axis (▶ Fig. 12.19). A secondary goal is partial grade reduction, which allows the proper placement of a cage/graft in the interbody L5-S1 space and compression of the instrumentation, resulting in a fixation system that is in compression rather that in distraction. Complete reduction of HGS is not necessary and is a potential cause of neurological impairment.[33] Distraction forces applied posteriorly should be avoided if possible as they will create a kyphotic moment at the L5-S1 junction. Sebaaly et al[15] have proposed that the simplest method to assess the quality of the reduction intraoperatively as well as postoperatively is by the measurement of L5I, which can be done even after the instrumentation is in place. Proper reduction of L5I to a value < 60° is a good indicator of proper restoration of sagittal balance (▶ Fig. 12.20).

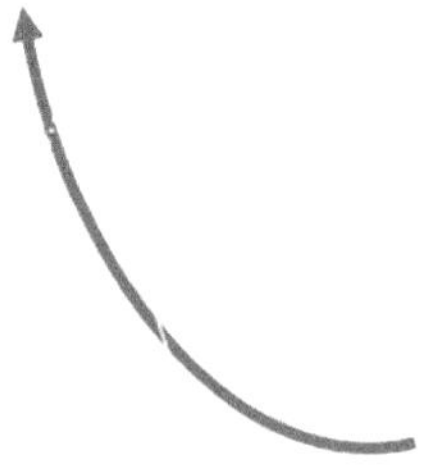

12.8 Conclusion

Global sagittal plane alignment is important to consider in both adult and pediatric patients with L5-S1 spondylolisthesis. Clinicians treating this disorder need to be aware that normal

Fig. 12.19 What to reduce: first the L5-S1 kyphosis, then partial slip grade reduction.

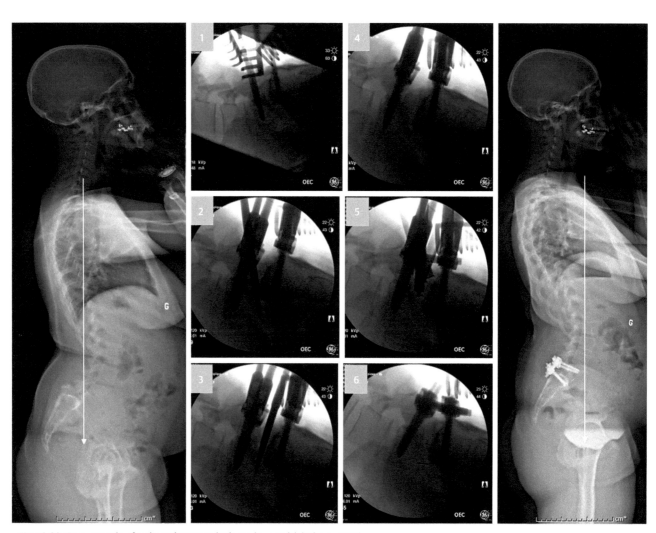

Fig. 12.20 Case example of a slip reduction in high-grade spondylolisthesis (HGS).

sagittal balance of the hip-spinopelvic axis is frequently disrupted and that it is insufficient to limit their evaluation and base their treatment plan strictly on the local L5-S1 area. Abnormal spinopelvic alignment alters the biomechanical stresses at the lumbosacral junction, and compensation mechanisms are developed to maintain an adequate posture. A classification based on sagittal alignment is proposed to help treatment decisions.

In patients with HGS associated with a postural abnormality, it is important to reduce and realign the spinal deformity, thus restoring global spinal alignment and improving the biomechanical environment for fusion. Recent evidence[26,27,28,29] supports the contention that reduction of HGS improves overall global hip-spinopelvic balance by correcting the local kyphotic deformity and partly reducing vertebral slippage, and that reduction is not associated with a greater risk of developing neurologic deficits compared with arthrodesis in situ.

References

[1] Mardjetko S, Albert T, Andersson G, et al. Spine/SRS spondylolisthesis summary statement. Spine. 2005; 30(6) Suppl:S3

[2] Deschênes S, Charron G, Beaudoin G, et al. Diagnostic imaging of spinal deformities: reducing patients radiation dose with a new slot-scanning X-ray imager. Spine. 2010; 35(9):989–994

[3] Fredrickson BE, Baker D, McHolick WJ, Yuan HA, Lubicky JP. The natural history of spondylolysis and spondylolisthesis. J Bone Joint Surg Am. 1984; 66 (5):699–707

[4] Tardieu C, Bonneau N, Hecquet J, et al. How is sagittal balance acquired during bipedal gait acquisition? Comparison of neonatal and adult pelves in 3D. Evolutionary implications. J Hum Evol. 2013; 6; 5(2):209–222

[5] Meyerding HW. Spondylolisthesis. Surg Gynecol Obstet. 1932; 54:371–377

[6] Wiltse LL, Newman PH, Macnab I. Classification of spondylolysis and spondylolisthesis. Clin Orthop Relat Res. 1976; 117:23–29

[7] Marchetti PC, Bartolozzi P. Classification of spondylolisthesis as a guideline for treatment. In: Bridwell KH, DeWald RL, Hammerberg KW, et al., eds. The Textbook of Spinal Surgery. 2nd ed. Philadelphia, PA: Lippincott-Raven; 1997:1211–1254

[8] Bourassa-Moreau E, Mac-Thiong J-M, Labelle H. Redefining the technique for the radiologic measurement of slip in spondylolisthesis. Spine. 2010; 35 (14):1401–1405

[9] Labelle H, Mac-Thiong JM. Sacro-pelvic morphology, spino-pelvic alignment and the Spinal Deformity Study Group classification. In: The Textbook of Spinal Surgery. Chap. 59. Philadelphia, PA: Lippincott Williams & Wilkins; 2011

[10] Labelle H, Mac-Thiong JM, Parent S. Pediatric spondylolisthesis. In: Chapman's Comprehensive Orthopaedic Surgery. Chap. 232. 4th ed. New Delhi, India: Jaypee Brothers; 2018

[11] Roussouly P, Labelle H, Berthonnaud E, Hu S, Brown C. The relationship between pelvic balance and a dome-shaped sacrum in L5-S1 spondylolisthesis. Podium presentation at: SRS Meeting, 2009, San Antonio, TX

[12] Labelle H, Roussouly P, Berthonnaud E, et al. Spondylolisthesis, pelvic incidence, and spinopelvic balance: a correlation study. Spine. 2004; 29 (18):2049–2054

[13] Wang Z, Parent S, Mac-Thiong JM, Petit Y, Labelle H. Influence of sacral morphology in developmental spondylolisthesis. Spine. 2008; 33(20):2185–2191

[14] Labelle H, Roussouly P, Berthonnaud E, Dimnet J, O'Brien M. The importance of spino-pelvic balance in L5-S1 developmental spondylolisthesis: a review of pertinent radiologic measurements. Spine. 2005; 30(6) Suppl:S27–S34

[15] Sebaaly A, El Rachkidi R, Grobost P, Burnier M, Labelle H, Roussouly P. L5 incidence: an important parameter for spinopelvic balance evaluation in high grade spondylolisthesis. Spine. 2018;18(8):1417–1423

[16] Roussouly P, Gollogly S, Berthonnaud E, Labelle H, Weidenbaum M. Sagittal alignment of the spine and pelvis in the presence of L5-S1 isthmic lysis and low-grade spondylolisthesis. Spine. 2006; 31(21):2484–2490

[17] Hresko MT, Labelle H, Roussouly P, Berthonnaud E. Classification of high-grade spondylolistheses based on pelvic version and spine balance: possible rationale for reduction. Spine. 2007; 32(20):2208–2213

[18] Mac-Thiong J-M, Wang Z, de Guise JA, Labelle H. Postural model of sagittal spino-pelvic alignment and its relevance for lumbosacral developmental spondylolisthesis. Spine. 2008; 33(21):2316–2325

[19] Tanguay F, Labelle H, Wang Z, Joncas J, de Guise JA, Mac-Thiong JM. Clinical significance of lumbosacral kyphosis in adolescent spondylolisthesis. Spine. 2012; 37(4):304–308

[20] Glavas P, Mac-Thiong J-M, Parent S, de Guise JA, Labelle H. Assessment of lumbosacral kyphosis in spondylolisthesis: a computer-assisted reliability study of six measurement techniques. Eur Spine J. 2009; 18(2):212–217

[21] Harroud A, Labelle H, Joncas J, Mac-Thiong JM. Global sagittal alignment and health-related quality of life in lumbosacral spondylolisthesis. Eur Spine J. 2013; 22(4):849–856

[22] Mac-Thiong JM, Parent S, Joncas J, Barchi S, Labelle H. The importance of proximal femoral angle on sagittal balance and quality of life in high-grade lumbosacral spondylolisthesis. Eur Spine J. 201 8; 27(8):2038–2043

[23] Labelle H, Mac-Thiong JM, Roussouly P. Spino-pelvic sagittal balance of spondylolisthesis: a review and classification. Eur Spine J. 2011; 20(5) Suppl 5:641–646

[24] Mac-Thiong JM, Duong L, Parent S, et al. Reliability of the Spinal Deformity Study Group classification of lumbosacral spondylolisthesis. Spine. 2012; 37 (2):E95–E102

[25] Transfeldt EE, Mehbod AA. Evidence-based medicine analysis of isthmic spondylolisthesis treatment including reduction versus fusion in situ for high-grade slips. Spine. 2007; 32(19) Suppl:S126–S129

[26] Longo UG, Loppini M, Romeo G, Maffulli N, Denaro V. Evidence-based surgical management of spondylolisthesis: reduction or arthrodesis in situ. J Bone Joint Surg Am. 2014; 96(1):53–58

[27] Mac-Thiong J-M, Labelle H, Parent S, et al. A prospective study of the improvement in health-related quality of life following surgical treatment of lumbosacral spondylolisthesis in young patients. Podium presentation at: SRS Annual Meeting, 2016, Milwaukee, WI

[28] Labelle H, Parent S, Mac-Thiong JM, et al. High grade spondylolisthesis in adolescents: reduction and circumferential fusion improves health related quality of life and sagittal balance. Podium presentation at: Scoliosis Research Society Annual Meeting, October 2018, Bologna, Italy

[29] Martiniani M, Lamartina C, Specchia N. "In situ" fusion or reduction in high-grade high dysplastic developmental spondylolisthesis (HDSS). Eur Spine J. 2012; 21 Suppl 1:S134–S140

[30] Agabegi SS, Fischgrund JS. Contemporary management of isthmic spondylolisthesis: pediatric and adult. Spine J. 2010; 10(6):530–543

[31] Labelle H, Roussouly P, Chopin D, Berthonnaud E, Hresko T, O'Brien M. Spino-pelvic alignment after surgical correction for developmental spondylolisthesis. Eur Spine J. 2008; 17(9):1170–1176

[32] Sailhan F, Gollogly S, Roussouly P. The radiographic results and neurologic complications of instrumented reduction and fusion of high-grade spondylolisthesis without decompression of the neural elements: a retrospective review of 44 patients. Spine. 2006; 31(2):161–169, discussion 170

[33] Petraco DM, Spivak JM, Cappadona JG, Kummer FJ, Neuwirth MG. An anatomic evaluation of L5 nerve stretch in spondylolisthesis reduction. Spine. 1996; 21(10):1133–1138, discussion 1139

[34] Mac-Thiong J-M, Labelle H, Berthonnaud E, Betz RR, Roussouly P. Sagittal spinopelvic balance in normal children and adolescents. Eur Spine J. 2007; 16 (2):227–234

[35] Berthonnaud E, Dimnet J, Roussouly P, Labelle H. Analysis of the sagittal balance of the spine and pelvis using shape and orientation parameters. J Spinal Disord Tech. 2005; 18(1):40–47

13 Degenerative Spondylolisthesis: Does the Sagittal Balance Matter?

Cédric Y. Barrey, Charles Peltier, Amir El Rahal, Théo Broussolle, and Pierre Roussouly

Abstract

This chapter focuses on the importance of considering the sagittal balance in the surgical treatment of lumbar degenerative spondylolisthesis (DS). The chapter includes epidemiology, prevalence, pathophysiology, imaging, and management of DS.

Keywords: degenerative spondylolisthesis, spinal stenosis, foraminal stenosis, posterior facets arthritis, L4-L5 discopathy, listhesis grade of slippage, Roussouly's classification, TLIF, posterior spinal fusion

13.1 General Considerations

13.1.1 Definition

Spondylolisthesis is defined as slippage of a vertebra in relation to the vertebra below (▶ Fig. 13.1). The slippage may be anterior, that is, anterolisthesis; posterior, that is, retrolisthesis; lateral, that is, laterolisthesis; or rotatory, that is, rotatory subluxation. Degenerative spondylolisthesis (DS) is most often associated with arthritic changes in the facet joints at the level of the listhesis. It differs from isthmic spondylolisthesis by the absence of a pars interarticularis defect and was first described as early as 1930 by Junghanns who introduced the term "pseudo-spondylolisthesis."[1] In 1950, MacNab[2] described spondylolisthesis "with the neural arch intact" as opposed to the spondylolisthesis of children and adolescents by isthmic lysis and, finally, Newman in 1963[3] proposed the term "degenerative spondylolisthesis" considering that DS was quasi-systematically associated with facet arthritis. In the lumbar spine, it usually occurs in patients over 50 years of age, with female predominance and ligament hyperlaxity as a predisposing factor. DS corresponds to type III according to the Wiltse[4] spondylolisthesis classification modified by the Scoliosis Research Society.[5]

13.1.2 Epidemiology and Prevalence

The DS is most commonly found at the L4-L5 level (80% to 85% of cases) in opposition to isthmic spondylolisthesis, which occurs most commonly at the L5-S1 level.[6] DS is rarely observed at L5-S1 for anatomical reasons. First, the frontal orientation of S1 facets represents a solid barrier to anteroposterior (AP) slippage and, second, there is an abundance of ligament structures around the L5-S1 complex with the presence of the strong iliolumbar ligaments. Prevalence is variable according to age and sex, augmented by a factor of 4 in the female population and is estimated to be ~ 10% after 60 years old for females (up to 43% referring to population-based studies).[7,8,9]

13.1.3 Imaging Findings

Positive diagnosis of DS is established on standards X-rays in a standing posture. The diagnosis is generally retained when the slippage is greater than 3 mm or when the slippage is measured to more than 10% according to the Meyerding classification. One must pay attention to the fact that around 20% of DS is undetected on magnetic resonance imaging (MRI).[10] Also, MRI typically underestimates the slippage by approximately 50%. Therefore, standing radiographs should be systematically performed for the management of lumbar degenerative disorders in addition to lying imaging modalities (computed tomography [CT] scan and/or MRI) (▶ Fig. 13.2).

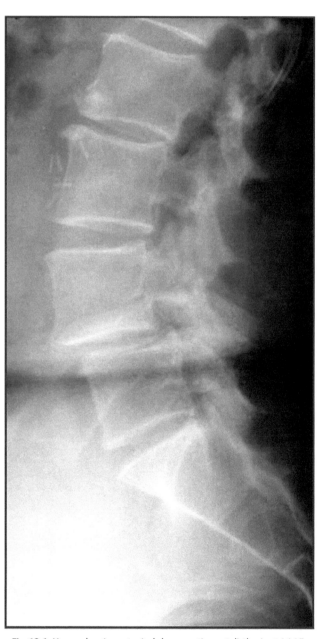

Fig. 13.1 X-rays showing a typical degenerative antelisthesis at L4-L5, low grade, with a slippage less than 25% (grade I according to Meyerding).

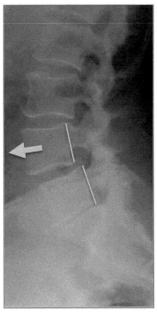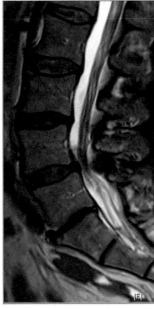

Fig. 13.2 Increase of the listhesis on standing X-rays in comparison with magnetic resonance imaging (MRI) findings. In 20% of cases, listhesis is undetected on lying imaging modalities (MRI and/or computed tomography scan).

13.2 Pathophysiology

Factors influencing the occurrence and/or progression of DS can be divided into general factors, regional factors (including the sagittal balance), and local factors.

13.2.1 General Factors

Genetic

It is unclear in the literature that genetical factors have been evoked to explain the increased frequency in certain populations and families without knowing precisely the role of posture and habitus. DS is more frequent in elderly Caucasian Americans, around 31% after 74 years old.[11] Prevalence estimates among women range from 8% in Denmark, 8.9% in Japan,[12] 12% in Thailand,[13] to ~ 25% in the United States.[14]

Obesity

Obesity seems to be a key factor with increasing stress on facet joints and disks. Schuller et al.[15] found a mean body mass index (BMI) in the DS group equal to 28 versus 24 in the control group without DS, and 70% of patients with DS presented with a BMI > 25. The continuous high load accelerates posterior disk and zygapophyseal degeneration and may, therefore, favor the development of DS.

Hormonal Factors

DS is constantly reported more frequently in women than men younger than 50 years old. Jacobsen[16] found a prevalence of DS in women of 8.3% versus only 2.7% for men. Otherwise, Enyo et al[6] reported a risk of female slip progression 3.5 times greater than in men because of joint laxity and instability. There is also

a high proportion of patients with ligament hyperlaxity; up to 65% of patients according to Postacchini. Cholewicki et al[17] found a risk of developing spondylolisthesis in women who experienced multiparity and hysterectomies.

Sanderson and Fraser[18] found an association between nulliparous and parous women and DS (28% vs. 16%) and the incidence of DS increased in parallel with the number of pregnancies. Many physiological changes during pregnancy, including relaxation of the pelvic and increase of the flexion moment on the lower back, play an essential role in the progression of listhesis.

Hyperlaxity

In the presence of hyperlaxity, Matsunaga et al[19] reported that the prevalence of DS was augmented by a factor of 8.

Age

Age represents one of the main factors in the natural history of DS, with a clear progressive increase in incidence after the age of 50 years old, which is greater in women than in men.[20]

13.2.2 Regional Anatomical Factors

Spinopelvic Alignment

We previously reported in 2004[21,22,23] that patients with DS were associated with a greater pelvic incidence (PI) compared to the normal population. Roussouly's spinopelvic morphotypes 3 and 4 represented more than 85% of DS patients versus only 60% in the control group. In our study, mean PI was measured at 60° versus only 52° for the control group.

PI and high lumbar lordosis represent important risk factors for the development of DS caused by stresses on the posterior elements and to the inclination of the L5 upper endplate. Since our work, many studies have confirmed the association between high PI and DS patients[21,22,24,25,26] with a mean PI of ~ 58°–60° in DS patients.

We assume that a high PI represents a risk factor for three main reasons:

1. High PI is associated with a high sacral slope (SS) and high inclination of the sacral plate and L5 endplates (inferior and superior L5 endplates). Because of gravity, the higher the slope, the higher the risk of slippage.
2. High PI is associated with hyperlordosis and stresses on the posterior structures of the lumbar spine, especially on posterior facets, which may favor degenerative changes of L4-L5 facets, making them less resistant to slippage.
3. Finally, high PI and hyperlordosis influence the geometry of the lumbar spine, reducing the space available for the posterior elements and making them more compact. By limiting the craniocaudal development of posterior arches, hyperlordosis reduces their ability to resist AP shear forces.

Further considerations about spinopelvic alignment and DS will be discussed in Section 3 of this chapter.

Sacralization of L5

Lumbosacral transition vertebra is the most common congenital anomaly of the lumbosacral spine with 8.1% in the general population,[27] but observed at high rates in DS at L4-L5 (up to 70%

according to Kong et al.[28]). Sacralization of L5 leads to a higher concentration of stresses on the L4-L5 segment with the risk of hypermobility.

Degenerative Ankylosis of L5-S1

For the same reasons as above, degenerative evolution of L5-S1 segment will result in hypermobility of the upper adjacent segment with the risk of developing a DS at this level.[7]

13.2.3 Local Factors

Local factors are represented by some specific anatomical variations of the involved vertebra at the index level.

Sagittal Orientation of the Facets

The facet joints play an essential role in segment balance and stability. The orientation of the facets may limit the amount of axial rotation and increase torsion resistance. Many authors[29,30,31,32,33] assume that the sagittal orientation of the facets at the index level is associated with a reduction of resistance to shear forces in the AP direction and may favor the occurrence of anterolisthesis. Sato et al[30] found that the sagittal orientation of the facet joints led to an increased risk of slippage as a result of greater and inadequately distributed stresses. Liu et al[29] in a literature review found a significant association

between sagitalization of facets and the appearance of DS. The transverse facet angle of more than 50° represents a significative factor of listhesis. This angle was found to be around 60° in the DS population versus 40° in the normal population.

Horizontalization of the Posterior Arch

Another anatomical variation that may favor the slippage is represented by a horizontal orientation of the posterior arch of the index vertebra. Once again, horizontalization of the posterior elements (lamina, facets) offers less resistance to AP shear forces with the risk to favor AP translation of the vertebra.[19,34]

Controversy

There is some controversy regarding the role played by the local anatomy in the development of DS as some authors[35] consider that these anatomical variations result mainly from the degenerative changes. They are mostly the consequence of the DS and not the primary cause.

13.3 Spinopelvic Alignment

Roussouly et al[36] (▶ Fig. 13.3) described a classification into four morphotypes of back depending on PI and SS. Type 1 is characterized by a SS of less than 35°, low PI, and, consequently, short

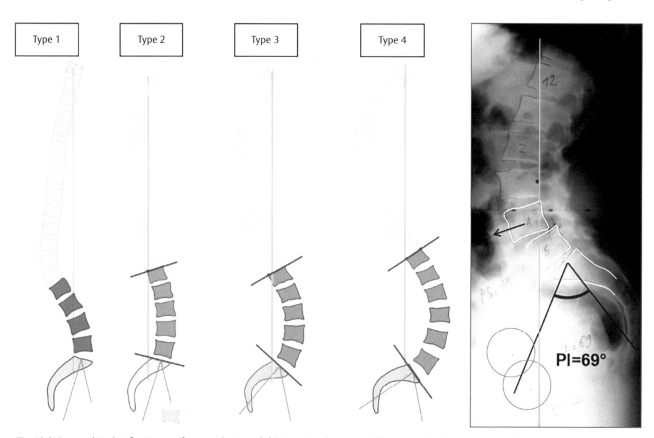

Fig. 13.3 Roussouly's classification into four morphotypes (left). Type 1 is characterized by a short lumbar lordosis and a long thoracolumbar kyphosis above, and types 2, 3, and 4 represent harmonious types with a progressive increase of pelvic incidence, sacral slope, and spinal curvatures from type 2 to type 4. Types 3 and 4 with pelvic incidence (PI) around 60°–70° (right) represent the typical predisposing morphotype for degenerative spondylolisthesis (DS).

lumbar lordosis, which predispose to arthritis of posterior elements (facets, spinous processes). Type 2, "flat" back, is characterized by low SS (<35°), low PI, and low lumbar lordosis that is longer and more harmonious and predisposes to premature disk degeneration. The type 3 back is the most common in the general population and is characterized by harmonious curves. The SS is between 35° and 45° and PI is around 50°–52°. Type 4 lordosis is characterized by a high PI with a pronounced SS (>45°) and by a compensation effect of marked sagittal curvatures that may cause spondylolisthesis or lumbar stenosis.

In the DS population, 85% of patients present with a morphotype 3 or 4 and mean PI ~ 60° (Barrey), which is significantly different from the normal population. Also, it has been reported that the lordosis was slightly reduced with a mean lack of lordosis ~ 10°. It was noted that the L1-S1 lordosis was not so reduced but that the lordosis was generally significantly reduced at the L4-S1 segment with compensation in the upper lumbar spine.[15,22] The disk degeneration associated with the anterior slippage at the index level results in a local loss of lordosis, which is needed for compensation in the upper lumbar spine (extension of L1-L4 segments). In most cases, the local loss of lordosis because of DS is limited, and the compensation provided by a slight extension of the adjacent spine above works very well.

The global balance is typically preserved even if some amount of pelvic compensation may be noted with increased PT and decreased SS. Most of the variations were regional except in the cases of multilevel DS with severe and global lumbar kyphosis (▶ Fig. 13.4).

It is also important to analyze the sagittal orientation of the slippage (▶ Fig. 13.4). This may occur in a neutral direction with the slippage progressing parallel to the superior endplate of L5. The slippage may be in extension, permitting local compensation of the lack of lordosis and thus limiting the consequences of the DS on the sagittal balance. The drawback of DS in extension is the risk of inducing canal stenosis and foraminal stenosis with the development of radicular symptoms. The latter situation is represented by the slippage in flexion, which is the worst situation regarding balance and generally associated with global sagittal imbalance. On the other hand, the slippage in flexion permits opening the canal, increasing the foramen size, and

decompressing the neurological structures. In the end, there is no perfect situation; both have consequences on balance on one side and the risk of canal stenosis on the other side. DS represents a degenerative disk disease (DDD) of the spine that exposes the patient to the risk of kyphosis and stenosis.

Finally, we must underline the situation of multilevel DS, which induces an important lack of lordosis in the lumbar spine because of multilevel slippages and multilevel DDD in the lumbar spine (▶ Fig. 13.5). They represent ~ 5%–8% of DS patients.[19] In this situation, the surgical strategy must restore adequately the lumbar lordosis and sagittal alignment and generally requires extensive instrumentation of the lumbar spine.

Similarly, when DS is associated with multilevel DDD, there is an additive effect of the segmental loss of lordosis, and, in the end, the deficit of lumbar lordosis is great even if not only a result of the DS. In the case of DS associated with multilevel DDD, especially at the level below (L5-S1) and above (L3-L4), the disease presents more as a degenerative lumbar kyphosis than a simple "one-level disease" with DS.

13.4 Natural History of Degenerative Spondylolisthesis

In DS, sliding rarely exceeds 30% (grades I–II). In contrast to isthmic lysis, the posterior arch in DS stays intact and, therefore, it limits the possibility for the vertebra to slip more than a few millimeters. High-grade DS is very rare, and low-grade sliding around 3 to 10 mm represents the rule for DS. Also, it has been observed that the slippage progresses in parallel with the disk degeneration and reaches its maximal grade when the disk is completely collapsed and ankylosed (similar to what is observed for isthmic listhesis) (▶ Fig. 13.6). Through a cohort of 145 nonsurgical patients with a minimum of 10 years followup (10 to 18 years), Matsunaga et al.[19] observed that the progression of slippage was typically minimal and more than 25% for 7% of patients only (n = 10). Also, the authors noted that the slippage progresses in almost all patients (96%, i.e., n = 49/51 patients) when the disk height was initially normal, confirming the fact that the slippage progresses in parallel with the disk degeneration.

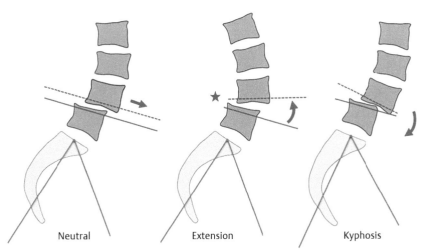

Neutral   Extension   Kyphosis

Fig. 13.4 Sagittal orientation of degenerative spondylolisthesis may be in neutral, extension, or kyphosis with different consequences in terms of alignment and compromise of neurological structures. Local extension permits rebalancing the patient but exposes him or her to the risk of nerve roots compression in the foramens. Local kyphosis increases the different parts of the canal but induces a severe situation regarding the balance.

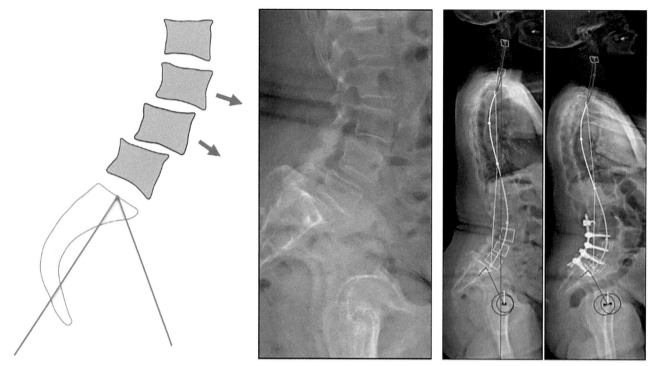

Fig. 13.5 Multilevel degenerative spondylolisthesis, observed in around 5%–8% of cases, results in a global imbalance with a kyphotic deformity of the lumbar spine. This situation generally requires extensive instrumentation of the spine to rebalance the patient.

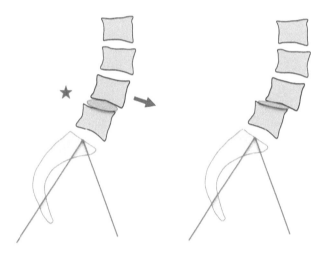

Fig. 13.6 Progression of the slippage in parallel to the progression of disk degeneration.

Seeing the degenerative lesions associated with DS and their sequence, it is possible to establish the natural history of DS, and this was published by our team in *Neurosurgery* in 2007[22] (▶ Fig. 13.7). First, there is a predisposing morphotype, and this was largely confirmed by several papers after our publication in 2004.[21,22,23,24,25,26] This favoring morphotype consists of Roussouly's morphotype type 3 or 4 characterized by an increased PI with a mean value of 60°. Also, the first anatomical lesion is represented by the degenerative subluxation of posterior facets. DS with normal facet joints are not the rule, and this was already observed by Newman in the 1960s. Also, at the

first stage, the disk may be normal, in contrast to the facets joints. Consequently, we may logically assume that the disease starts in the facet joints on a predisposing morphotype.

The slippage then progresses in parallel to the disk degeneration and results in segmental loss of lordosis. The combination of the anterior shift and the disk collapse induces a significant local kyphosis. This effect may be potentialized in the cases of adjacent DDD, especially at L5-S1. In most patients, the need for compensation is limited and slight pelvis back tilt (increased PT) with moderate extension of the upper lumbar spine is enough to keep the global balance of the spine (▶ Fig. 13.7).

Hyperextension of the upper lumbar spine (L1-L4 segments) in DS patients was reported in the literature[15,22] and, in some patients, may result in true instability and retrolisthesis. In general, compensation in the upper lumbar spine is observed when the loss of lordosis in the lower part (between L4 and sacrum) is significant and severe, and this is not specific for DS patients but all patients with kyphotic disease between L4 and the sacrum.

13.5 Degenerative Lesions Associated with Degenerative Spondylolisthesis

To describe the degenerative lesions associated with DS, we propose to refer to Kirkaldy-Willis stages, which divide the degenerative natural history of functional segment unit degeneration into three stages:
1. Dysfunction characterized by microlesions of the disk, capsules, and cartilages and normal imagery.

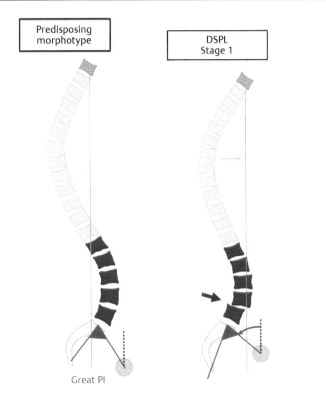
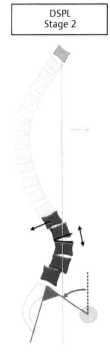

Fig. 13.7 Natural history of degenerative spondylolisthesis (DSPL). Existence of predisposing morphotype with progressive development of local loss of lordosis as a result of the slippage and disk degeneration. In most cases, the global balance is preserved, and only regional compensation takes place.[22] PI, Pelvic incidence.

2. Instability characterized by hyperlaxity, appearance of the slippage, and the risk to develop a synovial cyst. At this stage, the disk is still high, and the slippage is typically reduced between a standing and lying position. Instability results in a "dynamic" stenosis.
3. Restabilization characterized by the development of severe degenerative lesions of both the disks and facets with osteophytes and disk collapse. The slippage is typically fixed at this stage whatever the position of the patient.
   Restabilization results in a "fixed" stenosis.

13.5.1 Instability Stage

The instability, which can be defined by an abnormal displacement on dynamic X-rays, is not the rule and is rarely observed for DS. It corresponds to the initial phase of the degenerative process. Most authors consider more than 3 mm of translation and/or more than 15° of angular motion on dynamic X-rays as instability.

For low-grade listhesis at the initial phase, the slippage may completely reduce in a lying position, especially on MRI and CT scan imaging, and, therefore, standing X-rays always have to be performed. Chaput et al[10] found that around 20% of DS were not detected on lying MRI.

A synovial cyst develops during the early phase of DS and is synonymous with instability. It develops most frequently at L4-L5 and is associated with DS in 60% up to 90% of cases. The synovial cyst may contribute to nerve root compression when growing inside the canal, resulting especially into compression of the nerve root in the lateral recess. Central canal stenosis may occur in the case of a giant cyst. In 80% of patients with a synovial cyst, intra-articular fluid collection is observed on lying MRI. It has been reported that fluid collection in the

facets superior to 1.5 mm was highly predictive of the presence of DS.[10]

13.5.2 Restabilization

After the initial phase of hypermobility and hyperlaxity, the spinal unit is characterized by the progressive development of arthritic lesions and ankylosis. At this stage, the DS is no longer mobile, the disk is typically collapsed, and there is no motion on dynamic X-rays, either standing or lying down (▶ Fig. 13.8).

At this stage, hypertrophy and arthritic changes of the superior and inferior facets of the functional spinal unit result in the compression of the nerve root in the lateral part of the canal. The compression in the lateral recess may be consecutive to the anterior subluxation of the lower facet or by the hypertrophy of the superior facet. For L4-L5 DS, the L5 nerve root is typically compressed into the L5 lateral recess as a result of degenerative changes of L4-L5 facets (▶ Fig. 13.9). Lateral stenosis with respect of the central canal represents a frequent situation for DS (▶ Fig. 13.10).

In severe cases, the DS may result in both lateral and central stenosis of the canal. AP translation, hypertrophy of the yellow ligament, and bilateral hypertrophy of facets, may lead to central stenosis with the risk for the patient to develop chronic cauda equina syndrome (▶ Fig. 13.11). Otherwise, at the advanced stage of the degenerative process with complete disk collapse, DS is often associated with a foraminal stenosis at the level of the slippage. Thus, for L4-L5 DS, the foraminal stenosis is observed at L4-L5 with compression of the L4 nerve roots. Foraminal stenosis is multifactorial and consecutive to different mechanisms, including disk collapse, osteophytes from the superior facet, and/or AP translation of the vertebra.

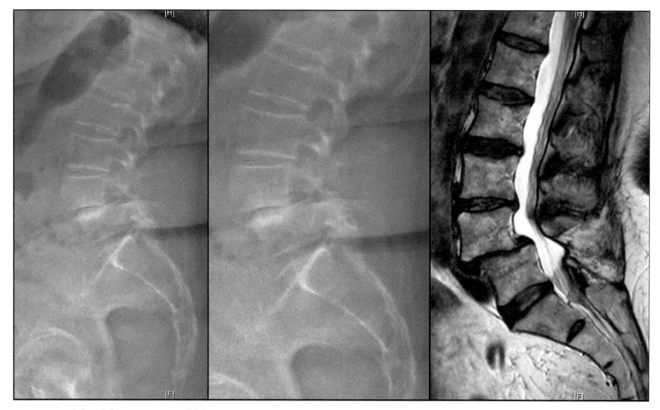

Fig. 13.8 Ankylosed degenerative spondylolisthesis. No variation is observed between standing X-rays and lying magnetic resonance imaging. The disk is completely collapsed.

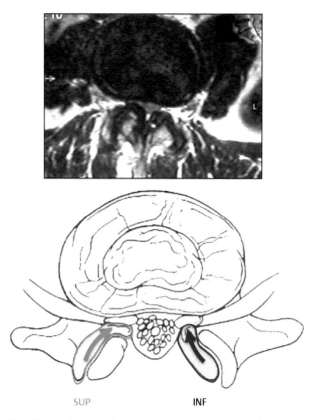

Fig. 13.9 Mechanisms of nerve roots compression into the lateral recess. This may be consecutive to the subluxation of the inferior (INF) facet (brown) but also to the hypertrophic arthritic changes of the superior (SUP) facet (blue).

SUP   INF

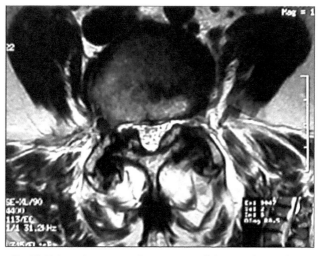

Fig. 13.10 Lateral stenosis with no stenosis of the central part of the canal. On the left side, compression is a result of the subluxation of the facet and, on the right side, compression is consecutive to the osteophytes coming from the superior facet.

13.6 Management of Degenerative Spondylolisthesis

13.6.1 General Considerations

DS represents a stenotic and kyphotic disease of the lumbar spine and, therefore, both these issues must be addressed during management, especially during surgical treatment.

Conservative treatment remains the first-line treatment in management in the absence of neurological deficit and severe stenosis. Matsunaga[19] studied the fate of 110 symptomatic patients for 10 years. He shows that, in patients with radiculalgia, conservative treatment combined with natural progression allows total cessation of pain in 86% of cases but with a recurrence rate of 35%. In the case of neurological deficit (cauda equina syndrome, sphincter disorders, motor weakness), surgery should be strongly considered.

13.6.2 Decompression Alone

There is no real consensus about DS surgery in the literature for symptomatic grade I associated with spinal stenosis regarding the need for systematic instrumentation of the spine.

Ghogawala et al[37] reported a randomized study (comparing spinal laminectomy alone versus associated with instrumented fusion with pedicular screws) that found no significant difference in terms of functional outcomes among patients with DS treated by decompression and fusion versus decompression alone but a greater score in SF-36 and a higher risk of slipping progression and reoperation (14% vs. 34%, respectively) in the case of isolated decompression. The study consisted of a multicenter randomized controlled study with 4 years follow-up and 66 patients included in the study.

The advantage of decompression alone is represented by its relative simplicity with a low complication rate because of the absence of implants,[38] but it should be reserved only for patients who cannot undergo fusion surgery. One must note that adequate nerve root decompression, even achieved minimally, implies partial facetectomy, which is associated with the risk of progression of slippage over time. In the case of decompression alone, the surgeon must be prepared to operate again on one-fourth of his or her patients during the first 2 years and predominantly at the same level as the index operation.[37,39,40]

The observational comparative study from the Norwegian registry[40] compared decompression versus decompression +

fusion with 260 patients in each group. The authors could not conclude that decompression was as good as fusion, observing that decompression alone was associated with more residual leg pain and back pain at 1 year postoperatively.

13.6.3 Posterior Fusion Techniques

The rationale to consider fusion as the first option is supported by the physiopathology and the natural history of the disease and by the data from the literature.[37,38,39,40] Traditionally, instrumented posterolateral fusion has been considered the gold standard for treating spondylolisthesis. It was initially described in 1953 by Cloward and has been continuously improved by more efficient fixation systems, especially since the introduction of pedicle screw-based fixation instrumentation. The main limitations of this technique are represented by the rates of fusion, which are lower compared to the interbody techniques, and by the difficulty to restore adequately the local lordosis (▶ Fig. 13.12).

The 90° interbody fusion techniques have increasingly gained popularity for treatment of spondylolisthesis because of the purported benefit of providing anterior column support, optimal bone grafting, and 360° fusion. It also allows restoration of a satisfactory local lordosis, which is an important point as DS represents a kyphotic disease of the lumbar spine. Not restoring the adequate balance may result in an increased incidence of adjacent syndromes.

13.6.4 Bilateral Transforaminal Lumbar Interbody Fusion

Our favored technique to treat DS is represented by the bilateral transforaminal lumbar interbody fusion (TLIF) using posterior lumbar interbody fusion (PLIF) cages (▶ Fig. 13.13). The patient is placed in the prone position. Surgical access to the intervertebral disk is obtained from a midline posterior direction through the intervertebral foramen after complete facetectomy

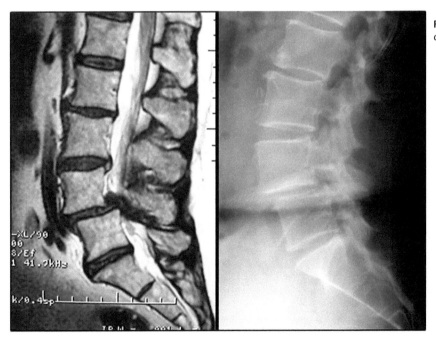

Fig. 13.11 Degenerative spondylolisthesis associated with a severe stenosis of the central canal.

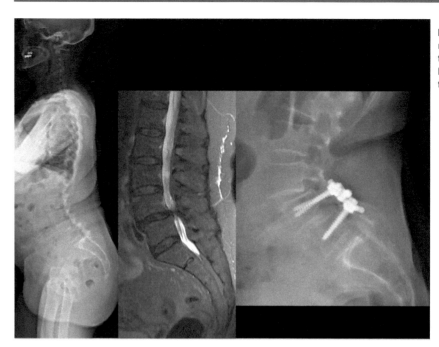

Fig. 13.12 Failure of posterolateral fusion to restore the segmental lordosis after instrumentation of L4-L5 degenerative spondylolisthesis. Because of the lack of anterior support, this technique should be avoided.

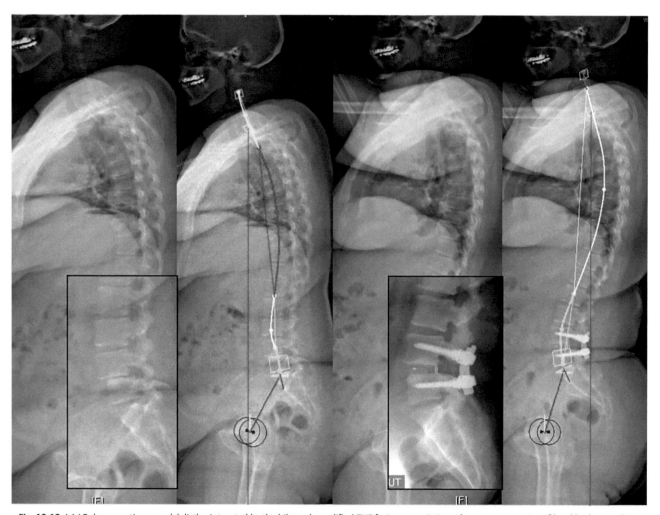

Fig. 13.13 L4-L5 degenerative spondylolisthesis treated by the bilateral, modified TLIF fusion, permitting adequate restoration of local lordosis with no need for an extensive instrumentation.

on each side. Once the spiny process and the laminas at the appropriate levels are identified, complete facet resection is achieved. The dura mater must be gently retracted medially to expose the lateral part of the disk. The endplates can then be prepared for implant or graft insertion. We use PLIF cages inserted bilaterally through the lateral part of the disk (typically 20 mm in length, 10° of lordosis, and 10 mm in height). Limited laminotomy is performed in some cases to facilitate cage implantation, but complete laminectomy is not necessary.

There are several advantages associated with this modified bilateral TLIF technique. First, this approach consists of the traditional posterior lumbar approach that most spine surgeons are well trained for and are comfortable in performing. A posterior exposure allows an excellent visualization of the nerve roots without compromising the blood supply to the graft. Placing anterior support allows adequate restoration of interbody height and local lordosis with a mean gain ~ 8°–10°, which is typically enough at L4-L5 (▶ Fig. 13.14). Also, posterior fusion surgery also allows a potential 360° fusion through a single incision.

Compared with the classical TLIF technique, our modified technique permits us to optimize the grafting and the biomechanical stability of the construct by placing two interbody cages and to ensure the adequate nerve root decompression with the bilateral approach.

Compared with the classical PLIF technique, our technique permits us to limit the risk of nerve root injury and dural tear as the cages are inserted through the lateral part of the canal and the foramens. In the literature, the risk of nerve damage is estimated to be 7.8% with PLIF versus 2% for TLIF, and the risk of dural tear is 17% versus 9%, respectively.

Compared with the extreme lateral interbody fusion/oblique lateral interbody fusion techniques, our technique permits us to decompress the lateral portion of the canal, especially the lateral recess, on both sides. Anterolateral techniques are efficient to restore the foraminal size or decompress the central canal but with poor effect on the lateral recess enlargement. Lateral recess is bordered by bony structures, including the facet, the pedicle, and osteophytes coming from the superior facet and, consequently, simple distraction is unlikely to decompress this area adequately, which is very frequently stenotic in DS. In our opinion, in most cases of DS, opening of the lateral recess should be achieved.

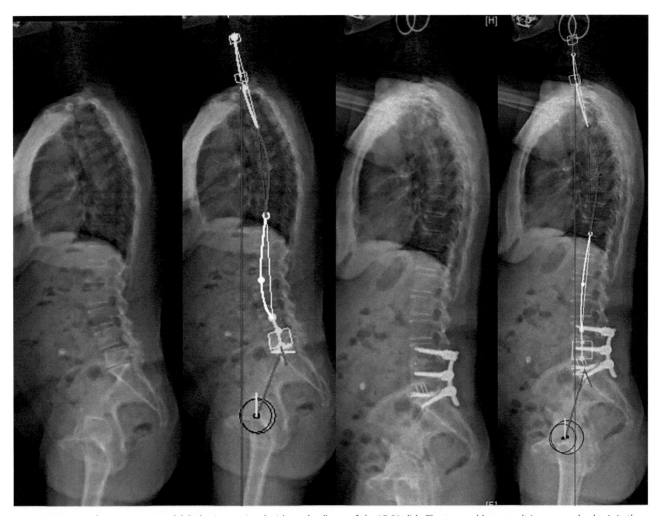

Fig. 13.14 L4-L5 degenerative spondylolisthesis associated with total collapse of the L5-S1 disk. The two problems result in a severe kyphosis in the lower lumbar part requiring adapted corrective surgery. The case was treated by combined surgery with anterior lumbar interbody fusion at L5-S1 and bilateral, modified transforaminal lumbar interbody fusion at L4-L5.

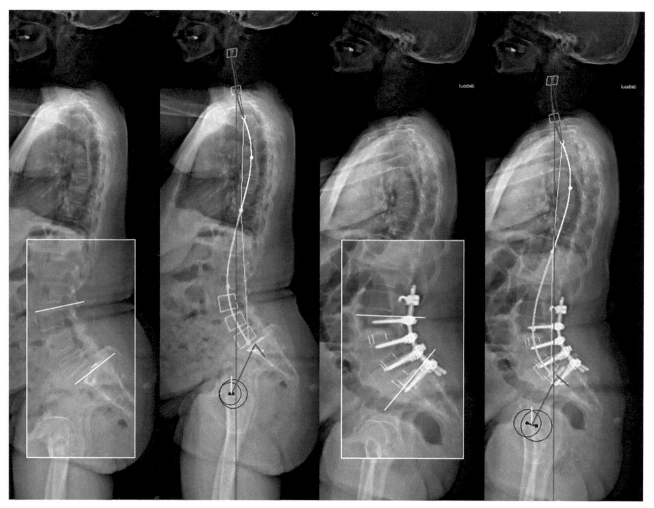

Fig. 13.15 Multilevel degenerative spondylolisthesis (L3-L4, L4-L5, and L5-S1) requiring extensive instrumentation of the lumbar spine (L2 sacrum) to correct the spinal deformity and rebalance the patient.

13.6.5 Complex Degenerative Spondylolisthesis

Three situations should be identified and separated as complex situations regarding the need for extensive surgery:
• Multilevel DS.
• DS with local kyphosis.
• DS associated with adjacent DDD.

All three of these situations result in a severe loss of lordosis, global sagittal imbalance requiring extensive corrective surgery (▶ Fig. 13.14, ▶ Fig. 13.15), and, in some cases, osteotomy surgery.

13.7 Conclusion

DS represents a stenotic and kyphotic degenerative disease of the lumbar spine. Surgical management of DS must deal with these two concerns. The stenosis affects predominantly the lateral part of the canal, that is, the lateral recess, because of the arthritic hypertrophy and subluxation of posterior facets. In general, direct opening of the lateral recess must be considered to achieve adequate nerve root decompression. Otherwise, in most cases, the local loss of lordosis caused by DS is limited, and the compensation provided by slight extension of the adjacent spine above works very well. The global balance is typically preserved, and, in such cases, limited stabilization of the DS represents the first surgical option permitting a solution to the problem regarding both the stenosis and local kyphosis. Our preferred option is the bilateral-modified TLIF technique as described in this chapter.

Situations at risk for global imbalance (complex DS) must be kept in mind and are represented by multilevel DS, DS associated with multilevel DDD, and DS associated with severe local kyphosis. These situations represent a spinal deformity generally requiring aggressive surgical treatment to rebalance the patient.

References

[1] Junghanns H. Spondylolisthesen ohne spalt im Zwishengelenkstuck. Arch Orthop Unfall-Chir. 1930; 29:118-1-27

[2] Macnab I. Spondylolisthesis with an intact neural arch; the so-called pseudo-spondylolisthesis. J Bone Joint Surg Br. 1950; 32-B(3):325-333

[3] Fitzgerald JA, Newman PH. Degenerative spondylolisthesis. J Bone Joint Surg Br. 1976; 58(2):184-192

[4] Wiltse LL, Newman PH, Macnab I. Classification of spondylolisis and spondylolisthesis. Clin Orthop Relat Res. 1976; 117:23-29

[5] Labelle H, Roussouly P, Berthonnaud E, et al. Spondylolisthesis, pelvic incidence, and spinopelvic balance: a correlation study. Spine. 2004; 29(18):2049-2054

[6] Enyo Y, Yoshimura N, Yamada H, Hashizume H, Yoshida M. Radiographic natural course of lumbar degenerative spondylolisthesis and its risk factors related to the progression and onset in a 15-year community-based cohort study: the Miyama study. J Orthop Sci. 2015; 20(6):978-984

[7] Rosenberg NJ. Degenerative spondylolisthesis. Predisposing factors. J Bone Joint Surg Am. 1975; 57(4):467-474

[8] Herkowitz HN. Spine update. Degenerative lumbar spondylolisthesis. Spine. 1995; 20(9):1084-1090

[9] Sengupta DK, Herkowitz HN. Degenerative spondylolisthesis: review of current trends and controversies. Spine. 2005; 30(6) Suppl:S71-S81

[10] Chaput C, Padon D, Rush J, Lenehan E, Rahm M. The significance of increased fluid signal on magnetic resonance imaging in lumbar facets in relationship to degenerative spondylolisthesis. Spine. 2007; 32(17):1883-1887

[11] Denard PJ, Holton KF, Miller J, et al. Lumbar spondylolisthesis among elderly men: prevalence, correlates, and progression. Spine. 2010; 35(10):1072-1078

[12] Chaiwanichsiri D, Jiamworakul A, Jitapunkul S. Lumbar disc degeneration in Thai elderly: a population-based study. J Med Assoc Thai. 2007; 90(11):2477-2481

[13] Horikawa K, Kasai Y, Yamakawa T, Sudo A, Uchida A. Prevalence of osteoarthritis, osteoporotic vertebral fractures, and spondylolisthesis among the elderly in a Japanese village. J Orthop Surg (Hong Kong). 2006; 14(1):9-12

[14] Kalichman L, Kim DH, Li L, Guermazi A, Berkin V, Hunter DJ. Spondylolysis and spondylolisthesis: prevalence and association with low back pain in the adult community-based population. Spine. 2009; 34(2):199-205

[15] Schuller S, Charles YP, Steib J-P. Sagittal spinopelvic alignment and body mass index in patients with degenerative spondylolisthesis. Eur Spine J. 2011; 20(5):713-719

[16] Jacobsen S, Sonne-Holm S, Rovsing H, Monrad H, Gebuhr P. Degenerative lumbar spondylolisthesis: an epidemiological perspective: the Copenhagen Osteoarthritis Study. Spine. 2007; 32(1):120-125

[17] Cholewicki J, Lee AS, Popovich JM, Jr, et al. Degenerative spondylolisthesis is related to multiparity and hysterectomies in older women. Spine. 2017; 42(21):1643-1647

[18] Sanderson PL, Fraser RD. The influence of pregnancy on the development of degenerative spondylolisthesis. J Bone Joint Surg Br. 1996; 78(6):951-954

[19] Matsunaga S, Ijiri K, Hayashi K. Nonsurgically managed patients with degenerative spondylolisthesis: a 10- to 18-year follow-up study. J Neurosurg. 2000; 93(2) Suppl:194-198

[20] Wang YXJ, Káplár Z, Deng M, Leung JCS. Lumbar degenerative spondylolisthesis epidemiology: a systematic review with a focus on gender-specific and age-specific prevalence. J Orthop Translat. 2016; 11:39-52

[21] Barrey C. Équilibre sagittal pelvi-rachidien et pathologies lombaires dégénératives: étude comparative à propos de 100 cas [Thèse] (in French); 2004

[22] Barrey C, Jund J, Perrin G, Roussouly P. Spinopelvic alignment of patients with degenerative spondylolisthesis. Neurosurgery. 2007; 61(5):981-986, discussion 986

[23] Barrey C, Jund J, Noseda O, Roussouly P. Sagittal balance of the pelvis-spine complex and lumbar degenerative diseases. A comparative study about 85 cases. Eur Spine J. 2007; 16(9):1459-1467

[24] Ferrero E, Ould-Slimane M, Gille O, Guigui P. Sagittal spinopelvic alignment in 654 degenerative spondylolisthesis. Eur Spine J. 2015; 24(6):1219-1227

[25] Morel E, Ilharreborde B, Lenoir T, et al. Sagittal balance of the spine and degenerative spondylolisthesis (in French). Rev Chir Orthop Reparatrice Appar Mot. 2005; 91(7):615-626

[26] Marty C, Boisaubert B, Descamps H, et al. The sagittal anatomy of the sacrum among young adults, infants, and spondylolisthesis patients. Eur Spine J. 2002; 11(2):119-125

[27] Sekharappa V, Amritanand R, Krishnan V, David KS. Lumbosacral transition vertebra: prevalence and its significance. Asian Spine J. 2014; 8(1):51-58

[28] Kong MH, He W, Tsai Y-D, et al. Relationship of facet tropism with degeneration and stability of functional spinal unit. Yonsei Med J. 2009; 50(5):624-629

[29] Liu Z, Duan Y, Rong X, Wang B, Chen H, Liu H. Variation of facet joint orientation and tropism in lumbar degenerative spondylolisthesis and disc herniation at L4-L5: a systematic review and meta-analysis. Clin Neurol Neurosurg. 2017; 161:41-47

[30] Sato K, Wakamatsu E, Yoshizumi A, Watanabe N, Irei O. The configuration of the laminas and facet joints in degenerative spondylolisthesis. A clinicoradiologic study. Spine. 1989; 14(11):1265-1271

[31] Kim NH, Lee JW. The relationship between isthmic and degenerative spondylolisthesis and the configuration of the lamina and facet joints. Eur Spine J. 1995; 4(3):139-144

[32] Boden SD, Riew KD, Yamaguchi K, Branch TP, Schellinger D, Wiesel SW. Orientation of the lumbar facet joints: association with degenerative disc disease. J Bone Joint Surg Am. 1996; 78(3):403-411

[33] Tassanawipas W, Chansriwong P, Mokkhavesa S. The orientation of facet joints and transverse articular dimension in degenerative spondylolisthesis. J Med Assoc Thai. 2005; 88 Suppl 3:S31-S34

[34] Nagaosa Y, Kikuchi S, Hasue M, Sato S. Pathoanatomic mechanisms of degenerative spondylolisthesis. A radiographic study. Spine. 1998; 23(13):1447-1451

[35] Love TW, Fagan AB, Fraser RD. Degenerative spondylolisthesis. Developmental or acquired? J Bone Joint Surg Br. 1999; 81(4):670-674

[36] Roussouly P, Gollogly S, Berthonnaud E, Dimnet J. Classification of the normal variation in the sagittal alignment of the human lumbar spine and pelvis in the standing position. Spine. 2005; 30(3):346-353

[37] Ghogawala Z, Dziura J, Butler WE, et al. Laminectomy plus fusion versus laminectomy alone for lumbar spondylolisthesis. N Engl J Med. 2016; 374(15):1424-1434

[38] Epstein NE. A review: reduced reoperation rate for multilevel lumbar laminectomies with noninstrumented versus instrumented fusions. Surg Neurol Int. 2016; 7 Suppl 13:S337-S346

[39] Ahmad S, Hamad A, Bhalla A, Turner S, Balain B, Jaffray D. The outcome of decompression alone for lumbar spinal stenosis with degenerative spondylolisthesis. Eur Spine J. 2017; 26(2):414-419

[40] Austevoll IM, Gjestad R, Brox JI, et al. The effectiveness of decompression alone compared with additional fusion for lumbar spinal stenosis with degenerative spondylolisthesis: a pragmatic comparative non-inferiority observational study from the Norwegian Registry for Spine Surgery. Eur Spine J. 2017; 26(2):404-413

14 The Degenerative Aging Spine: A Challenge for Contemporaneous Societies

Jean-Charles Le Huec, Wendy Thompson, Amélie Leglise, Marion Petit, and Thibault Cloché

Abstract

Degenerative disk disease of the nonscoliotic spine in the elderly is dominated by vertebral canal stenosis and osteoporotic fracture, which aggravates sagittal imbalance in most cases as a result of collapsed disks. While the treatment of cervical stenosis has few iatrogenic effects, the treatment of lumbar stenosis benefits greatly from new minimally invasive techniques. When the origins of sagittal forward bending are clearly positional with antalgic imbalance, limited surgery may suffice to compensate imbalance, which may be less efficient on the muscular level, but less risky for fragile patients. The overall analysis of sagittal balance using the recently described odontoid-hip axis angle (angle between the line joining the tip of the odontoid process to the center of femoral heads and the vertical line) is useful to establish a compromise, with the help of preoperative planning software like the KEOPS analyzer (SMAIO), of which the reliability is still to be improved by the use of data banks. Chevron osteotomies and posterior subtraction osteotomies are the commonly used surgical techniques to restore lordosis and global balance in spine, including supplemental interbody devices. Analysis of compensatory mechanisms during standing and walking are important to determine the length of the fusion and avoid proximal junctional problems.

Keywords: canal stenosis, degenerative spine, global balance, imbalance, kyphosis, lordosis, OD-HA, osteotomy

14.1 Introduction

Degenerative disk disease (DDD) in the elderly is an increasingly important problem for health systems worldwide. The osteoarticular system, of which the spine is an essential part, together with the cardiovascular system, grant functional autonomy. In fact, the aging of the population results in two phenomena: the first is the increase in the number of people over 60, with their pathologies and desire to remain healthy (growing old staying autonomous and healthy); the second is the increase in the costs of maintaining quality of life despite the decrease in funding contributions. This problem is far beyond the scope of this chapter as it involves societal choices.

DDD combines two problems: on the one hand, disk degeneration causing loss of cervical and lumbar lordosis and increasing thoracic kyphosis,[1] and on the other hand, consequences on the neurologic system as a result of narrowing of the vertebral canal and foramina. The first problem seems inevitable and probably depends largely on individual genetics, as suggested by Battié et al.[2] The second problem is responsible for pain and neurological deficits, the extent of which determines the loss of autonomy, which is associated with osteoporosis, fostering cuneiform collapse of the vertebrae by both thoracic and lumbar compression fractures. All these developments or events aggravate the overall kyphosis by a progressive anterior imbalance of the torso.[3] The aging of

Junghans' functional unit of the spine, whether cervical or lumbar, is essentially manifested by a narrowing of the spinal canal. Narrowing takes place either in the center of the canal or in the foramina, or in both. It is responsible for various symptoms: single-, multiradicular, or medullary. Moreover, the combination of cervical and lumbar damage affects 30% of patients.[4]

All in all, the characteristic pathologies of the elderly can be grouped under different headings:

- The narrowed central canal, whether cervical or lumbar, with its neurological consequences on the upper and lower limbs, is often accompanied by deformities: less in cervical deformities that resemble vertebral ankyloses and much more in lumbar deformities with narrowing as result of arthrosis.
- Kyphotic deformation caused by disk degeneration aggravated by osteoporotic compression fractures causes loss of sagittal balance. In this chapter, only nonscoliotic arthrogenic kyphoses will be analyzed.

We shall describe these two themes, and for each, clinical and paraclinical evaluations as well as the most appropriate therapeutic options.

14.2 Spinal Narrowing of Degenerative Origin with Loss of Normal Spine Shape at the Cervical Level

The most common pathology is cervicobrachial neuralgia characterized by typical pain most commonly found in elderly patients with disk osteophytes compressing the nerve root in the foramen. This must be distinguished from soft hernia neuralgia, more common in young patients.

The diagnosis is based on a clinical examination, without particular tests, to determine whether radicular pain is typical or incomplete. The paraclinical examinations are based on magnetic resonance imaging (MRI) that may reveal a narrowing, but it is mainly on axial and sagittal computed tomography (CT) sections that the disk-osteophytic nature of the stenosis can be confirmed (▶ Fig. 14.1). Electromyography is often useful when there are neurologic impairment symptoms indicating an acute phase.

In diagnosing, it is necessary to inspect for soft hernias as well as carpal tunnel and Guyon symptoms, which are quite common in older patients, while keeping in mind potential shoulder pathologies. The treatment is based on prescription of analgesics (level I, II, or III) and nonsteroidal anti-inflammatory drugs, in accordance with the precautions and contraindications applicable to the elderly and patients with multicomorbidity, but also through rest by wearing a surgical collar and by physiotherapy (self-stretching exercises and stress-relieving massages). A CT-guided infiltration can help overcome an acute phase, but has little or no effect in cases with calcified hernias and posterior osteophytes.

Surgery is only required when there are neurological radicular disorders or when pain increases over more than 6 to 8 weeks despite suitable medical treatment. Treatment is usually a standard diskectomy-arthrodesis via the anterior sternocleidomastoid approach.[5] In rare cases, the posterior approach is indicated, but the calcified nature of the hernias and the median prolongation of the osteophytes makes this surgery increasingly risky. The restoration of lordosis during the arthrodesis is still a matter of debate. Based on the work of Le Huec,[6] lordosis is physiological in only 50% of cases. It therefore seems advisable to measure the C7 slope before any cervical arthrodesis. If the C7 slope is less than 20°, a neutral fixation is preferable. If greater than 20°, the cervical spine is naturally in lordosis and it therefore makes sense to maintain the native curvature by arthrodesis. Surgery involving several levels is problematic because the risk of developing an adjacent syndrome is not negligible. Whereas there are presently no guidelines available, maintaining good posterior cervical muscle strength is undoubtedly the best prevention.

Myelopathy as a result of osteoarthrosis of the cervical spine is a common phenomenon. It is all the more important when there is a C2-C7 cervical kyphosis, which presses the spinal cord against the corporal osteophytes, even in the absence of ossification of the posterior longitudinal ligament.

The standard clinical picture associates certain signs

- To the upper limbs with parasthesia of the hands, more or less systemic with clumsiness (difficulty buttoning clothes, sewing, tinkering, etc.).
- To the lower limbs that with gait fatigue. This fatigue is often wrongly labeled because of the lack of any characteristic radicular signs, patients describing a general weakness, often with a reduced walking perimeter, but also sometimes with an erratic or spastic gait.
- To the urinary sphincter, often present but wrongly diagnosed as dysuria.

However, this standard clinical picture is not the most commonly observed, and the clinical presentations may combine several elements (posterior cord compression, amyotrophic, sphincteral, etc.). The presence of pyramidal signs can be noted, with a positive Hoffmann sign and a unilateral or bilateral Babinski sign.

Possible complications are mostly the Schneider syndrome or suspended spinal cord syndrome, which can ensue from a benign trauma or a low-impact fall, rather than the classic whiplash mechanism following a road accident. The clinical diagnosis is based on frontal and lateral radiography, but above all on MRI, which will reveal a narrowing of the cervical central canal caused by osteophytes at several levels, accompanied by myelopathy, well-illustrated by a T2 hypersignal on the MRI (▶ Fig. 14.2). The treatment of these changes has not yet been clearly coded.

Management of osteoarthritic cervical myelopathies is based on surgical decompression, which has proved more efficient than conservative treatment.[7] Surgery does not always reduce clinical signs, but permits stabilization of lesions. The choice of technique depends on the patient's age and general state, the number of segments affected by stenosis, and, last, the sagittal profile of the spine. Therefore, the treatment must be adapted according to the following criteria[8]:

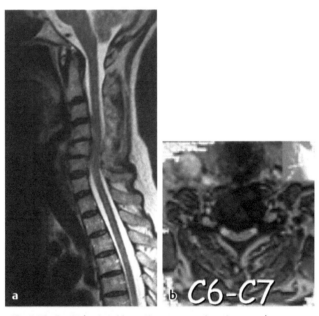

Fig. 14.1 Cervical spine. Magnetic resonance imaging reveals a narrowing. (a) Sagittal view; (b) axial view.

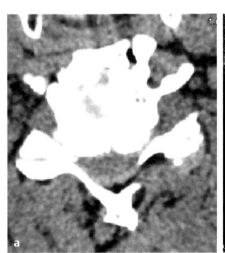
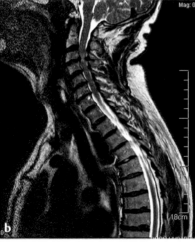

Fig. 14.2 (a) Cervical central canal as a result of osteophytosis clearly seen on a computed tomography scan; and (b) myelomalacia, well-illustrated by a T2 hypersignal using magnetic resonance imaging.

- If the spine is lordotic, with a central stenosis at more than three levels, "open-door" laminoplasty and reconstruction is the technique of choice. However, caution should be taken at the C5-C6 level, where a risk of paresis or paralysis of both roots exists through elongation when the spinal cord is released backward.
- If the spine is lordotic with stenosis at one to three levels, then the anterior approach with corporectomy, grafting, and fusion is satisfactory (▶ Fig. 14.3).
- If the spine is kyphotic with a central stenosis, an anterior approach is also preferable, with a corporectomy at one or two levels; if more than two levels of corporectomy are required, an intermediate vertebra must be retained to ensure a stable assembly. In fact, corpectomies at more than two levels have a much higher incidence of failure. Lordosis may be restored by the anterior approach using a sufficiently long graft or expandable cages. Occasionally, this anterior approach is insufficient and can be supplemented by posterior facet screws.

These criteria are no more than a decision-making framework. The advantages and disadvantages of each of these methods are not clearly agreed on and remain the subject of numerous studies.

14.2.1 At the Lumbar Level

The most common pathology is intermittent radicular claudication. The diagnosis is based on the general clinical experience of radiculalgia. It must be differentiated from vascular pathology. The palpation of the distal pulse must be systematic because in elderly patients the two pathologies may be interlinked.

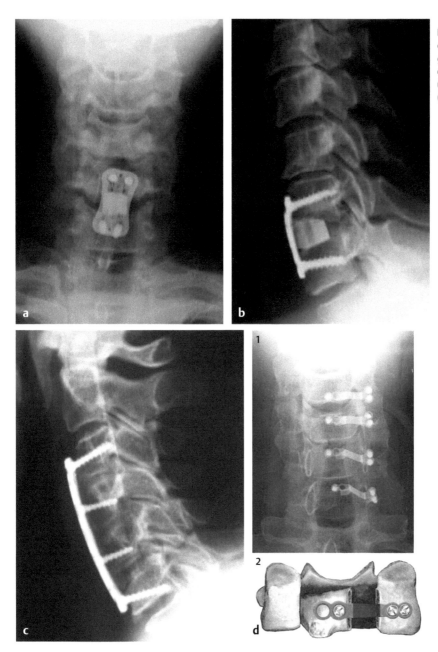

Fig. 14.3 (a) Anterior approach; (b) X-ray control of anterior approach with large diskectomy, grafting, and osteosynthesis; (c) X-ray control of corpectomy with iliac crest reconstruction; and (d) posterior laminoplasty for cervical stenosis: (1) X-ray image, and (2) principle of laminoplasty.

However, a posture in lumbar kyphosis to relieve pain, as well as its metameric topography, both help determine the diagnosis. The use of a cane to attend consultation often indicates the patient's need to compensate for the kyphosis necessary to increase the width of the central canal and the foramina. This analgesic kyphotic posture must be differentiated from a fixed kyphosis, irreducible in the supine position, and from a kyphosis caused by muscular insufficiency as with camptocormia. Radiography, MRI, and CT are standard examinations to confirm this central canal and/or foraminal stenosis, sometimes associated with disk inflammation and especially with vacuum disks caused by degenerative collapse (▶ Fig. 14.4).

Treatment is mostly surgical. In fact, conservative treatment is not without merit, but is less effective than surgery for reducing pain and improving quality of life.[9] Decompression is the technique[10] mostly associated with stabilization, depending on the extent of the facet resection needed to free the roots. An analysis of their sagittal balance is therefore an important factor in determining whether or not to operate on these patients. The use of minimally invasive techniques is highly desirable as they are not very destabilizing. The tube technique, with or without an endoscope or microscope, is the method of choice for operating on a single level. Differentiation of a voluntary kyphosis for dynamic widening of the canal is essential because a simple decompression, best assessed by the patient's odontoid-hip axis angle (OD-HA), and the absence of pelvic retroversion will suffice. Postoperatively, the patient will regain a satisfactory overall balance.[11] If the kyphotic posture is related to pathology such as multilevel kyphogenic DDD, ankylosing spondylitis, or major muscular insufficiency, then stabilization and correction of the deformity will be needed as described hereafter. In the second situation, the patient has pelvic retroversion and other compensatory mechanisms visible on the full standing X-rays.[12]

14.3 Pure Kyphotic Degenerative Deformities

Kyphotic degenerative deformities can be considered as two schematic types. The first is degenerative scoliosis associated with kyphosis and coronal deformation, resulting in a 3D phenomenon of vertebral twist (dealt with in another chapter). The second is pure degenerative kyphosis, aggravated by (1) the presence of osteoporotic compression fractures, and (2) muscular insufficiency of the posterior chains. The diagnosis of kyphosis is clinical and is based on an overall analysis of the patient.

14.3.1 Static Standing Analysis

This basic clinical semiology is often overlooked because on arrival, patients provide their own radiographs. The clinician should inspect for an anterior imbalance by initiating a walk on crutches or a difficult walk requiring support (caddy sign), which would reveal a limited walking perimeter because of pain and radicular claudication. These patients often complain of pain in the front of the thighs, often defined as cruralgia, when in fact it is quadriceps muscle pain fatigue related to permanent knee flexion attempting to restore sagittal balance, and thereby to compensate the overall kyphosis (▶ Fig. 14.5). This is a common mistake, sometimes resulting in surgery at the L3-L4 and L4-L5 levels as soon as a more or less obvious narrowing of the central canal or foramina is observed on radiographs. Static analysis is important and the patient should be instructed to maintain the static vertical position for as long as possible. Posterior muscular insufficiency is thereby quickly detected, and the same applies when patients are in the prone, face-down position, unable to raise their torsos. It is also important to differentiate the progressive analgesic posture in kyphosis—that of a dynamic narrow lumbar canal not accompanied by pelvic retroversion—from arthrogenic lumbar kyphosis, where there is pelvic retroversion with hip extension, compensating for fixed kyphosis. An even better diagnosis will be obtained on a walking mat, using dynamic analysis.

14.3.2 Dynamic Analysis during Gait

Recently, Shiba et al.[13] performed a three-dimensional gait analysis in patients with degenerative lumbar kyphosis. They demonstrated that loss of global sagittal alignment was underestimated on static images. In fact, anterior imbalance appears or increases as soon as the step is initiated and progresses along the passage of the step. This is explained by the compensation

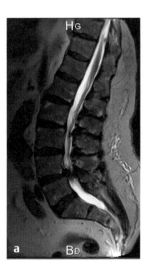
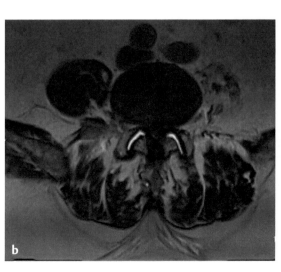

Fig. 14.4 Lumbar spine: central canal and foraminal stenosis, associated (a) with disk Modic changes using magnetic resonance imaging, and (b) with vacuum disks on a computed tomography scan.

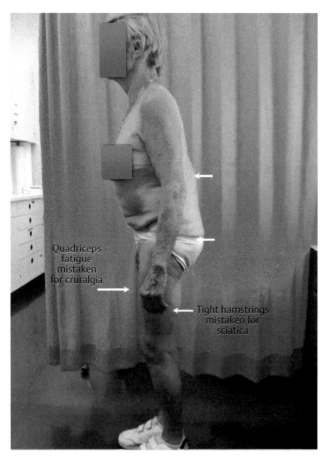

Fig. 14.5 Quadriceps muscle pain fatigue related to permanent knee flexion in an attempt to restore sagittal balance, and thereby to compensate the overall kyphosis.

phenomena involved in anterior imbalance. Indeed, one of the first compensatory phenomena occurs at the pelvic level, involving the extensor hip muscles, which participate in pelvic retroversion. During gait, the hip extensor muscles contract for the stance phase and no longer contribute to pelvic retroversion, which results in net pelvic anteversion. Anterior imbalance is then no longer compensated for and increases from the heel strike. This tendency to lean forward during gait is greater when the posterior spinal muscles have atrophied and no longer maintain the torso vertically. In a study of degenerative flat backs, Lee et al.[14] demonstrated the existence of two groups of patients defined by their pelvic tilt (PT) during gait. The first group could maintain pelvic retroversion, whereas the second group could not. These findings indicate that, during gait, patients who could maintain pelvic retroversion (approximately 80%) would benefit from surgical correction, unlike those with pelvic anteversion. Bae et al.[15] recently proposed imaging the entire vertebral column after 10 minutes of gait, to reveal any major anterior imbalance that may be compensated for on static images taken at rest.

14.3.3 Image Analysis

Long cassette radiographs of the entire spine, including the femoral heads, can be made everywhere and are absolutely indispensable for these patients. The low radiation system (EOS imaging, France)[16] is increasingly becoming the examination of choice, because it allows simultaneous acquisition of frontal and lateral images and 3D reconstruction, which eliminates distortions when the image is acquired with pelvic rotation. The measurements are thus simultaneously comparable for the same patient (▶ Fig. 14.6).

Here, spinal analysis focuses on the lateral view, although not of course ignoring frontal analysis. Apart from segmental arthrosis imaging, compensation phenomena must be inspected for at every level (ante- and retrolisthesis, "leaning back sign"; ▶ Fig. 14.7). Reciprocal expulsion of the articular facets is common. Retrolisthesis with anterior disk widening is a classic compensation phenomenon above a level that has lost lordosis. The "leaning back sign" described by Le Huec and Faundez[17] is a variant to be considered, as it points to the existence of an adjacent hypermobile disk with anterolisthesis, anterior widening of the disk, and slippage of the posteroinferior corner of the vertebra suprajacent to the endplate of the vertebra below it (▶ Fig. 14.7). This phenomenon is often accompanied by irritation of the outgoing root.

The analysis of sagittal balance will include all the standard criteria (▶ Fig. 14.6): pelvic incidence (PI), PT and sacral slope, lumbar lordosis L1-S1 and distal lordosis L4-S1, thoracic kyphosis, the C2-C7 angle, the C7 plumb line (sagittal vertical axis), the spinosacral angle, and the Barrey index. These measurements enable investigation of compensation phenomena caused by loss of lumbar lordosis or thoracic hyperkyphosis, by comparing them with theoretical values in the asymptomatic normal population. Le Huec,[18] using 3D full spine analysis, has thus been able to establish two useful formulas, explaining the theoretical reference values for lumbar lordosis and PT as a function of PI.

Theoretical lordosis L1-S1 = 0.54 PI + 28°
Theoretical PT = 0.4 PI – 11°

These formulas, based on a substantial sample for all PI values, are important as they can correct former errors caused by oversimplistic formulas established from small samples[19] and that lead to completely inappropriate interpretations for patient with PI higher than 70°. Thus, to affirm[20] that a PT < 20° is a target systematically associated with good results is completely false. For example, a person with a low PI of 35° would normally have a PT of ~ 3°, and a PT measuring 20° would represent a major compensation probably associated with knee flexion (small PI with flexion of the knees and a PT of 18°; ▶ Fig. 14.8). Similarly, an asymptomatic healthy person with a PI of 80° will have a PT of around 23°. The PT is an adaptive parameter that reflects the rotation of the pelvis around the femoral heads. An overall analysis of sagittal balance must include the cervical spine supporting the head. In a normal state of equilibrium, this is always been located above the pelvis. Analyses of the gravity line[21] showed that, in healthy persons, it passes through the femoral head, making it an essential reference point, and by an upper marker that may be the posterior edge of the sella turcica or the middle of the external auditory ducts or, what is an even easier reference, the tip of the odontoid process. These three reference points are very close to each other and correspond to the head's center of gravity.[22] The OD-HA described by Amabile et al.[23] (▶ Fig. 14.9) is a quick way to analyze overall balance

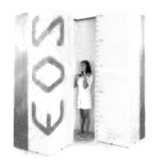

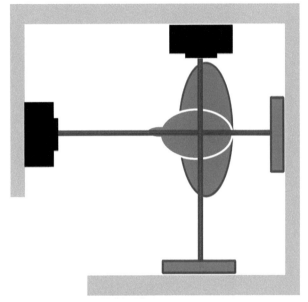

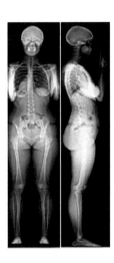

Fig. 14.6 EOS imaging allows simultaneous acquisition of frontal and lateral images and 3D reconstruction.

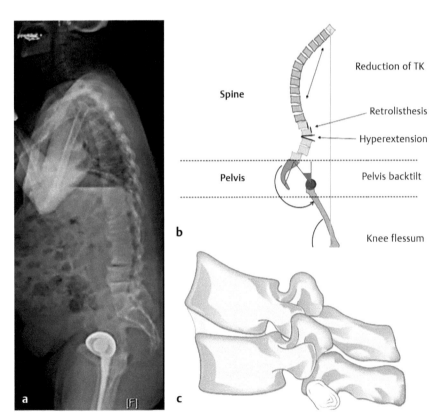

Reduction of TK

Spine

Retrolisthesis

Hyperextension

Pelvis

Pelvis backtilt

Knee flessum

Fig. 14.7 (a) X-ray: segmental compensation phenomena must be inspected for at every level: **(b)** antelisthesis, hyperextension, retrolisthesis; and **(c)** leaning back sign: antelisthesis with anterior disk opening. TK, Thoracic kyphosis.

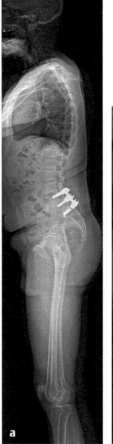
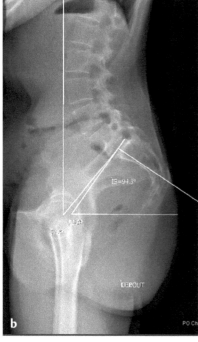

Fig. 14.8 (a) Small pelvic incidence value with high pelvic tilt value (18°) in a totally imbalanced patient; and (b) high pelvic incidence value with a pelvic tilt value of 34°, which is absolutely normal for this well-balanced patient.

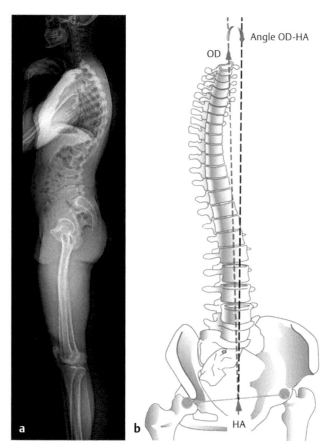

Fig. 14.9 Odontoid-hip axis angle (OD-HA): (a) normal value, and (b) drawing showing the measurement.

inclusive of the head. This angle connecting the tip of the odontoid process to the center of the femoral head and the plumb line passing through the femoral head is between 0° and -5° in an asymptomatic population of young persons or aged over 50.[11] This article demonstrates that in persons over 50 there are compensatory phenomena related to disk degeneration (loss of lordosis, increase in average PT, increase in cervical lordosis), although the OD-HA remains normal in asymptomatic individuals. It is of course important to check that there is no flexion of the knees. The most common problem to be solved is the analysis of the extent of the correction to be made to restore a satisfactory balance. This value is determined by calculating the full balanced integrated index,[24] which will determine the overall correction needed to restore balance in the sagittal plane by linking it to the potential compensation relating to knee flexion.

14.3.4 Vertebral Compression Fracture Is Extremely Common[25]

The "vertebral compression fracture" may be an acute phenomenon with osteoporotic fracture, without neurological

disorders. It typically consists of A3 fractures as classified by the AO, causing a moderate local kyphosis of 10° to 15°, but it can also rapidly worsen or even result in bone necrosis. MRI enables diagnosis of a recent fracture.

There may be progressive microtraumas, with increasing kyphosis responsible for respiratory repercussions, especially when there are multiple and long-standing compressions that the MRI will also reveal. When in doubt, always look for metastases using scintigraphy and/or an MRI or positron emission tomography/CT.

14.3.5 Dynamic and Cushioned Radiographs

Flexion/extension radiographs using the Putto protocol[26] and lateral radiographs cushioned at the apex of the kyphosis enable analysis of the passive reducibility of kyphoses and therefore the extent of the residual correction to be performed —sometimes to decrease it by 50%—which changes the entire correction strategy.

14.3.6 MRI and Other Imaging Examinations

MRI is useful for detecting associated bone pathologies and neurological compressions. The CT scan is useful for analysis of osteophytes and the phenomena of vacuum disks, which are synonymous with disk mobility. Osteodensitometry reveals the extent of osteoporosis, confirming the need for medical treatment. It also helps to prevent bad anchoring of screws, thereby justifying the use of fenestrated cemented screws or other technical devices/solutions during surgery.

14.4 The Treatment of Arthrogenic Kyphoses

The treatment of kyphotic degenerative pathologies must take into account various criteria:
- The patient's age and associated comorbidities.
- Associated surgery.
- Imbalance correction, sometimes requiring major surgery such as posterior subtraction osteotomy, but which must also take into account the desired objectives in an elderly patient.

The patient's age and associated comorbidities may significantly restrict therapeutic options. Osteoporosis should be evaluated, which need not exclude surgery. Parkinson's disease and camptocormia require a long construct and the patient must be informed of the risks of complications. General complications can affect up to 20% of cases or even more, up to 40%.[27,28]

Associated surgery such as a narrow canal treatment, the combination of an intervertebral arthrodesis at the L5-S1 level by anterior lumbar interbody fusion or lateral between L2 and L5 (lateral lumbar interbody fusion) are useful in avoiding pseudarthrosis and loss of corrections. Mechanical complications can affect 10% of long construct.[27]

14.4.1 Imbalance Correction

An analgesic posture linked to a narrow dynamic canal will self-correct after the root or canal is freed, which must be sparing with the recalibration principle. Most common is the treatment of nearly permanent radicular syndromes while correcting kyphosis, which cannot be done with the patient in the supine position. This typically requires arthrodesis to restore physiological curvatures, and thereby permit standing in an efficient polygon.

When the problem is located on two or three lumbar segments, especially between L3 and S1, transforaminal lumbar interbody fusion (TLIF) surgery with adaptive restoration of segmental lordosis is fairly easy by referencing the normative values described in this chapter. This is only valid if preoperative measurements of the corrected lordosis are made either with radiography or on a digital flat-screen monitor or the use of a control with certain smart phone applications, including an inclinometer.

Correction of major thoracolumbar kyphosis requires planning:
- Dynamic and cushioned imaging shows the reducibility of the kyphosis and therefore the suitability of a customized correction using multilevel chevron osteotomies and associated TLIFs. This often allows a gain of 6° to 10° per level. If lumbar kyphosis is fixed (previous arthrodesis or ankylosing disease), a posterior pedicle subtraction osteotomy (PSO) of the vertebral body is often the only possible way to restore lordosis consistent with PI (▶ Fig. 14.10a, b).

- The effects of segmental corrections on overall balance must also be anticipated. Currently, software (KEOPS analyzer [SMAIO]) (▶ Fig. 14.10c) simulates a correction by implementing cages, inter- or transpedicular osteotomy, etc. This is a very interesting advance in surgical planning, and assessing whether to allow the patient certain compensatory options, thereby determining the extent of correction in kyphosis surgery. This planning is particularly useful in frail elderly subjects where there is often a need to compromise between a "perfect" curvature and an acceptable restoration of the OD-HA to normative values including some compensatory mechanisms. A PSO results in an average bleeding of 1.5 L for an average correction of 30°.[29] This may be a reason to refuse this type of intervention in certain patients. It is then necessary to adopt a "small means" policy so as to regain a compensated balance permitting an acceptable autonomy. The use of flexible corsets to prevent thoracic collapse and daily muscle exercises associated with cardiorespiratory rehabilitation can improve the quality of life in the elderly, whose expectations are often modest, but whose main purpose is to retain even limited autonomy. Measurement of OD-HA is a good way to anticipate the occurrence of proximal junctional kyphosis, especially in the case of intermediate fusion construct ending around the thrombolumbar junction.

The special case of elderly Parkinson's patients with degenerative kyphosis is a major problem, which is also true for those suffering from camptocormia as a result of insufficiency of the posterior muscular chains. Short constructs are certain to fail, and one should not hesitate to go as far as the upper thoracic level.[30] Installing four to six upper thoracic pedicular screws, strutted and connected to the standard lumbar assembly, obviates the need to place screws at all stages.

Reinforcement vertebroplasty has been suggested in some cases of severe osteoporosis proximate to junctional areas. Initially described by Galibert and Deramond[31] for the treatment of vertebral angiomas, the use of vertebroplasty has widened with the "balloon technique," in this case called kyphoplasty.[32] Halting of the thoracic kyphosis and strengthening the spinal muscles through regular physical work improves the quality of life.[33]

14.5 Conclusion

Degenerative disk pathology of the nonscoliotic vertebral column is a kyphogenic disease and, in the elderly, is worsened by spinal stenosis and osteoporotic fractures that systematically increase sagittal imbalance caused by disk collapse. The treatment of cervical stenosis is not iatrogenic and lumbar stenosis benefits greatly from new minimally invasive techniques. When sagittal imbalance is of an obvious segmental or more global origin like muscle insufficiency, limited surgery may suffice to obtain a compensated balance in some cases. Although certainly less efficient on the muscular plane, it is generally less risky in a fragile patient. The overall analysis of balance by reference to the OD-HA and with the help of preoperative planning software (though its reliability needs further improvement), is a good way to reach a compromise.

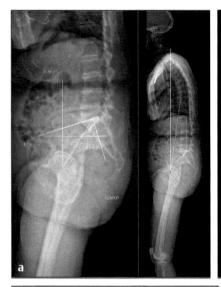
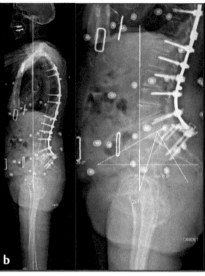

Fig. 14.10 (a) Preoperative kyphosis; (b) postoperative correction using a pedicle subtraction osteotomy (PSO) and multiple chevron osteotomy; and (c) KEOPS sagittal analyzer for preoperative planning.

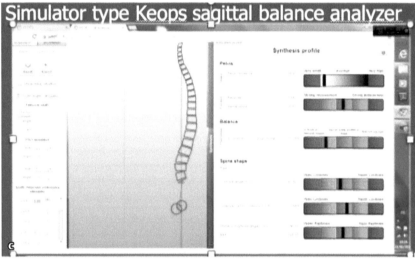

References

[1] Yılmaz E, Çıkrıkçıoğlu HY, Baydur H. The effect of functional disability and quality of life on decision to have surgery in patients with lumbar disc herniation. Orthop Nurs. 2018; 37(4):246–252

[2] Battié MC, Videman T, Parent E. Lumbar disc degeneration: epidemiology and genetic influences. Spine. 2004; 29(23):2679–2690

[3] Le Huec JC, Aunoble S, Sibilla F, Saddiki R, Bertrand F, Pellet N. Pathologie rachidienne de la personne âgée fragile. In: Terver S, Martins-Condé F, Leblanc B, eds. Orthopédie-traumatologie de la personne âgée fragile. Paris, France: Springer; 2013:359–372. https://doi.org/10.1007/978-2-8178-0377-7_29. Accessed October 14, 2018

[4] Kong L, Bai J, Zhang B, Shen Y, Tian D. Predictive factors of symptomatic lumbar canal stenosis in patients after surgery for cervical spondylotic myelopathy. Ther Clin Risk Manag. 2018; 14:483–488

[5] Lassale B, Guigui P, Delecourt C. Voies d'abord du rachis. Available from: http://www.em-premium.com.docelec.u-bordeaux.fr/article/21006/resulta-trecherche/3. Accessed October 24, 2018

[6] Le Huec JC, Demezon H, Aunoble S. Sagittal parameters of global cervical balance using EOS imaging: normative values from a prospective cohort of asymptomatic volunteers. Eur Spine J. 2015; 24(1):63–71

[7] Edwards CC, II, Riew KD, Anderson PA, Hilibrand AS, Vaccaro AF. Cervical myelopathy: current diagnostic and treatment strategies. Spine J. 2003; 3 (1):68–81

[8] Wang B, Lü G, Kuang L. Anterior cervical discectomy and fusion with stand-alone anchored cages versus posterior laminectomy and fusion for four-level cervical spondylotic myelopathy: a retrospective study with 2-year follow-up. BMC Musculoskelet Disord. 2018; 19(1):216

[9] Covaro A, Vilà-Canet G, de Frutos AG, Ubierna MT, Ciccolo F, Caceres E. Management of degenerative lumbar spinal stenosis: an evidence-based review. EFORT Open Rev. 2017; 1(7):267–274

[10] Weinstein JN, Lurie JD, Tosteson TD, et al. Surgical compared with nonoperative treatment for lumbar degenerative spondylolisthesis. Four-year results in the Spine Patient Outcomes Research Trial (SPORT) randomized and observational cohorts. J Bone Joint Surg Am. 2009; 91(6):1295–1304

[11] Amabile C, Le Huec J-C, Skalli W. Invariance of head-pelvis alignment and compensatory mechanisms for asymptomatic adults older than 49 years. Eur Spine J. 2018; 27(2):458–466

[12] Barrey C, Roussouly P, Le Huec JC, D'Acunzi G, Perrin G. Compensatory mechanisms contributing to keep the sagittal balance of the spine. Eur Spine J. 2013; 22 Suppl 6:S834–S841

[13] Shiba Y, Taneichi H, Inami S, Moridaira H, Takeuchi D, Nohara Y. Dynamic global sagittal alignment evaluated by three-dimensional gait analysis in patients with degenerative lumbar kyphoscoliosis. Eur Spine J. 2016; 25 (8):2572–2579

[14] Lee CS, Lee CK, Kim YT, Hong YM, Yoo JH. Dynamic sagittal imbalance of the spine in degenerative flat back: significance of pelvic tilt in surgical treatment. Spine. 2001; 26(18):2029–2035

[15] Bae J, Theologis AA, Jang J-S, Lee S-H, Deviren V. Impact of fatigue on maintenance of upright posture: dynamic assessment of sagittal spinal deformity parameters after walking 10 minutes. Spine. 2017; 42(10):733–739

[16] Dubousset J, Charpak G, Dorion I, et al. A new 2D and 3D imaging approach to musculoskeletal physiology and pathology with low-dose radiation and the

standing position: the EOS system. Bull Acad Natl Med. 2005; 189(2):287–297, discussion 297–300

[17] Faundez A-A, Cogniet A, Racloz G, Tsoupras A, Le Huec JC. Spondylolisthésis dégénératif lombaire; 2017. Available from: http://www.em-premium.com.docelec.u-bordeaux.fr/article/1100628. Accessed September 16, 2018

[18] Le Huec JC, Hasegawa K. Normative values for the spine shape parameters using 3D standing analysis from a database of 268 asymptomatic Caucasian and Japanese subjects. Eur Spine J. 2016; 25(11):3630–3637

[19] Schwab F, Lafage V, Patel A, Farcy J-P. Sagittal plane considerations and the pelvis in the adult patient. Spine. 2009; 34(17):1828–1833

[20] Scheer JK, Lafage R, Schwab FJ, et al. Under correction of sagittal deformities based on age-adjusted alignment thresholds leads to worse health-related quality of life whereas over correction provides no additional benefit. Spine. 2018; 43(6):388–393

[21] Schwab F, Lafage V, Boyce R, Skalli W, Farcy J-P. Gravity line analysis in adult volunteers: age-related correlation with spinal parameters, pelvic parameters, and foot position. Spine. 2006; 31(25):E959–E967

[22] Vital JM, Senegas J. Anatomical bases of the study of the constraints to which the cervical spine is subject in the sagittal plane. A study of the center of gravity of the head. Surg Radiol Anat. 1986; 8(3):169–173

[23] Amabile C, Pillet H, Lafage V, Barrey C, Vital J-M, Skalli W. A new quasi-invariant parameter characterizing the postural alignment of young asymptomatic adults. Eur Spine J. 2016; 25(11):3666–3674

[24] Le Huec JC, Leijssen P, Duarte M, Aunoble S. Thoracolumbar imbalance analysis for osteotomy planification using a new method: FBI technique. Eur Spine J. 2011; 20 Suppl 5:669–680

[25] Majd ME, Farley S, Holt RT. Preliminary outcomes and efficacy of the first 360 consecutive kyphoplasties for the treatment of painful osteoporotic vertebral compression fractures. Spine J. 2005; 5(3):244–255

[26] Putto E, Tallroth K. Extension-flexion radiographs for motion studies of the lumbar spine. A comparison of two methods. Spine. 1990; 15(2):107–110

[27] Le Huec JC, Cogniet A, Demezon H, Rigal J, Saddiki R, Aunoble S. Insufficient restoration of lumbar lordosis and FBI index following pedicle subtraction osteotomy is an indicator of likely mechanical complication. Eur Spine J. 2015; 24 Suppl 1:S112–S120

[28] Faundez A, Le Huec JC, Hansen LV, Poh Ling F, Gehrchen M. Optimizing pedicle subtraction osteotomy techniques: a new reduction plier to increase technical safety and angular reduction efficiency. Oper Neurosurg (Hagerstown). 2018. DOI: 10.1093/ons/opy086

[29] Choi HY, Hyun S-J, Kim K-J, Jahng T-A, Kim H-J. Surgical and radiographic outcomes after pedicle subtraction osteotomy according to surgeon's experience. Spine. 2017; 42(13):E795–E801

[30] Guigui P, Lambert P, Lassale B, Deburge A. Long-term outcome at adjacent levels of lumbar arthrodesis (in French). Rev Chir Orthop Reparatrice Appar Mot. 1997; 83(8):685–696

[31] Galibert P, Deramond H, Rosat P, Le Gars D. Preliminary note on the treatment of vertebral angioma by percutaneous acrylic vertebroplasty. Neurochirurgie. 1987; 33(2):166–168

[32] Garfin SR, Yuan HA, Reiley MA. New technologies in spine: kyphoplasty and vertebroplasty for the treatment of painful osteoporotic compression fractures. Spine. 2001; 26(14):1511–1515

[33] Senthil P, Sudhakar S, Radhakrishnan R, Jeyakumar S. Efficacy of corrective exercise strategy in subjects with hyperkyphosis. J Back Musculoskeletal Rehabil. 2017; 30(6):1285–1289

15 Scheuermann's Kyphosis

Stefan Parent, Abdulmajeed Alzakri, and Hubert Labelle

Abstract

Scheuermann's kyphosis is defined by an increased kyphosis with increased anterior vertebral wedging of more than 5° over three consecutive levels. The prevalence of the condition varies from 1% to 8% and affects males more than females. Various etiologies have been proposed, and it is considered to be a form of juvenile osteochondrosis of the spine. Treatment is aimed at limiting progression with most curves responding well to physiotherapy and bracing. In immature patients with significant curves and significant back pain, surgical correction can be entertained. Surgical correction should be tailored to the patient's pelvic morphology and sagittal balance. Posterior-based instrumentation and fusion can lead to adequate correction by shortening of the posterior spine length and compression. Overcorrection can lead to significant junctional issues and poor outcomes. Long-term results are usually good with patients achieving similar outcomes with appropriate treatment.

Keywords: back pain, kyphosis, physical therapy modalities, prevalence, Scheuermann's disease, spine, surgery

15.1 Introduction

In 1921, Holger Scheuermann differentiated painful and fixed dorsal hyperkyphosis deformity from postural kyphosis, and he called it "osteochonritis deformans juvenilis dorsi."[1] The thoracic spine is the most commonly affected region, but involvement of the thoracolumbar and lumbar spine in the disease has been previously documented.[2] Patients with Scheuermann's kyphosis (SK) had more intense lower back pain, less range of trunk motion, and an abnormal pulmonary function test when the kyphosis was more than 100°.[3] The round back associated with back pain often causes concern among patients, parents, and physicians. There have been many reports that this condition leads, in adulthood, to backache; embarrassment about physical appearance; interruption of work; disability; severe, progressive deformity; tightness of the hamstrings or other muscles; spondylolisthesis; disk degeneration; and interference with recreational activities.[4]

15.1.1 Epidemiology

SK is the most common cause of fixed painful structural kyphosis deformity in the thoracic and thoracolumbar spine among adolescents.[5] The prevalence is 1% to 8% in the United States, the male-to-female ratio is at least 2:1 and is most commonly diagnosed in adolescents at 12–17 years of age.[6]

15.1.2 Etiology

The definitive cause of SK remains uncertain. The heritability in Scheuermann's disease is 0.74, but the mode of transmission has not yet been defined.[7] Other factors that have also been implicated in Scheuermann's disease development are idiopathic juvenile osteoporosis, elevated growth hormone levels, dural cysts, spondylolysis, vitamin D deficiency, spinal deformities, and infections.[8,9,10] Mechanical hyperpressure on growth cartilage has been proposed as a possible etiology and is based on the weak mechanical interface between stiff bone and the resilient disk. Patients usually present with a higher body mass index and are more active individuals.[11]

15.1.3 Histopathology

Histological analysis shows endplate irregularities, narrowed intervertebral disks, a thickened anterior longitudinal ligament (ALL), and Schmorl's nodes. It is considered to be a form of juvenile osteochondrosis of the spine whereby defective growth of the cartilage endplate leads to disorganized endochondral ossification. The microscopic findings include markedly irregular endplates and endplate disruption with protrusion of disk material into the vertebral body. The ring apophysis does not show avascular necrosis. The intervertebral disk is interpreted as normal both by routine histology and electron microscopy.[12]

15.1.4 History and Physical Exam

The family usually attributes the deformity to poor posture, which delays the diagnosis and treatment. SK is a structural deformity of the thoracic or thoracolumbar spine, which appears before puberty and progresses to become symptomatic during growth.[8,13,14] The patient usually seeks medical attention between the age of 8 and 12 years old, and those who attend later usually present with more severe and rigid deformity. The initial reason for consultation in adolescents is the cosmetic deformity and in adults because of increased pain. The pain is usually located at the paravertebral region, just caudal to the apex of the kyphosis.[15,16] The compensatory cervical and lumbar hyperlordosis could also be a cause of pain. Some patients presented with lumbosacral spondylosis or spondylolisthesis because of increasing stress on the pars intraarticular.[5,8,14,16]

In rare severe cases, neurological symptoms may appear in the form of radicular pain with progressive weakness of the lower limbs, even spastic paraparesis.[10,13,14,15] The neurological symptoms could be secondary to the onset of thoracic disk herniation, dural cysts, or by spinal traction and compression mechanisms in the apex of the kyphosis in cases of severe deformity. Cardiopulmonary symptoms are uncommon among patients with Scheuermann's disease.[5,8,14,15,16,17,18]

15.1.5 Differential Diagnosis

It is crucial to differentiate the SK from postural kyphosis, which is nonrigid, nonprogressive, and correctable in the hyperextension or supine position. The apical vertebrae and adjacent disks have a normal appearance without wedging, irregularities of the endplate, or premature degeneration of the disk.

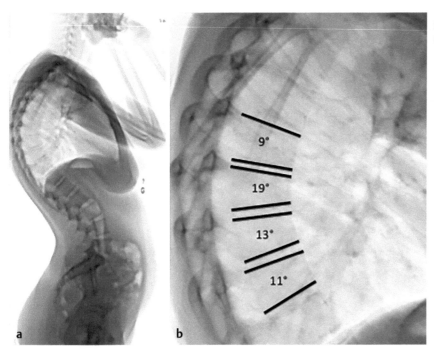

Fig. 15.1 (a,b) Simple lateral radiograph of an adolescent patient with Scheuermann's disease.

15.1.6 Radiological Features

The average normal thoracic kyphosis among asymptomatic adolescents is 44° ± 10.9° (measuring from T1 to T12).[19] However, the relevant literature reflects the existence of a wide variability for what could be considered normal sagittal balance in asymptomatic individuals.

The diagnosis of Scheuermann's disease is obtained by lateral spine radiography with the patient standing. To measure the angle of kyphosis, the final cranial and caudal vertebrae included in the deformity must be selected. The measurement of the wedging degree is obtained from the angle of intersection of the tangents on the upper and lower plates of each vertebral body. The diagnostic criterion establishes a level of wedging over 5° in at least three consecutive vertebrae in the apex of kyphosis (▶ Fig. 15.1). Other common findings in radiology include the presence of Schmorl's nodes, irregularity, and thinning of the vertebral endplates and disk space impingement (▶ Fig. 15.2). In the classical type I disease, the apex of kyphosis is located between T6 and T9. In type II, the apex of kyphosis is located in the thoracolumbar junction.[5,8,9,10,14,15]

Pelvic incidence (PI) is a key regulator of sagittal balance in normal individuals. Lumbar lordosis usually closely correlates with PI with increasing lordosis seen in patients with higher PI.[20] Intuitively, higher thoracic kyphosis and higher lordosis could be related to a higher PI. SK is, however, not considered a normal state, and therefore, sagittal balance is often disrupted.

Recently, the sagittal spinopelvic alignment in adolescents associated with SK has been studied. Jiang et al reported that SK patients had significantly lower PI and pelvic tilt. They found different compensation mechanisms in these patients to keep their sagittal spinopelvic alignment. A significant correlation was noticed between thoracic kyphosis and cervical lordosis in Scheuermann's thoracic kyphosis (STK) patients and also

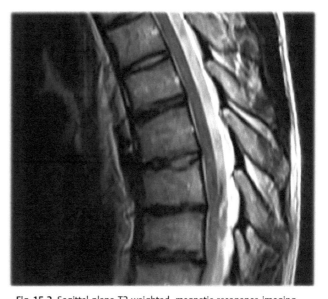

Fig. 15.2 Sagittal plane T2 weighted, magnetic resonance imaging. Other common findings in radiology include the presence of Schmorl hernias, irregularity, and thinning of the vertebral plates and diskal space impingement.

between thoracic kyphosis and lumbar lordosis in both STK and Scheuermann's thoracolumbar kyphosis patients.[21,22,23]

15.2 Possible Etiology Based on Roussouly's Classification of Spinopelvic Morphotype

If in Scheuerman's disease, PI is lower than in the normal population, type 1 and type 2 of Roussouly's classification are predominant because of their direct relation with low PI (<50°).[24]

Type 1 is characterized by thoracolumbar kyphosis and, in the elderly, with occurrence of disk degeneration at the thoracolumbar level. We could then conclude that thoracolumbar SK with low PI have a type 1 shape and that low PI played a role in this thoracolumbar localization (▶ Fig. 15.3a).

In Roussouly's type 2 (global flat back) the shape may induce in adults early lumbar distal degeneration and, later, in the elderly, multilevel degeneration and degenerative lumbar kyphosis. The same mechanism could explain lumbar Scheuerman kyphosis by distal lumbar hyperpressure in very flat back with small PI during growth. Very severe lumbar SK is always linked to a very low PI and in some cases in low pathological PI (< 30°), which is unknown in asymptomatic populations (▶ Fig. 15.3c). This situation is quite impossible to treat adequately because of the inability to restore a normal spinal balance. Pelvises with such a low PI are very difficult to balance. The spine is on a very straight edge without any possibility of creating balance by pelvic rotation. Scheuermann's disease with low PI has a very limited mechanism for pelvic compensation by retroversion.

Cases with high PI (> 50°) correspond to Roussouly's type 3 and 4. Type 4 mainly is characterized by a higher angle of lordosis that may correlate with a higher angle of thoracic kyphosis (▶ Fig. 15.3b, d). This disposition may induce Scheuermann's disease at the thoracic level. The thoracic hyperkyphosis is compensated for by lumbar hyperextension. A longer area of lordosis, as in type 4, allows this compensation easily and could potentially be less painful, at least in younger patients where the spine is more flexible.

In conclusion, PI seems to be a strong determinant for Scheuermann severity and localization, and has to be taken into consideration for treatment strategy.[24]

15.3 Natural History

The group of patients with SK presented with a higher frequency of back pain, greater concern for their physical appearance, and generally had fewer physical jobs or occupations. In general, thoracolumbar deformity (type II) caused greater functional limitations than thoracic hyperkyphosis. Up to 38% of patients reported suffering a level of pain that caused a significant alteration in their activities of daily living. Adults with more severe deformities as a result of untreated Scheuermann's disease may present with severe back pain secondary to degenerative spondylosis, which could result in severe functional limitations.[5,12,22]

Lonner et al have studied the preoperative health-related quality of life in patients with SK. They noticed that patients with SK had significantly lower scores in all domains of the SRS-22 Patient Questionnaire than the normal population. Patients with SK with a thoracolumbar apex reported significantly lower mean scores in the pain domain than those with a thoracic apex. There is a significant negative correlation between all domains of the SRS-22 and T5-T12 kyphosis; the self-image domain demonstrated the highest correlation $(r = 0.37)$.[25]

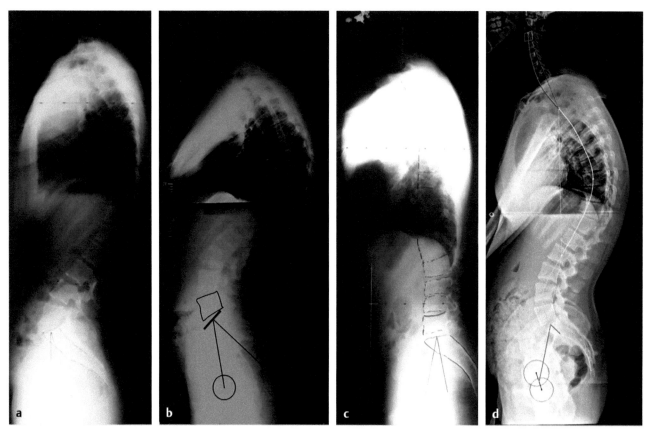

Fig. 15.3 (a) Thoracolumbar Scheuermann, type 1 shape with pelvic incidence (PI) < 20°. (b) Thoracic Scheuermann, anteverted type 4, PI = 25°. Thoracic kyphosis is compensated for by a very anteverted pelvis (pelvic tilt = -15°) to adapt sacral slope. (c) Lumbar Scheuermann, type 2 global flat back with PI = 15°. (d) Thoracic Scheuermann, type 4 with PI = 60°.

15.4 Treatment

15.4.1 Physiotherapy

Adolescents with immature skeletons who present with a slight increase in normal kyphosis, with values of up to 60° and no evidence of worsening of the deformity, will require only regular clinical and radiological follow-up until they reach skeletal maturity. Exercises that can help to relieve the symptoms are those aimed at improving balance and posture through progressive stretching of the thigh and chest muscles, as well as strengthening of the abdominal and dorsal muscles. Physical therapy exercises can also help during the initial developmental stages of hip flexion contractures and increased lumbar lordosis associated with thoracic kyphosis. Physical therapy can sometimes produce a noticeable improvement in the symptoms, but it will not produce any effect on the magnitude of the deformity. Performing regular exercises is also recommended for those patients treated with thoracolumbosacral orthosis.[8,9,10,24,26]

15.4.2 Orthosis

Treatment with orthosis can be effective in patients with hyperkyphosis less than 65°, with an initial in-brace correction of the deformity of more than 15° and the presence of skeletal immaturity with at least 1 year of the remaining growth. Boys can typically be treated until the age of 18 years. The brace should be worn for between 16 and 23 hours each day for 18 months, followed by wearing it for a part of each day for an additional 18 months with gradual weaning.[25,26] Both the Milwaukee brace and thoracolumbosacral orthosis, adding a pressure point on the sternum as one of the three points, have shown effectiveness for the correction of thoracic hyperkyphosis.[27,28]

15.4.3 Surgery

Surgical treatment should be considered in the presence of severe and progressive deformity (above 80°), especially if the patient is still in a growth phase, after failure of treatment with orthoses to control the progression of hyperkyphosis, in the presence of disabling pain resistant to conservative treatment for at least 6 months, or with neurological involvement as result of medullary compression at the apex of the kyphosis.[22,29,30,31] Sagittal imbalance has also been proposed as an indication for surgery. Improvement in quality of life is not correlated to the amount of kyphosis reduction.[32]

Biomechanical Principle of Correction

Throughout the development of the kyphosis curve, the anterior spine undergoes a gradual shortening in relation to the posterior spine, and the spinal cord must adjust to the length difference between both columns. As the deformity progresses, the bone gradually becomes compressed at the apex of the kyphosis. The correction of hyperkyphosis produces a sudden stretching of the anterior column, involving a risk of neurological damage caused by sudden stretching of the spinal cord. Therefore, it is necessary to perform a shortening of the posterior column through multiple segmental osteotomies at the apex of the hyperkyphosis to achieve a balanced correction between the anterior and posterior columns and thus avoid stretching of the spinal cord.[5]

Surgical Technique

There is a lack of consensus on the surgical approach for the management of SK. Current controversies include the need to add an anterior release compared to the single posterior approach, the selection of optimal superior and inferior levels for instrumented arthrodesis, the use of hybrid instrumentation instead of only transpedicular screws, and the type of posterior column shortening to be employed: segmental facetectomies, Ponte-type, Smith-Petersen-type, or posterior closing wedge osteotomy.

Selection of Fusion Levels

Proximal junctional kyphosis is defined as kyphosis measured from one segment cephalad, to the upper end instrumented vertebrae, to the proximal instrumented vertebrae with an abnormal value defined as > 10°. Distal junctional kyphosis is defined as kyphosis measured from one segment caudal to the end instrumented vertebrae to the distal instrumented vertebrae with an abnormal value defined as > 10° of kyphosis.[33] Junctional kyphosis developed in patients whose fusion ended short of the first lordotic segment and sagittal stable vertebra (the most proximal lumbar vertebral body touched by the vertical line from the posterior–superior corner of the sacrum) or when fusion started short of the proximal vertebra in the measured kyphosis.[34,35] Lonner et al reported on a series of 78 patients with SK treated operatively; the rate of proximal and distal junctional kyphosis occurred in 25 (32.1%) and 4 (5.1%), respectively. The development of a proximal junctional kyphosis correlated directly with kyphosis at follow-up and indirectly with the percent correction.[25]

The anterior approach enables a complete diskectomy and offers the possibility of releasing the ALL as well as placing grafts between vertebral bodies under compression conditions. Double approaches are usually reserved for cases of very rigid and severe deformities that are not corrected by forced trunk hyperextension, and especially in the presence of bone ankylosis of the posterior column with ossification of the ALL at the apex of the hyperkyphosis. The anterior approach can be performed either by open thoracotomy or, with better results and less surgical morbidity but with less capacity to obtain a complete diskectomy, by thoracoscopy.[8,15,36,37] In recent years, there has been a shift toward using a posterior-only approach for the correction of SK. This is in part a result of the reduction maneuver used (shortening the posterior column) and a better understanding of sagittal balance. Care should be taken to avoid excessive kyphosis reduction which may, in turn, create abnormal stresses both proximally and distally to the fusion mass, resulting in proximal or distal junctional kyphosis.

Degree of Deformity Correction

Proximal junctional kyphosis was associated with overcorrection (greater than 50% reduction in preoperative kyphosis)

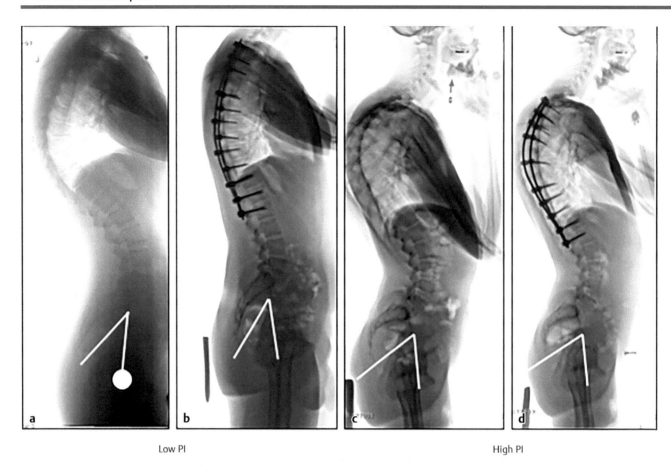

Low PI   High PI

Fig. 15.4 Surgical strategies for different pelvic morphology: **(a)** preoperative patient with low pelvic incidence (PI) and lower thoracic Scheuermann's kyphosis (SK), **(b)** postoperative correction showing kyphosis reduction with reciprocal reduction in lumbar lordosis in harmony with pelvic incidence, **(c)** preoperative thoracic SK with high pelvic incidence, and **(d)** postoperative correction with less aggressive correction respecting the sagittal pelvic profile thereby preventing junctional kyphosis.

of the kyphotic deformity.[34] In patients with low PI, the surgical management should aim at a correction within the high normal kyphosis range of 40° to 50°, but in patients with high PI, care should be taken to avoid aggressive reduction of the kyphosis as this could lead to junctional issues (▶ Fig. 15.4). Consequently, particularly in flexible adolescents and young adults, an anterior release is not necessary to provide optimal results.[38,39]

15.4.4 Complications

The analysis of complications published by the Morbidity and Mortality Committee of the Scoliosis Research Society on 683 surgical procedures for the treatment of Scheuermann's disease conducted between 2001 and 2004 reported a total incidence of complications of 14.5%. The overall incidence of surgical complications was more common in adults (21.7%) compared to patients in their teens (11.8%). There were no significant differences in complication rates between posterior spinal fusion (PSF) and PSF with same-day anterior spinal fusion (ASF/PSF) procedures.[40] The main reported surgical complications are wound infection (3.8%), implant-related complications (2.5%), spinal cord injury (0.6%), and dural tear (0.3%).

15.4.5 Prognosis

Personalized treatment based on the patient's age, spinal deformity, and back pain can lead to similar long-term outcomes for patients with SK. Neurological deterioration is rare, but patients with significant curves who choose nonsurgical management should be monitored regularly for progression of the curve. Similar functional outcomes can be achieved at long-term follow-up.[28]

References

[1] Scheuermann HW. The classic: kyphosis dorsalis juvenilis. Clin Orthop Relat Res. 1977; 128:5–7

[2] Blumenthal SL, Roach J, Herring JA. Lumbar Scheuermann's. A clinical series and classification. Spine. 1987; 12(9):929–932

[3] Murray PM, Weinstein SL, Spratt KF. The natural history and long-term follow-up of Scheuermann kyphosis. J Bone Joint Surg Am. 1993; 75(2): 236–248

[4] Bradford DS, Moe JH, Montalvo FJ, Winter RB. Scheuermann's kyphosis and roundback deformity. Results of Milwaukee brace treatment. J Bone Joint Surg Am. 1974; 56(4):740–758

[5] Tsirikos AI, Jain AK. Scheuermann's kyphosis; current controversies. J Bone Joint Surg Br. 2011; 93(7):857–864

[6] Fisk JW, Baigent ML, Hill PD. Incidence of Scheuermann's disease. Preliminary report. Am J Phys Med. 1982; 61(1):32–35

[7] Damborg F, Engell V, Nielsen J, Kyvik KO, Andersen MØ, Thomsen K. Genetic epidemiology of Scheuermann's disease. Acta Orthop. 2011; 82(5):602–605

[8] Tsirikos AI. Scheuermann's kyphosis: an update. J Surg Orthop Adv. 2009; 18(3):122–128

[9] Lowe TG. Scheuermann disease. J Bone Joint Surg Am. 1990; 72(6):940–945

[10] Papagelopoulos PJ, Mavrogenis AF, Savvidou OD, Mitsiokapa EA, Themistocleous GS, Soucacos PN. Current concepts in Scheuermann's kyphosis. Orthopedics. 2008; 31(1):52–58, quiz 59–60

[11] Lonner BS, Toombs CS, Husain QM, et al. Body mass index in adolescent spinal deformity: comparison of Scheuermann's kyphosis, adolescent idiopathic scoliosis, and normal controls. Spine Deform. 2015; 3(4):318–326

[12] Bradford DS, Moe JH. Scheuermann's juvenile kyphosis. A histologic study. Clin Orthop Relat Res. 1975; 110:45–53

[13] Lowe TG, Line BG. Evidence based medicine: analysis of Scheuermann kyphosis. Spine. 2007; 32(19) Suppl:S115–S119

[14] Ali RM, Green DW, Patel TC. Scheuermann's kyphosis. Curr Opin Pediatr. 1999; 11(1):70–75

[15] Tribus CB. Scheuermann's kyphosis in adolescents and adults: diagnosis and management. J Am Acad Orthop Surg. 1998; 6(1):36–43

[16] Wood KB, Melikian R, Villamil F. Adult Scheuermann kyphosis: evaluation, management, and new developments. J Am Acad Orthop Surg. 2012; 20(2):113–121

[17] Putz C, Stierle I, Grieser T, et al. Progressive spastic paraplegia: the combination of Scheuermann's disease, a short-segmented kyphosis and dysplastic thoracic spinous processes. Spinal Cord. 2009; 47(7):570–572

[18] Kapetanos GA, Hantzidis PT, Anagnostidis KS, Kirkos JM. Thoracic cord compression caused by disk herniation in Scheuermann's disease: a case report and review of the literature. Eur Spine J. 2006; 15 Suppl 5:553–558

[19] Mac-Thiong J-M, Labelle H, Berthonnaud E, Betz RR, Roussouly P. Sagittal spinopelvic balance in normal children and adolescents. Eur Spine J. 2007; 16(2):227–234

[20] Legaye J, Duval-Beaupère G, Hecquet J, Marty C. Pelvic incidence: a fundamental pelvic parameter for three-dimensional regulation of spinal sagittal curves. Eur Spine J. 1998; 7(2):99–103

[21] Tyrakowski M, Mardjetko S, Siemionow K. Radiographic spinopelvic parameters in skeletally mature patients with Scheuermann disease. Spine. 2014; 39(18):E1080–E1085

[22] Jiang L, Qiu Y, Xu L, et al. Sagittal spinopelvic alignment in adolescents associated with Scheuermann's kyphosis: a comparison with normal population. Eur Spine J. 2014; 23(7):1420–1426

[23] Sorensen KH. Scheuermann's Juvenile Kyphosis; Clinical Appearances, Radiography, Aetiology, and Prognosis. Copenhagen, Denmark: Munksgaard; 1964

[24] Roussouly P, Gollogly S, Berthonnaud E, Dimnet J. Classification of the normal variation in the sagittal alignment of the human lumbar spine and pelvis in the standing position. Spine. 2005; 30(3):346–353

[25] Lonner BS, Newton P, Betz R, et al. Operative management of Scheuermann's kyphosis in 78 patients: radiographic outcomes, complications, and technique. Spine. 2007; 32(24):2644–2652

[26] Bradford DS, Ahmed KB, Moe JH, Winter RB, Lonstein JE. The surgical management of patients with Scheuermann's disease: a review of twenty-four cases managed by combined anterior and posterior spine fusion. J Bone Joint Surg Am. 1980; 62(5):705–712

[27] Wenger DR, Frick SL. Scheuermann kyphosis. Spine. 1999; 24(24):2630–2639

[28] Soo CL, Noble PC, Esses SI. Scheuermann kyphosis: long-term follow-up. Spine J. 2002; 2(1):49–56

[29] Weiss H-R, Turnbull D, Bohr S. Brace treatment for patients with Scheuermann's disease—a review of the literature and first experiences with a new brace design. Scoliosis. 2009; 4:22

[30] Sachs B, Bradford D, Winter R, Lonstein J, Moe J, Willson S. Scheuermann kyphosis. Follow-up of Milwaukee-brace treatment. J Bone Joint Surg Am. 1987; 69(1):50–57

[31] Riddle EC, Bowen JR, Shah SA, Moran EF, Lawall H, Jr. The duPont kyphosis brace for the treatment of adolescent Scheuermann kyphosis. J South Orthop Assoc. 2003; 12(3):135–140

[32] Lonner B, Yoo A, Terran JS, et al. Effect of spinal deformity on adolescent quality of life: comparison of operative Scheuermann kyphosis, adolescent idiopathic scoliosis, and normal controls. Spine. 2013; 38(12):1049–1055

[33] O'Brien MF, Lenke LG. Spinal Deformity Study Group Radiographic Measurement Manual. Memphis, TN: Medtronic Sofamor Danek; 2004

[34] Lowe TG, Kasten MD. An analysis of sagittal curves and balance after Cotrel-Dubousset instrumentation for kyphosis secondary to Scheuermann's disease. A review of 32 patients. Spine. 1994; 19(15):1680–1685

[35] Cho K-J, Lenke LG, Bridwell KH, Kamiya M, Sides B. Selection of the optimal distal fusion level in posterior instrumentation and fusion for thoracic hyperkyphosis: the sagittal stable vertebra concept. Spine. 2009; 34(8):765–770

[36] Lowe TG. Scheuermann's kyphosis. Neurosurg Clin N Am. 2007; 18(2):305–315

[37] Herrera-Soto JA, Parikh SN, Al-Sayyad MJ, Crawford AH. Experience with combined video-assisted thoracoscopic surgery (VATS) anterior spinal release and posterior spinal fusion in Scheuermann's kyphosis. Spine. 2005; 30(19):2176–2181

[38] Hosman AJ, Langeloo DD, de Kleuver M, Anderson PG, Veth RP, Slot GH. Analysis of the sagittal plane after surgical management for Scheuermann's disease: a view on overcorrection and the use of an anterior release. Spine. 2002; 27(2):167–175

[39] Lonner BS, Parent S, Shah SA, et al. Reciprocal changes in sagittal alignment with operative treatment of adolescent Scheuermann kyphosis—prospective evaluation of 96 patients. Spine Deform. 2018; 6(2):177–184

[40] Coe JD, Smith JS, Berven S, et al. Complications of spinal fusion for Scheuermann kyphosis: a report of the scoliosis research society morbidity and mortality committee. Spine. 2010; 35(1):99–103

16 Cervical Sagittal Alignment and Cervicarthrosis

Darryl Lau and Christopher P. Ames

Abstract

The cervical spine is very complex, allowing the widest range of motion, and inherently is more susceptible to degeneration, injury, and dysfunction. Cervical kyphosis, a sagittal deformity, is the most common deformity in this region. Severe cervical kyphosis can lead to debilitating neck pain, difficulties with eating, inability to maintain horizontal gaze, imbalanced gait, and restrictions of activities of daily living. In addition, cervical deformities can result in spinal cord compression and clinical signs of myelopathy. All patients should undergo standing scoliosis X-rays to evaluate for regional cervical and overall global spinal alignment. Flexion–extension films are critical to evaluate for fixed deformities. On radiographs, clinically significant cervical parameters measurements include cervical lordosis, cervical sagittal vertical axis (cSVA), and chin-brow vertical angle. More novel parameters include neck tilt, thoracic inlet angle, T1-slope, C2 pelvic tilt, and craniocervical angle. There is a paucity of studies looking at these parameters and its association of clinical outcomes. However, among these cervical measurements, loss of cervical lordosis and greater cSVA results in poorer outcomes based on health-related quality of life (HRQoL) outcomes. Traditionally, it is presumed that restoring cervical lordosis provided the most optimal outcomes, but there is emerging evidence that obtaining cSVA of less than 40 mm may result in better HRQoL outcomes. The decisions regarding the approach, extent of osteotomy, and construct size is unique to each case and dependent on a variety of factors. The correction of fixed hyperkyphotic cervical deformities can be quite challenging, but utilizing combined anterior–posterior osteotomy (multilevel Smith-Petersen osteotomy) or posterior-only-based osteotomy (pedicle subtraction osteotomy) has proven to be effective. Cervical traction preoperatively may be utilized. Managing complications and guiding these patients through their perioperative course is imperative to providing them the most optimal outcome possible.

Keywords: cervical, deformity, kyphosis, osteotomy

16.1 Introduction

There has been new and engaging research in the understanding of how sagittal and coronal spinal imbalance affects patient function and satisfaction. The most robust data concentrates on spinal pelvic parameters in the thoracolumbar spine. More recently, there has been an accumulation of data demonstrating the importance of balance in the cervical spine (i.e., cervical sagittal alignment impacts quality of life). Each spinal region is unique because of their anatomical features and physiologic functions. Unlike the more rigid thoracic and lumbar spine, the cervical spine is very complex; it allows the widest range of motion while needing to support the head in a neutral position to allow horizontal gaze. Because of this complex nature, the cervical spine is inherently more susceptible to degeneration, injury, and dysfunction.[1] Cervical kyphosis, a

sagittal deformity, is the most common deformity in this region and is secondary to a multitude of etiologies: inflammatory spondyloarthropathies (ankylosing spondylitis and diffuse idiopathic skeletal hyperostosis), myopathies, degenerative disease, traumatic injuries, pathologic fractures, and iatrogenic causes (postlaminectomy kyphosis).[1,2,3,4,5]

16.2 Relationship between Sagittal Deformity and Cervical Myelopathy

Traditionally, cervical myelopathy is thought to be secondary to cervical stenosis and spondylosis. However, there is evidence suggesting that abnormal cervical sagittal alignment accounts for many cases of myelopathy. Abnormal cervical sagittal alignment, with the majority of cases being loss of lordosis or kyphosis, can lead to spinal cord injury and clinical myelopathy.[6] In cadaver models and animal studies, increased sagittal alignment (kyphosis) results in spinal cord tension and flattening, which leads to increased intramedullary pressure within the spinal cord.[7,8,9,10] The end result of high intramedullary pressure is ischemia, demyelination, neuronal apoptosis, and injury.[10] In the setting of cervical kyphosis, the spinal cord can be further injured by being forced over the posterior aspect of the vertebral body causing direct mechanical pressure onto the spinal cord. This impingement causes direct injury to the underlying spinal tracts, most notably the corticospinal tracts that are located in the anterior portion of the spinal cord. This mechanical pressure can further result in greater tension within the spinal cord and contribute to even higher intramedullary pressures.[2,11] This direct mechanical pressure onto the spinal cord has been observed in patients with cervical sagittal malalignment during flexion–extension studies on electrophysiology and magnetic resonance imaging (MRI).[12,13,14]

Cervical kyphosis is often a progressive process and can become quite severe if left untreated. The structural malalignment itself can result in significant patient dysfunction. These dysfunctions include debilitating neck pain, difficulties with eating (infrequently requiring a feeding tube in severe cases), inability in maintaining horizontal gaze (look straight), imbalanced gait, and restrictions of activities of daily living.[15] With regard to specific locations of pain other than the neck, patients that maintain a forward head posture can have increased incidence of interscapular head pains.

16.3 Cervical Spinal Curvature and Alignment Parameters

16.3.1 Cervical Lordosis

There are three general methods to measuring cervical lordosis: Cobb angle, the Harrison posterior tangent method, and

Jackson physiological stress lines.[1,16] Cobb angle is the clinical mainstay given its easy-to-use format and good intra- and interrater reliability.[17,18] To measure cervical sagittal Cobb angle, either C1 to C7 or C2 to C7 can be used. The angle subtended between perpendicular lines drawn from the caudal line (C1 or C2) and rostral line (C7) is the cervical sagittal Cobb angle. The caudal line at C1 is drawn extending from the anterior tubercle of C1 to the posterior margin of the spinous process. If C2 is used, a line parallel to the inferior endplate of C2 vertebral body is drawn.[1,16] The rostral line is drawn parallel to the superior endplate of C7. The method of measuring the C2 to C7 sagittal Cobb angle is shown in ▶ Fig. 16.1. The Harrison posterior tangent method involves drawing parallel lines to the posterior surfaces of all cervical vertebral bodies from C2 to C7 and then summing up the segmental angles for an overall cervical curvature angle.[1,16] The cervical lordosis measured by the Jackson physiological stress lines is performed by drawing parallel lines to the posterior surface of C2 and C7; the angle between those lines is the cervical lordosis measurement.

16.3.2 Cervical Sagittal Alignment

Like global sagittal alignment, regional cervical sagittal alignment can also be quantified as the cervical sagittal vertical axis (cSVA).[1] cSVA is a regional measurement of sagittal alignment. This is the distance between a plumb line dropped from the centroid of C2 (or odontoid) and the posterior superior aspect of the C7 vertebral body (▶ Fig. 16.2). Another method of assessing regional cervical sagittal alignment is to use the

center of gravity (COG) of the head (COG-cSVA) rather than the C2 centroid. To measure COG-cSVA, a plumb line is drawn from the anterior portion of the external auditory canal and the distance from the posterior–superior aspect of C7 is measured.[1] The most commonly used method is the cSVA because past studies have shown that this parameter is directly correlated with health-related quality of life (HRQoL) outcomes (i.e., greater cSVA is associated with worse outcomes especially when greater than 40 mm).[19]

16.3.3 Chin-Brow Vertical Angle

The chin-brow vertical angle (CBVA) is a measurement of horizontal gaze. This is an important parameter as horizontal gaze is essential for many of the activities of everyday life and ambulation.[20,21,22] The CBVA is measured by drawing a line from the patient's brow to chin and a vertical line. The angle subtended between those two lines is the CBVA (▶ Fig. 16.3).[1]

16.3.4 Neck Tilt, Thoracic Inlet Angle, and T1 Slope

More investigational and novel methods of quantifying sagittal alignment in the cervical spine include neck tilt (NT), thoracic inlet angle (TIA), and T1 slope.[1] NT is defined as an angle

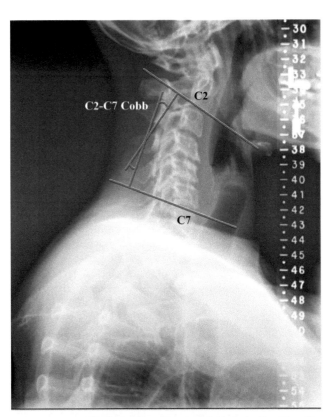

Fig. 16.1 Cervical lordosis: C2 to C7 sagittal Cobb angle. The C2 to C7 sagittal Cobb angle is subtended between perpendicular lines drawn from the caudal line at C2 and rostral line at C7.

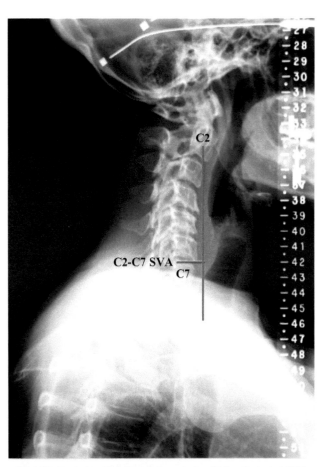

Fig. 16.2 Cervical sagittal alignment: cervical sagittal vertical axis (cSVA). The cSVA is the distance between a plumb line dropped from the centroid of C2 and the posterior superior aspect of the C7 vertebral body.

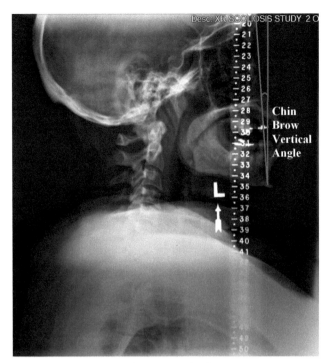

Fig. 16.3 Chin-brow vertical angle. The chin-brow vertical is the angle subtended by a line from the patient's brow to chin and a vertical line.

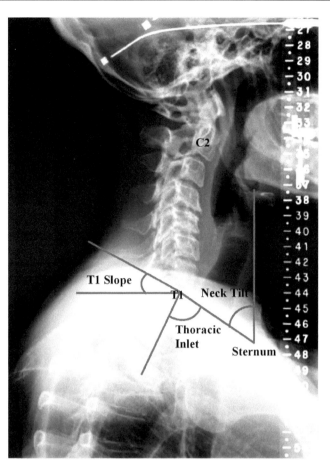

Fig. 16.4 Neck tilt, thoracic inlet angle, and T1-slope. Neck tilt is the angle between two lines both originating from the upper end of the sternum with one being a vertical line and the other connecting to the center of the T1 endplate. Thoracic inlet angle is the angle between a line originating from the center of the T1 endplate that is perpendicular to the T1 endplate and a line from the center of the T1 endplate to the upper end of the sternum. T1 slope is the angle measured between a horizontal plane and a line parallel to the T1 endplate.

between two lines both originating from the upper end of the sternum with one being a vertical line and the other connecting to the center of the T1 endplate. The TIA is defined as the angle between a line originating from the center of the T1 endplate that is perpendicular to the T1 endplate and a line from the center of the T1 endplate to the upper end of the sternum. T1 slope is the angle measured between a horizontal plane and a line parallel to the T1 endplate. T1 slope is significant because it is a surrogate for the amount of subaxial lordosis required to maintain the COG of the head in a balanced position. Hence, this parameter may guide and predict physiological alignment following deformity correction.[23] Examples of these three measurements can be seen in ▶ Fig. 16.4.

16.3.5 C2 Pelvic Tilt

A novel measurement that has been shown to be valuable in preoperative evaluation of cervical deformity is C2 pelvic tilt (C2PT). C2PT considers the relationship of T1 slope and cervical lordosis with the extent of pelvic retroversion. C2PT is the sum of C2 tilt and pelvic tilt. C2 tilt is defined as an angle subtended by a line drawn parallel on the posterior aspect of the C2 vertebral body and a vertical line (▶ Fig. 16.5).[24] Pelvic tilt is the angle formed by the intersection of a line drawn from the middle of the S1 endplate and a vertical line from the femoral head if aligned or bicoxofemoral axis (midpoint between the femoral heads) (▶ Fig. 16.5). The C2PT angle can be measured by extending the line parallel to the posterior edge of the C2 vertebral body until it intersects the line that is extended from the femoral head to the midpoint of the superior endplate of S1 (▶ Fig. 16.5).

16.3.6 Craniocervical Angle

Craniocervical angle (CCA) is a measurement that considers cervical compensation and sagittal inclination. CCA is the angle subtended by a line from the hard palate to the opisthion (McGregor's line) and a line from the hard palate to the center of C7 vertebral body (▶ Fig. 16.6).[24] As cervical deformity worsens, the CCA value gets smaller, and a CCA of less than 45° may be an indicator of the presence of a large cervical deformity.

16.4 Normative Cervical Curve and Alignment

Cervical sagittal curve is closely related to cervical sagittal alignment. The difference between the two is that cervical sagittal curve is a regional measurement while cervical sagittal alignment considers global spinal balance (thoracic, lumbar, and sacral spine). Normal or mean cervical lordosis can be quite

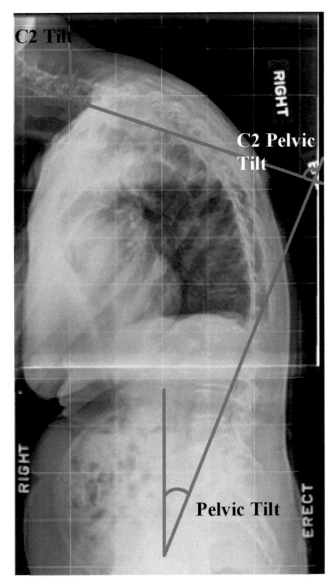

Fig. 16.5 C2 pelvic tilt. C2 pelvic tilt is the sum of C2 tilt and pelvic tilt. C2 tilt is the angle subtended by a line drawn parallel on the posterior aspect of the C2 vertebral body and a vertical line.

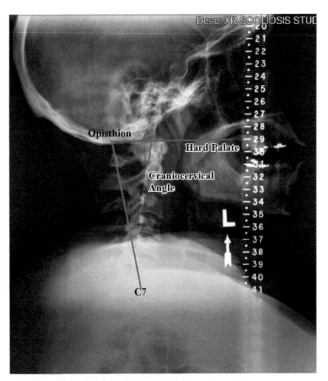

Fig. 16.6 Craniocervical angle. Craniocervical angle is the angle subtended by a line from hard palate to the opisthion (and a line from the hard palate to the center of C7 vertebral body).

16.5 Cervical Sagittal Alignment and Quality of Life Outcomes

Studies regarding the relationship between cervical sagittal curve and alignment are few relative to the number of studies concentrating on the thoracolumbar spine. The available studies mostly concentrate on regional cervical sagittal curve and its relation to neck pain. Based on past surgical cohort studies, loss of cervical lordosis or presence of kyphosis (based on sagittal Cobb angle measurements) have been associated with increased neck pain.[29] The findings from studies evaluating the association between regional cervical sagittal curve and HRQoL outcomes are very limited. There are mixed results and findings of whether regional cervical sagittal curves correlate with clinical outcomes and postoperative functional status.[30,31] Some studies suggest that changes in regional cervical curve does not correlate significantly with clinical outcomes.[32] The studies of cervical alignment via cSVA are even fever. There is only one study looking into the relationship of cSVA and HRQoL outcomes.[19] In that study, cSVA correlated negatively with SF-36 physical component scores and positively correlated with neck disability scores; increased sagittal cervical imbalance led to lower SF-36 physical component scores and increase neck pain scores, especially when cSVA is greater than 40 mm. There is clearly a dire need of prospective studies assessing the association of cervical parameters with functional outcomes. Studies

variable depending on age and gender. According to past studies of asymptomatic patients, normative regional cervical lordosis from C1 to C7 in adults was 41.8°.[1,25] Most of the cervical lordosis occurs at the C1-C2 junction (mean of 32.2°), while other individual cervical levels only contribute approximately 1° to 2° of additional lordosis.[1,25,26] It is also important to keep in mind that a mild physiologic cervical kyphosis is present in up to 34% of asymptomatic individuals, especially in younger individuals.[27,28] Cervical sagittal alignment is dependent on the global spinal curvature and the anatomy of the cervicothoracic junction, because the body tries to maintain a neutral upright posture and horizontal gaze. In asymptomatic adults, mean cSVA has been reported to be 15.6 mm.

on other cervical parameters need to be assessed: cSVA, CBVA, T1 slope, TIA, NT, C2PT, and CCA.

16.6 Preoperative Evaluation and Considerations

All patients should undergo standing scoliosis X-rays to evaluate for regional cervical and overall global spinal alignment. Flexion–extension films can be obtained to determine whether a patient's deformity is mobile or rigid as this dictates the type of surgery that needs to be performed. Computed tomography and MRI should be performed to appreciate bony anatomy and assess for compression of neural elements (spinal cord and nerve roots), respectively. In the evaluation of a patient with cervical kyphosis that is a candidate for surgical correction of their deformity, it is essential to ensure that their cervical curve is not compensatory to deformities in other areas of the spine or even a normal physiologic feature, especially among younger individuals that have negative thoracolumbar SVA.[33] Because the cervical spine is the most mobile, it has the capacity to undergo "reciprocal changes" to its alignment to compensate for deformities affecting the thoracic and lumbar spine.[33,34,35] A method of determining whether a thoracolumbar deformity is contributing cervical malalignment is to measure the T1 slope; if the T1 slope is greater than 30° then likely a thoracolumbar deformity is present.[36,37] In addition, the relationship of cervical sagittal Cobb and T1 slope has been reported to be important in identification of a true cervical deformity; the difference between T1 slope and cervical Cobb greater than 17° suggests the presence of a cervical sagittal deformity, even if a concurrent thoracic or lumber deformity is present.

In deciding the specific surgery to be performed, there needs to be an understanding of the severity of the cervical deformity and how much correction needs to be achieved. There is emerging but little data regarding defining the optimal cervical lordosis and sagittal alignment that needs to be achieved. In the past, the general goal was to aim for normal regional cervical lordosis following deformity correction.[5] But, more recently, other cervical parameters are being considered and more frequently being used to guide the extent of deformity correction. cSVA and CBVA are examples.[19,22] It is suggested that a cSVA of less than 40 mm may result in better HRQoL outcomes. It is important to also evaluate TIA and T1 slope as these parameters have been suggested to be able to predict sagittal balance, outcomes, and guide deformity corrections.[23] There seems to be an important relationship between the two parameters, and ideal balance is achieved when TIA is equal to the T1 slope. This is similar to the lumbosacral region in which the pelvic incidence equals the sacral slope plus the pelvic tilt.

16.7 Surgical Options for Correction of Cervical Sagittal Deformities

The decisions regarding the approach, extent of osteotomy, and construct size is unique to each case and dependent on a variety of factors. There is no consensus even among senior spinal deformity surgeons in how to treat a specific entity, especially for

mild-to-moderate cervical deformities. For a kyphotic apex in the lower cervical and cervicothoracic junction and chin-to-chest deformities more than 80% of expert surgeons would recommend a posterior-only approach and more than 70% would recommend either pedicle subtraction osteotomy (PSO) or vertebral body resection (VCR).[38] There was a lack of a consensus in how many levels should be instrumented. There is agreement that understanding the etiology of the cervical sagittal deformity is critical in being successful to achieve a balanced correction. Other important factors that need to be considered are the rigidity and morphologic type of the deformity. Fixed deformities should be divided as ankylosed or not ankylosed. Patients who are ankylosed anteriorly should undergo anterior osteotomies and release followed by posterior instrumentation (anterior then posterior). If a patient is ankylosed posteriorly, a posterior osteotomy and release should first be performed followed by an anterior release and then posterior instrumentation (posterior then anterior then posterior). In patients with both ankyloses anterior and posterior, a PSO is recommended. In patients that are fixed but not ankylosed, they should generally be approached anteriorly with possible posterior instrumentation. For patients who have flexible cervical deformities, a variety of approaches and surgeries can be performed.[39]

The type of osteotomy and spinal releases required is dependent on whether the spine is rigid and how much correction needs to be obtained. Ames et al classifies seven different types of osteotomies that can be used on the cervical spine (as seen in ▶ Table 16.1).[40]

Table 16.1 Cervical osteotomy classification

Spine type	Cervical osteotomy grade	Technique
Flexible	1	Partial joint resection including partial resection of the uncinate joints and/or partial removal of the posterior facets
Flexible	2	Removal of both the inferior and superior articular facets
Rigid	3	Corpectomy
Rigid	4	Corpectomy with associated complete resection of the uncinate joints laterally to the transverse foramen
Rigid/ankylosed	5	Complete resection of the posterior elements (lamina, spinous process, and facets), closure of the posterior defect, and controlled fracture of the ankylosed anterior column
Rigid/ankylosed	6	Pedicle subtraction osteotomy (complete removal of the lamina, spinous process, facets, and pedicles at the desired level), followed by creation of a closing wedge osteotomy in the vertebral body
Rigid/ankylosed	7	Complete vertebrectomy (removal of the vertebral body and uncinate joints anteriorly, and complete removal of the facets, lamina, and spinous process posteriorly)

The extent and ability to surgically correct cervical sagittal deformities, specifically kyphotic deformities, varies based on a variety of reasons: intent to correct, surgical techniques, and patient characteristics.[29,41] Preoperative cervical traction for 24 to 72 hours is a viable option in patients with severe kyphosis, and some surgeons would argue for leaving patients in traction for even longer periods of time. Traction is beneficial in patients with fixed kyphotic deformities and can be maintained intraoperatively if needed.[42] The disadvantages to preoperative cervical traction are patient discomfort and unfamiliarity of its use at some institutions.

The extent of correction vary by techniques and approaches: 11° to 32° with anterior approaches,[43,44,45,46,47] 23° to 54° with posterior approaches,[48,49,50,51,52,53,54,55] and 24° to 61° with a combined approach.[4,56,57] There is a trend for a greater correction when a posterior or a combined anterior–posterior approach to osteotomy is taken.[40] An anterior osteotomy combined with posterior Smith-Petersen osteotomy (SPO) can provide similar correction as a lower cervical or upper thoracic PSO.[58]

Anterior approaches to the cervical spine can offer the ability to perform multilevel diskectomies and/or corpectomies. Significant kyphosis correction can be achieved during anterior column reconstruction with distraction and placement of large lordotic cages.[29] Expandable cages can offer additional distraction as well.[59] The reported ranges of global cervical curvature correction from a standard single-level corpectomy ranges from -1.0° to 5.0° and two-level diskectomy ranges from 1.6° to 8.0°.[60,61,62] But with more aggressive controlled distraction, more cervical kyphosis correction can be achieved. The main issues with an anterior-alone approach are the risks for dysphagia (rate as high as 50% at 1 month), vocal cord injury, and inability to release cervical deformities associated with fixed posterior elements.[63,64,65] In cases were anterior column reconstruction is warranted and posterior elements are fixed, a posterior-anterior-posterior approach may be warranted to release the three spinal columns.

Unlike the thoracic or lumbar spine, posterior-based VCR or corpectomies are extremely difficult. There have been reports of cases in which posterior transpedicular corpectomies and anterior column reconstruction were performed, but this approach has not been widely adapted.[66] Posterior-based osteotomies are viable options for the correction of severe sagittal deformities in the cervical spine. Traditionally, for fixed cervical kyphotic deformities, SPOs were used in the cervical spine; this was oftentimes supplemented by a controlled wedge fracture at C7 to restore sagittal balance.[67,68,69] This technique is very effective in patients with inflammatory spondylitis. More recently, there has been interest and contemporary studies of using PSO for cervical deformity correction. The cervicothoracic PSO is taut to offer greater controlled closure, stronger biomechanical stability, and avoid the anterior open wedge defects compared to the traditional cervical SPO.[70,71] Cervical PSO is a technique that can offer correction for fixed coronal deformities

as well.[72] Most cervicothoracic junction PSOs are performed at T1, T2, or T3.[73] With regard to kyphosis deformity correction, cervicothoracic PSO offers a mean C2-C7 SVA correction of 2.2 to 4.5 cm, cervical sagittal Cobb of 10.1 to 19.0°, and CBVA of 36.7°.[20,73] Patients who undergo cervicothoracic PSO have been shown to gain significant benefits with regard to neck disability index, neck visual analogue pain scores, and SF-36 physical component summary scores.[20] The cervicothoracic PSO is an extremely powerful technique for correction of fixed cervical sagittal deformities but also is associated with high complication rates up to 56.5% (major and minor).[73] The most common complications encountered within 90 days include neurological deficits (spinal cord and nerve root involvement), wound infections, distal junctional issues, and cardiorespiratory failure.

▶ Fig. 16.5 shows a case example of an 82-year-old female who had undergone prior cervical laminectomy with onlay fusion who presented with a progressive rigid cervical kyphosis, resulting in debilitating neck pain and significant functional disability (▶ Fig. 16.7a). Her preoperative C2-C7 sagittal Cobb was -20° (kyphosis), C2-C7 SVA of positive 80 mm, a T1 slope of 71°, and a TIA of 89°. She underwent a T1 PSO and posterior spinal fixation/fusion with C4 to C6 lateral mass screws, C7 pedicle screws, and T2 to T4 pedicle screws. Her postoperative cervical parameters were C2-C7 sagittal Cobb of 21° (lordosis), C2-C7 SVA 35 mm, a T1 slope of 56°, and a TIA of 86° (▶ Fig. 16.7b). This patient has a concurrent sagittal lumbar deformity as well with loss of lumbar lordosis.

16.8 Conclusion

The cervical spine is a relatively mobile and complex segment compared to the thoracic and lumbar spine. Therefore, a variety of pathologies can result in significant deformities causing significant imbalance and dysfunction. Cervical sagittal deformity, cervical kyphosis in particular, is associated with the pathogenesis of spinal cord injury and myelopathy. In the evaluation of patients with cervical sagittal deformities, 3-foot standing scoliosis X-rays are essential to ensure their cervical deformity is not compensatory secondary to a separate deformity in other spinal regions. Cervical spinal parameters most commonly assessed and utilized as a guide for surgical deformity correction include C2-C7 sagittal Cobb angle, cSVA, CBVA, and T1-slope. Patients with abnormal parameters have poor functional status, and correction of their deformity seems to improve HRQoL outcomes. The correction of fixed hyperkyphotic cervical deformities can be quite challenging but utilizing combined anterior–posterior osteotomy (multilevel SPO) or posterior-only-based osteotomy has proven to be effective. Managing complications and guiding these patients through their perioperative course is imperative to providing them the most optimal outcome possible.

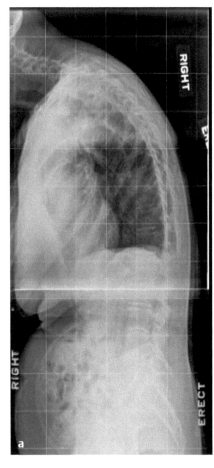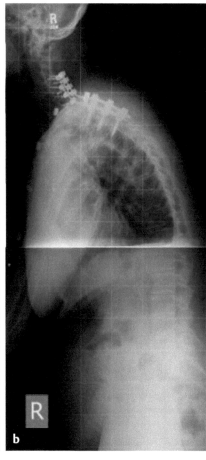

Fig. 16.7 Case example: T1 pedicle subtraction osteotomy. **(a)** Preoperative standing X-rays demonstrated loss of lordosis and sagittal imbalance: C2-C7 sagittal Cobb of -20° (kyphosis), C2-C7 sagittal vertical axis (SVA) of positive 80 mm, T1 slope of 71°, and thoracic inlet angle (TIA) 89°. **(b)** Postoperative standing X-rays shows normalized parameters: C2-C7 sagittal Cobb of 21° (lordosis), C2-C7 SVA of 35 mm, T1 slope of 56°, and TIA of 86°.

References

[1] Ames CP, Blondel B, Scheer JK, et al. Cervical radiographical alignment: comprehensive assessment techniques and potential importance in cervical myelopathy. Spine. 2013; 38(22) Suppl 1:S149–S160

[2] Albert TJ, Vacarro A. Postlaminectomy kyphosis. Spine. 1998; 23(24): 2738–2745

[3] Kaptain GJ, Simmons NE, Replogle RE, Pobereskin L. Incidence and outcome of kyphotic deformity following laminectomy for cervical spondylotic myelopathy. J Neurosurg. 2000; 93(2) Suppl:199–204

[4] O'Shaughnessy BA, Liu JC, Hsieh PC, Koski TR, Ganju A, Ondra SL. Surgical treatment of fixed cervical kyphosis with myelopathy. Spine. 2008; 33 (7):771–778

[5] Steinmetz MP, Stewart TJ, Kager CD, Benzel EC, Vaccaro AR. Cervical deformity correction. Neurosurgery. 2007; 60(1) Suppl 1:S90–S97

[6] Grosso MJ, Hwang R, Mroz T, Benzel E, Steinmetz MP. Relationship between degree of focal kyphosis correction and neurological outcomes for patients undergoing cervical deformity correction surgery. J Neurosurg Spine. 2013; 18(6):537–544

[7] Chavanne A, Pettigrew DB, Holtz JR, Dollin N, Kuntz C, IV. Spinal cord intramedullary pressure in cervical kyphotic deformity: a cadaveric study. Spine. 2011; 36(20):1619–1626

[8] Iida H, Tachibana S. Spinal cord intramedullary pressure: direct cord traction test. Neurol Med Chir (Tokyo). 1995; 35(2):75–77

[9] Jarzem PF, Quance DR, Doyle DJ, Begin LR, Kostuik JP. Spinal cord tissue pressure during spinal cord distraction in dogs. Spine. 1992; 17(8) Suppl: S227–S234

[10] Shimizu K, Nakamura M, Nishikawa Y, Hijikata S, Chiba K, Toyama Y. Spinal kyphosis causes demyelination and neuronal loss in the spinal cord: a new model of kyphotic deformity using juvenile Japanese small game fowls. Spine. 2005; 30(21):2388–2392

[11] Deutsch H, Haid RW, Rodts GE, Mummaneni PV. Postlaminectomy cervical deformity. Neurosurg Focus. 2003; 15(3):E5

[12] Kato Y, Imajo Y, Kanchiku T, Kojima T, Kataoka H, Taguchi T. Dynamic electrophysiological examination of cervical flexion myelopathy. J Neurosurg Spine. 2008; 9(2):180–185

[13] Miura J, Doita M, Miyata K, et al. Dynamic evaluation of the spinal cord in patients with cervical spondylotic myelopathy using a kinematic magnetic resonance imaging technique. J Spinal Disord Tech. 2009; 22(1):8–13

[14] Zhang L, Zeitoun D, Rangel A, Lazennec JY, Catonné Y, Pascal-Moussellard H. Preoperative evaluation of the cervical spondylotic myelopathy with flexion-extension magnetic resonance imaging: about a prospective study of fifty patients. Spine. 2011; 36(17):E1134–E1139

[15] Griegel-Morris P, Larson K, Mueller-Klaus K, Oatis CA. Incidence of common postural abnormalities in the cervical, shoulder, and thoracic regions and their association with pain in two age groups of healthy subjects. Phys Ther. 1992; 72(6):425–431

[16] Harrison DE, Harrison DD, Cailliet R, Troyanovich SJ, Janik TJ, Holland B. Cobb method or Harrison posterior tangent method: which to choose for lateral cervical radiographic analysis. Spine. 2000; 25(16):2072–2078

[17] Polly DW, Jr, Kilkelly FX, McHale KA, Asplund LM, Mulligan M, Chang AS. Measurement of lumbar lordosis. Evaluation of intraobserver, interobserver, and technique variability. Spine. 1996; 21(13):1530–1535, discussion 1535–1536

[18] Singer KP, Jones TJ, Breidahl PD. A comparison of radiographic and computer-assisted measurements of thoracic and thoracolumbar sagittal curvature. Skeletal Radiol. 1990; 19(1):21–26

[19] Tang JA, Scheer JK, Smith JS, et al. ISSG. The impact of standing regional cervical sagittal alignment on outcomes in posterior cervical fusion surgery. Neurosurgery. 2012; 71(3):662–669, discussion 669

[20] Deviren V, Scheer JK, Ames CP. Technique of cervicothoracic junction pedicle subtraction osteotomy for cervical sagittal imbalance: report of 11 cases. J Neurosurg Spine. 2011; 15(2):174–181

[21] Kim KT, Lee SH, Son ES, Kwack YH, Chun YS, Lee JH. Surgical treatment of "chin-on-pubis" deformity in a patient with ankylosing spondylitis: a case report of consecutive cervical, thoracic, and lumbar corrective osteotomies. Spine. 2012; 37(16):E1017–E1021

[22] Suk KS, Kim KT, Lee SH, Kim JM. Significance of chin-brow vertical angle in correction of kyphotic deformity of ankylosing spondylitis patients. Spine. 2003; 28(17):2001–2005

[23] Lee SH, Kim KT, Seo EM, Suk KS, Kwack YH, Son ES. The influence of thoracic inlet alignment on the craniocervical sagittal balance in asymptomatic adults. J Spinal Disord Tech. 2012; 25(2):E41–E47

[24] Bess S, Protopsaltis TS, Lafage V, et al. Clinical and radiographic evaluation of adult spinal deformity. Clin Spine Surg. 2016; 29(1):6–16

[25] Hardacker JW, Shuford RF, Capicotto PN, Pryor PW. Radiographic standing cervical segmental alignment in adult volunteers without neck symptoms. Spine. 1997; 22(13):1472–1480, discussion 1480

[26] Jackson RP, McManus AC. Radiographic analysis of sagittal plane alignment and balance in standing volunteers and patients with low back pain matched for age, sex, and size. A prospective controlled clinical study. Spine. 1994; 19 (14):1611–1618

[27] Kuntz C, IV, Levin LS, Ondra SL, Shaffrey CI, Morgan CJ. Neutral upright sagittal spinal alignment from the occiput to the pelvis in asymptomatic adults: a review and resynthesis of the literature. J Neurosurg Spine. 2007; 6(2): 104–112

[28] Le Huec JC, Demezon H, Aunoble S. Sagittal parameters of global cervical balance using EOS imaging: normative values from a prospective cohort of asymptomatic volunteers. Eur Spine J. 2015; 24(1):63–71

[29] Lau D, Ziewacz JE, Le H, Wadhwa R, Mummaneni PV. A controlled anterior sequential interbody dilation technique for correction of cervical kyphosis. J Neurosurg Spine. 2015; 23(3):263–273

[30] Guérin P, Obeid I, Gille O, et al. Sagittal alignment after single cervical disc arthroplasty. J Spinal Disord Tech. 2012; 25(1):10–16

[31] Jagannathan J, Shaffrey CI, Oskouian RJ, et al. Radiographic and clinical outcomes following single-level anterior cervical discectomy and allograft fusion without plate placement or cervical collar. J Neurosurg Spine. 2008; 8(5):420–428

[32] Villavicencio AT, Babuska JM, Ashton A, et al. Prospective, randomized, double-blind clinical study evaluating the correlation of clinical outcomes and cervical sagittal alignment. Neurosurgery. 2011; 68(5):1309–1316, discussion 1316

[33] Oh T, Scheer JK, Eastlack R, et al. Cervical compensatory alignment changes following correction of adult thoracic deformity: a multicenter experience in 57 patients with a 2-year follow-up. J Neurosurg Spine. 2015; 22(6):658–665

[34] Protopsaltis TS, Scheer JK, Terran JS, et al. How the neck affects the back: changes in regional cervical sagittal alignment correlate to HRQOL improvement in adult thoracolumbar deformity patients at 2-year follow-up. J Neurosurg Spine. 2015; 23(2):153–158

[35] Smith JS, Shaffrey CI, Lafage V, et al. Spontaneous improvement of cervical alignment after correction of global sagittal balance following pedicle subtraction osteotomy. J Neurosurg Spine. 2012; 17(4):300–307

[36] Knott PT, Mardjetko SM, Techy F. The use of the T1 sagittal angle in predicting overall sagittal balance of the spine. Spine J. 2010; 10(11):994–998

[37] Protopsaltis T, Schwab F, Bronsard N, et al. TheT1 pelvic angle, a novel radiographic measure of global sagittal deformity, accounts for both spinal inclination and pelvic tilt and correlates with health-related quality of life. J Bone Joint Surg Am. 2014; 96(19):1631–1640

[38] Smith JS, Klineberg E, Shaffrey CI, et al. Assessment of surgical treatment strategies for moderate to severe cervical spinal deformity reveals marked variation in approaches, osteotomies, and fusion levels. World Neurosurg. 2016; 91:228–237

[39] Hann S, Chalouhi N, Madineni R, et al. An algorithmic strategy for selecting a surgical approach in cervical deformity correction. Neurosurg Focus. 2014; 36(5):E5

[40] Ames CP, Smith JS, Scheer JK, et al. A standardized nomenclature for cervical spine soft-tissue release and osteotomy for deformity correction: clinical article. J Neurosurg Spine. 2013; 19(3):269–278

[41] Etame AB, Wang AC, Than KD, La Marca F, Park P. Outcomes after surgery for cervical spine deformity: review of the literature. Neurosurg Focus. 2010; 28 (3):E14

[42] Zhang H, Liu S, Guo C, et al. Posterior surgery assisted by halo ring traction for the treatment of severe rigid nonangular cervical kyphosis. Orthopedics. 2010; 33(4):33

[43] Ferch RD, Shad A, Cadoux-Hudson TA, Teddy PJ. Anterior correction of cervical kyphotic deformity: effects on myelopathy, neck pain, and sagittal alignment. J Neurosurg. 2004; 100(1) Suppl Spine:13–19

[44] Herman JM, Sonntag VK. Cervical corpectomy and plate fixation for postlaminectomy kyphosis. J Neurosurg. 1994; 80(6):963–970

[45] Song KJ, Johnson JS, Choi BR, Wang JC, Lee KB. Anterior fusion alone compared with combined anterior and posterior fusion for the treatment of degenerative cervical kyphosis. J Bone Joint Surg Br. 2010; 92(11):1548–1552

[46] Steinmetz MP, Kager CD, Benzel EC. Ventral correction of postsurgical cervical kyphosis. J Neurosurg. 2003; 98(1) Suppl:1–7

[47] Zdeblick TA, Bohlman HH. Cervical kyphosis and myelopathy. Treatment by anterior corpectomy and strut-grafting. J Bone Joint Surg Am. 1989; 71 (2):170–182

[48] Abumi K, Shono Y, Taneichi H, Ito M, Kaneda K. Correction of cervical kyphosis using pedicle screw fixation systems. Spine. 1999; 24(22):2389–2396

[49] Belanger TA, Milam RA, IV, Roh JS, Bohlman HH. Cervicothoracic extension osteotomy for chin-on-chest deformity in ankylosing spondylitis. J Bone Joint Surg Am. 2005; 87(8):1732–1738

[50] Gerling MC, Bohlman HH. Dropped head deformity due to cervical myopathy: surgical treatment outcomes and complications spanning twenty years. Spine. 2008; 33(20):E739–E745

[51] Langeloo DD, Journee HL, Pavlov PW, de Kleuver M. Cervical osteotomy in ankylosing spondylitis: evaluation of new developments. Eur Spine J. 2006; 15(4):493–500

[52] Lee SH, Kim KT, Suk KS, Kim MH, Park DH, Kim KJ. A sterile-freehand reduction technique for corrective osteotomy of fixed cervical kyphosis. Spine. 2012; 37(26):2145–2150

[53] McMaster MJ. Osteotomy of the cervical spine in ankylosing spondylitis. J Bone Joint Surg Br. 1997; 79(2):197–203

[54] Simmons ED, DiStefano RJ, Zheng Y, Simmons EH. Thirty-six years experience of cervical extension osteotomy in ankylosing spondylitis: techniques and outcomes. Spine. 2006; 31(26):3006–3012

[55] Tokala DP, Lam KS, Freeman BJ, Webb JK. C7 decancellisation closing wedge osteotomy for the correction of fixed cervico-thoracic kyphosis. Eur Spine J. 2007; 16(9):1471–1478

[56] Mummaneni PV, Dhall SS, Rodts GE, Haid RW. Circumferential fusion for cervical kyphotic deformity. J Neurosurg Spine. 2008; 9(6):515–521

[57] Nottmeier EW, Deen HG, Patel N, Birch B. Cervical kyphotic deformity correction using 360-degree reconstruction. J Spinal Disord Tech. 2009; 22(6):385–391

[58] Kim HJ, Piyaskulkaew C, Riew KD. Comparison of Smith-Petersen osteotomy versus pedicle subtraction osteotomy versus anterior-posterior osteotomy types for the correction of cervical spine deformities. Spine. 2015; 40(3):143–146

[59] Perrini P, Gambacciani C, Martini C, Montemurro N, Lepori P. Anterior cervical corpectomy for cervical spondylotic myelopathy: Reconstruction with expandable cylindrical cage versus iliac crest autograft. A retrospective study. Clin Neurol Neurosurg. 2015; 139:258–263

[60] Burkhardt JK, Mannion AF, Marbacher S, et al. A comparative effectiveness study of patient-rated and radiographic outcome after 2 types of decompression with fusion for spondylotic myelopathy: anterior cervical discectomy versus corpectomy. Neurosurg Focus. 2013; 35(1):E4

[61] Lin Q, Zhou X, Wang X, Cao P, Tsai N, Yuan W. A comparison of anterior cervical discectomy and corpectomy in patients with multilevel cervical spondylotic myelopathy. Eur Spine J. 2012; 21(3):474–481

[62] Oh MC, Zhang HY, Park JY, Kim KS. Two-level anterior cervical discectomy versus one-level corpectomy in cervical spondylotic myelopathy. Spine. 2009; 34(7):692–696

[63] Bazaz R, Lee MJ, Yoo JU. Incidence of dysphagia after anterior cervical spine surgery: a prospective study. Spine. 2002; 27(22):2453–2458

[64] Singh K, Marquez-Lara A, Nandyala SV, Patel AA, Fineberg SJ. Incidence and risk factors for dysphagia after anterior cervical fusion. Spine. 2013; 38 (21):1820–1825

[65] Zeng JH, Zhong ZM, Chen JT. Early dysphagia complicating anterior cervical spine surgery: incidence and risk factors. Arch Orthop Trauma Surg. 2013; 133(8):1067–1071

[66] Ames CP, Wang VY, Deviren V, Vrionis FD. Posterior transpedicular corpectomy and reconstruction of the axial vertebra for metastatic tumor. J Neurosurg Spine. 2009; 10(2):111–116

[67] Law WA. Osteotomy of the cervical spine. J Bone Joint Surg Br. 1959; 41-B:640–641

[68] Simmons EH. The surgical correction of flexion deformity of the cervical spine in ankylosing spondylitis. Clin Orthop Relat Res. 1972; 86(86):132–143

[69] Urist MR. Osteotomy of the cervical spine; report of a case of ankylosing rheumatoid spondylitis. J Bone Joint Surg Am. 1958; 40-A(4):833–843

[70] Chin KR, Ahn J. Controlled cervical extension osteotomy for ankylosing spondylitis utilizing the Jackson operating table: technical note. Spine. 2007; 32 (17):1926–1929

[71] Scheer JK, Tang JA, Buckley JM, et al. Biomechanical analysis of osteotomy type and rod diameter for treatment of cervicothoracic kyphosis. Spine. 2011; 36(8):E519–E523

[72] Theologis AA, Bellevue KD, Qamirani E, Ames CP, Deviren V. Asymmetric C7 pedicle subtraction osteotomy for correction of rigid cervical coronal imbalance secondary to post-traumatic heterotopic ossification: a case report, description of a novel surgical technique, and literature review. Eur Spine J. 2017; 26 Suppl 1:141–145

[73] Smith JS, Shaffrey CI, Lafage R, et al. ISSG. Three-column osteotomy for correction of cervical and cervicothoracic deformities: alignment changes and early complications in a multicenter prospective series of 23 patients. Eur Spine J. 2017; 26(8):2128–2137

17 Advantages and Limitations of the SRS-Schwab Classification for Adult Spinal Deformity

Hideyuki Arima, Leah Y. Carreon, and Steven D. Glassman

Abstract

Adult spinal deformity (ASD) is a term that encompasses various primary and degenerative conditions that contribute to an altered three-dimensional structure of the spine. ASD may influence the progression and impact on otherwise normal aging changes in the spine. This complexity makes it difficult to easily describe or classify diagnosis and treatment of adult spinal deformity. Aided by research efforts examining sagittal spinopelvic alignment and balance, our understanding of the pathology of spinal deformity has greatly advanced. Importantly, we have learned that positive sagittal spinal alignment is strongly associated with poor health-related quality of life and low back pain. The Scoliosis Research Society (SRS)-Schwab classification of adult spinal deformity has focused the attention of surgeons and researchers on global sagittal imbalance; and this has contributed to improvement of treatment outcomes. As a result, global research efforts regarding adult spinal deformity has grown, and are helping to improve clinical practice. However, there are also limitations to a radiographic classification that only indirectly assesses clinical symptoms. This is particularly relevant, as adult deformities mainly occur in middle-aged and elderly people, in whom neurological symptoms caused by spinal stenosis are a critical element of diagnosis and treatment. In this chapter, we review the importance of sagittal balance in adult spinal deformities, regarding the advantages and limitations of using the SRS-Schwab classification.

Keywords: adult spinal deformity, age, classification, ethnicity, health-related quality of life, outcomes, pelvis, spinopelvic alignment, sagittal alignment, SRS-Schwab classification

17.1 Introduction

Adult spinal deformity is a broad diagnostic classification that encompasses a complex group of spinal pathologies with various clinical presentations. With longer life expectancy and an increasing proportion of healthy older individuals, there is an increasing population presenting with adult spinal deformity. Schwab and colleagues reported a prevalence of adult spinal deformity as high as 68% in those older than 60 years.[1] Although some cases are asymptomatic or can be treated nonsurgically, a substantial number of patients present for corrective surgery because of pain and disability. To optimize surgical treatment, it is necessary to understand the existing pathology, the surgical indications, have a comprehensive preoperative plan to restore both spinal sagittal and coronal plane alignment, and spinopelvic alignment, as well as address neurologic compromise. In adult spinal deformity, a lack of understanding of the underlying pathology and poor surgical planning leads to poor outcomes or revision surgery.[2,3,4,5,6,7] Historically, restoration of the coronal plane was considered of prime importance in the correction of spinal deformities. However, several studies have demonstrated that, in adult spinal deformity, sagittal spinal imbalance, a deformity of the spine in the sagittal plane, has a greater impact on health-related quality of life than the spinal deformity in the coronal plane.[8,9] Moreover, patients with adult spinal deformity often have other issues associated with their deformity such as spinal stenosis with radicular or claudication-type pain and osteoporosis.[10,11,12,13,14,15]

The Scoliosis Research Society-Schwab (SRS-Schwab) adult spinal deformity classification gives weight to sagittal plane evaluation by using the pelvic tilt (PT), sagittal vertical axis (SVA), and the mismatch between pelvic incidence (PI) and lumbar lordosis (PI minus lumbar lordosis [LL]).[16] This classification is very useful in terms of raising awareness of the importance of spinopelvic alignment among surgeons and researchers. In this chapter, we discuss the advantages and limits of using SRS-Schwab classification in surgical planning in patients with adult spinal deformity.

17.2 Sagittal Spinopelvic Alignment

17.2.1 History

Before the 1980s, many studies focused mainly on thoracic kyphosis and/or lumbar lordosis.[17,18,19,20] In 1991, Itoi[15] investigated for the first time the relationship between postural deformities to include both the spine and lower extremities. In 1994, Jackson[21] reported the measurement method of sagittal balance using C7 sagittal plumb line. At the same time, research on sagittal morphology of pelvis was being actively conducted in Europe.[22,23,24,25] In 1998, Legaye et al[26] proposed PI as a key anatomic pelvic parameter that is predictive of the sagittal balance of the spine. Since then, the importance of spinal global sagittal alignment and balance including the pelvis has been extensively studied.[27,28,29,30,31] This has revealed that the sagittal morphology and inclination of the pelvis are important components in human standing alignment.[31]

17.2.2 Imaging Studies

Standard evaluation of spinopelvic alignment is performed by using full-length 36-inch standing posteroanterior and lateral radiographs of the spine and pelvis. The SRS recommends that patients should stand with their knees locked, feet shoulder-width apart, looking straight ahead with their elbows bent and knuckles in the supraclavicular fossa bilaterally.[32] This will place the patient's arms at approximately a 45° angle to the vertical axis of the body. The position of the arms at the time the radiograph is taken can have a bearing on sagittal alignment.[33] If a leg length discrepancy of greater than 2 cm is present, a shoe lift should be used.[32] The lateral radiograph should include C0 and both femoral heads at a minimum, and sagittal alignment and balance should be measured with the patient ideally standing fully erect with the knees and hips in full extension to counteract compensatory mechanisms.[34] Because of the importance of sagittal alignment of lower extremities including the hip joint and knee joints has been recently clarified, full-length standing lateral radiographs of lower extremities should also be evaluated when available.

17.2.3 Sagittal Spinopelvic Parameters

Pelvic Parameters

Three pelvic parameters have been defined: PI is an individual-specific morphologic pelvic parameter that has been demonstrated to define lumbar alignment.[26] PI is a shape parameter that is not affected by changes in the alignment of the lower extremities.[35] The PT is a positional and dynamic pelvic parameter that measures pelvic retroversion. In some cases, this parameter has been demonstrated to act as a compensatory

mechanism to maintain an upright posture. The sacral slope (SS) quantifies the sagittal sacral inclination and completes the geometric relationship "PI = PT + SS"[36] (▸ Fig. 17.1a).

Global Sagittal Alignment

SVA is usually used to determine the global sagittal spinal alignment (▸ Fig. 17.1b).[21,37] This is identified by a plumb line dropped from C7 to the anterior edge of the sacral endplate. If compensated by posture, such as knee flexion and pelvic retroversion, SVA may be underestimated.[38,39] Recently, T1-pelvic angle (TPA) and global tilt (GT) have been proposed as novel global spinopelvic parameters (▸ Fig. 17.1c).[38,40] TPA is defined as the angle subtended by a line from the femoral heads to the center of the T1 vertebral body and a line from the femoral heads to the center of the superior sacral endplate. GT is the superior sacral endplate to the center of the C7 vertebral body and a line from the femoral heads to the center of the superior

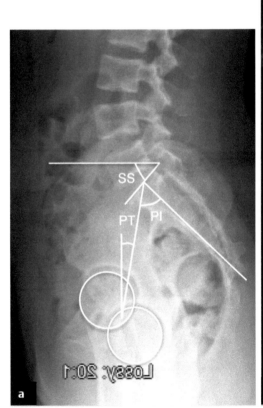
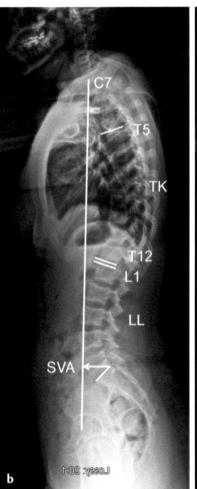
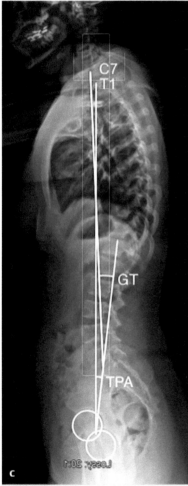

Fig. 17.1 Radiographic representation of spinopelvic parameters using full-length 36-inch standing lateral radiographs of the spine and pelvis. **(a)** Sacral slope (SS) defined as the angle between the horizontal and the sacral plate. Pelvic tilt (PT) defined by the angle subtended by a vertical reference line originating from the center of the femoral heads and the midpoint of the sacral endplate. Pelvic incidence (PI) defined as the angle between the perpendicular to the sacral plate at its midpoint and the line connecting this point to the femoral heads axis. Pelvic parameters complete the geometric relationship "PI = PT + SS." **(b)** Thoracic kyphosis (TK) measured from the superior endplate of T5 to the inferior endplate of T12. Lumbar lordosis measured from the superior endplate of L1 to the superior endplate of S1. Sagittal vertical axis (SVA) defined as the horizontal offset from the posterosuperior corner of S1 to the vertebral body of C7. **(c)** T1 pelvic angle (TPA) is defined as the angle subtended by a line from the femoral heads to the center of the T1 vertebral body and a line from the femoral heads to the center of the superior sacral endplate. Global tilt (GT) is defined as the angle subtended by a line from the center of the superior sacral endplate to the center of the C7 vertebral body and a line from the femoral heads to the center of the superior sacral endplate.

sacral endplate. Both novel parameters combine trunk ante-version and pelvic retroversion as one parameter to assess global spinal deformity.[39]

17.3 Sagittal Imbalance

17.3.1 Cone of Economy

Abnormal posture in the sagittal plane has been demonstrated to cause significant impairments in the elderly.[8,14] Sagittal balance in normal asymptomatic individuals is a state of congruence among the spine, pelvis, and lower extremities to achieve an economic posture, placing the axis of gravity in a physiologic position.[26,41,42,43,44] This concept is clearly illustrated by Dubousset's "cone of economy."[43] Increasing positive sagittal imbalance causes the body to assume a position toward the periphery of the cone, which results in increased muscular effort and energy expenditure causing pain, fatigue, and disability. If the body is shifted beyond the periphery of the cone, external supports such as a cane, crutch, or walker may be required to maintain balance.[11,43]

17.3.2 Cause of Sagittal Malalignment

The causes of sagittal spine imbalance are multifactorial and range from iatrogenic causes to genetic and metabolic causes.[34] Sagittal imbalance of the spine is mainly related to any underlying pathology causing loss of LL such as multilevel degenerative disk disease, ankylosing spondylitis, diffuse idiopathic skeletal hyperostosis, flat back syndrome following spinal fusion surgery, osteoporosis, tumor, trauma, or infection.[2,11,34,45,46] Bridwell and colleagues classified sagittal imbalance into primary or secondary causes. The most common primary cause of sagittal imbalance is multilevel disk degeneration. Secondary causes are iatrogenic in nature and are related to previous spinal fusion surgeries. The classic secondary type is a flat back syndrome following the Harrington operation for adolescent idiopathic scoliosis.[47,48] However, the most frequent cause of secondary sagittal imbalance is that following lumbar spinal fusion (e.g., posterior lumbar interbody fusion, transforaminal lumbar interbody fusion, and posterolateral fusion) with inadequate restoration of sagittal alignment.[11,12,49] Other secondary causes of sagittal plane deformity include posttraumatic kyphosis that can be divided into the following two types: fixed kyphosis following major spinal fractures/dislocations that occurs in relatively young individuals; and vertebral collapse or pseudarthrosis that occurs in elderly with severe osteoporosis.[11]

17.3.3 Sagittal Imbalance and Health-Related Quality of Life

In sagittal imbalance, spinal malalignment generally causes back pain and postural abnormalities. Patients may also present with difficulty in maintaining a standing posture caused by fatigue of the back muscles, neurologic symptoms caused by coexisting spinal stenosis, gastrointestinal symptoms caused by a decrease in the abdominal cavity volume, and mental health issues resulting from anxiety about pain and deformity.

In the assessment of health-related quality of life for patient with adult spinal deformity, surgeons use a common patient-reported outcome such as 36-Item Short Form Survey (SF-36),[1,50,51,52] the Short Form-12 (SF-12),[8,9] EuroQol 5D (EQ-5D), Oswestry Disability Index (ODI),[9,51,53] and the SRS-22r instrument.[54] The SRS-22r has been found to be reliable, valid, and responsive to change in patients undergoing surgery for patients with adult spinal deformity.[54,55,56] These clinical studies revealed that health-related quality of life in patients with adult spinal deformity is lower than normal controls[1,52] or patients with other common chronic conditions.[57] It is very important to evaluate the clinical symptoms of adult spinal deformity patients with the health-related quality of life questionnaire, but it is equally important to objectively evaluate the spine deformity when considering surgical treatment. To establish objective surgical criteria, the relationship between radiographic parameters and clinical outcome has been extensively studied. As a result, previous studies demonstrated that the global positive balance in the sagittal plane rather than imbalance in the coronal plane was significantly associated with deterioration of the health-related quality of life.[8] Among various spinopelvic parameters, PI minus LL, SVA, and PT were detected as key parameters related to pain and low back disability.[58]

17.4 SRS-Schwab Classification

17.4.1 The Establishment of SRS-Schwab Classification

At the same time that the Lenke classification was developed to guide treatment of patients with adolescent idiopathic scoliosis, an initial classification of adult spinal deformity was first reported in 2006.[59,60] Concurrently, the importance of spinopelvic alignments and balance was being elucidated.[31,36,41,58,61,62,63,64] From these studies, Schwab and colleagues proposed radiographic parameter thresholds that were predictive of an Oswestry disability score of 40. These were PI minus LL greater than 11°, PT greater than 22°, and SVA greater than 46 mm.[16] The SRS-Schwab classification of adult spinal deformity was established by incorporating these sagittal spinopelvic threshold values into a comprehensive classification[16] (▶ Fig. 17.2). A primary feature of this classification is that the sagittal plane morphology is subdivided using two spinopelvic parameters (PI minus LL and PT) and SVA evaluating global sagittal alignment. Coronal Cobb angles less than 30° are not considered as coronal deformity.

17.4.2 Evaluation of Coronal Curve

Evaluation of the coronal curve is as follows: Type T, patients with a thoracic major curve of greater than 30° (apical level of

Coronal Curve Types
T: Thoracic only with lumbar curve < 30°
L: TL / Lumbar only with thoracic curve < 30°
D: Double curve with T and TL/L curve > 30°
N: No major coronal deformity all coronal curves < 30°

Sagittal Modifiers
PI minus LL 0: within 10° +: moderate = 10°-20° ++: marked > 20°
Global Alignment 0: SVA < 4 cm +: SVA = 4-9.5 cm ++: SVA > 9.5 cm
Pelvic Tilt 0: PT < 20° +: PT = 20°-30° ++: PT > 30°

Fig. 17.2 The SRS-Schwab classification includes four coronal curves types and three sagittal modifiers. PI-LL, Pelvic incidence–lumbar lordosis mismatch; PT, pelvic tilt; SVA, sagittal vertical axis.[16]

T9 or higher); type L, patients with a lumbar or thoracolumbar major curve of greater than 30° (apical level of T10 or lower); type D, patients with a double major curve, with each curve greater than 30°; and type N, patients with no coronal curve greater than 30° (i.e., no major coronal deformity). This classification is very simple in terms of the coronal plane deformity compared with the former Schwab adult scoliosis classification and the earlier SRS classification for adult spinal deformity.[59,60]

17.4.3 Evaluation of Sagittal Modifiers

Sagittal plane modifiers (PI minus LL, SVA, and PT) were classified into three grades for each parameter.

PI Minus LL

- Patients with a PI-LL value of less than 10° are classified with a PI-LL modifier "0."
- Patients with a PI-LL value between 10° and 20° are classified with a PI-LL modifier "+."
- Patients with a PI-LL value of greater than 20° are classified with a PI-LL modifier "++."

PT

- Patients with a PT of less than 20° are classified with a PT modifier "0."
- Patients with a PT between 20° and 30° are classified with a PT modifier "+."
- Patients with a PT of greater than 30° are classified with a PT modifier "++."

SVA

- Patients with an SVA of less than 40 mm are classified with an SVA modifier "0."
- Patients with an SVA between 40 and 95 mm are classified with an SVA modifier "+."
- Patients with an SVA of greater than 95 mm are classified with an SVA modifier "++."

17.5 Advantage of SRS-Schwab Classification

17.5.1 Understanding of Importance of Sagittal Plane Evaluation

The SRS-Schwab classification has led surgeons to recognize that sagittal parameters such as PI minus LL, SVA, and PT are very important. This classification is reliable and valid.[65,66] As a result, it was found that the L curve modifier in the coronal plane and abnormalities in any of the sagittal modifiers resulted in deterioration of health-related quality of life.[65] This classification has sagittal plane modifiers that are relatively simple and substantially correlated to clinical symptoms. This classification is currently the most widely accepted method for classification of adult spinal deformity. Because the sagittal modifiers have an objective and specific cut-off value, they are a useful indicator to grasp the severity of spinal deformity when surgeons perform surgical treatment for patients with adult spinal deformity. Especially, regarding research, there has been a clear benefit to this classification. Having a classification that allows for common recognition makes it possible to conduct global comparative research about baseline differences and surgical outcomes.

17.5.2 Clinical Relevance of SRS-Schwab Classification

Recent studies have reported the potential benefits of surgical treatment for adult spinal deformity.[67,68,69] However, clinical decision-making, as to which patients will benefit from surgical treatment or nonsurgical treatment, continues to be debated. As it has been demonstrated that the SRS-Schwab classification reflects severity of disease state based on multiple measures of health-related quality of life, this classification may be useful clinically in surgical decision-making.[65] Moreover, improvement in the SRS-Schwab classification sagittal modifiers grade (PT, SVA, and PI-LL mismatch) after surgery has been shown to be associated with significant improvement in health-related quality of life.[70] Studies have demonstrated that patients with improvement of PT, SVA, or PI-LL modifiers were more likely to achieve minimal clinically important difference values for ODI, SRS-22 activity, and SRS-22 pain (PI-LL only).[70]

17.5.3 Ethnic Differences Using SRS-Schwab Classification

Adult spinal deformity is a common problem not only in North America but also in developed countries in Europe and Asia. Therefore, it is desirable that classification of adult spinal deformity is appropriate not only for patients in the United States but also in other ethnic groups. Ames and colleagues examined the differences between adult spinal deformity patients between the United States and Japan, and examined whether the SRS-Schwab classification is valid in other ethnic groups.[53] This study found no statistically significant difference between the United States and Japan regarding the distribution of the coronal plane deformity. However, in the sagittal plane, the Japanese group showed that the pelvis tended to be more retroverted than the American group, and the American group had a more positive sagittal global alignment compared to the Japanese group. Interestingly, within the same sagittal modifier group, health-related quality of life was worse in the North American group than in the Japanese group. In this way, this classification makes it possible to compare between different cultural groups and is considered to be useful for research in the future.

17.6 Limitation of SRS-Schwab Classification

17.6.1 Lack of Clinical Evaluation

Ideally, classification systems of diseases should be designed to guide treatment. As the new SRS-Schwab classification is based on radiographic evaluation alone, without consideration of the patients' clinical presentation, the value of the classification to guide surgical decision-making is limited. The symptoms of patients with adult spinal deformity include muscle fatigue resulting from spinal deformity, lower back pain, balance failure accompanying a global forward shift, and walking disturbance. In addition, these deformities mainly occur in the elderly such that neurological symptoms as a result of spinal stenosis are not uncommon. Therefore, when spine surgeons consider the surgical strategies for patients with adult spinal deformity, it is necessary to evaluate whether the symptoms are primarily a result of spinal deformity and/or from spinal stenosis in the setting of adult spinal deformity.[71]

17.6.2 Influence of Age and Ethnicity

The SRS-Schwab classification is considered most applicable to patients with adult spinal deformity around age 50, when considering the average age of the population from which the thresholds were calculated.[16] Some studies have shown that the SRS-Schwab classification may not be valid in adult spinal deformity patients who are relatively younger or older.[72] In addition, it has been demonstrated that health-related quality of life varies depending on age and ethnicity.[53,73] Therefore, it may be necessary to set stricter radiographic threshold values for young patients and more tolerant threshold values for elderly patients.[72] Furthermore, considering differences in pelvic morphology and recognition of pain and disorder among ethnic groups, it may be necessary to adjust the threshold values of sagittal modifiers in each ethnic group.[53]

17.6.3 Other Issues

The validity in terms of reproducibility (particularly based upon premarked films) for this SRS-Schwab classification[16] does not imply validity in terms of predicting outcomes based on use of the system. And, a previous report pointed out that the consistent interrater agreement for this classification was too low to support the use of an entire grade as a stand-alone parameter.[74,75]

PI is considered the key parameter among the radiographic spinopelvic measures.[26,34,76,77] The PI has been known to increase until the age of maturity and then stabilize.[78,79,80,81] The PI value was considered as a constant for each individual because of the rigidity of the pelvis. However, Legaye reported recently that PI may increase with aging changes.[82] Lee also reported recently that PI increased in all patients with surgically corrected, adult sagittal deformity, following surgical correction of fixed LL.[83] In this way, even the basic components related to the sagittal spinopelvic alignment are still not yet fully clarified.

Patients with adult spinal deformity are usually evaluated with full-length static standing radiographic films. However, some patients with relatively good sagittal alignment on a standing radiograph walk with their trunk leaning forward.[84] The hip extensor muscles most involved in pelvic retroversion in a static state are used for hip joint extension during walking.[12,85] Therefore, the sagittal imbalance becomes worse in the dynamic state than in the static state. Taking these results into account, it is considered that dynamic assessment is necessary to avoid underestimation of the severity of sagittal imbalance detected by standing full-length radiographic measurement.

17.7 Conclusion

The new SRS-Schwab classification for adult spinal deformity has enhanced common recognition of global sagittal imbalance among surgeons and researchers, which has greatly contributed to improvement of treatment outcomes. As a result, international research has progressed and it is helping to improve clinical practice. However, there are also some limitations such as not including the clinical symptoms of spinal stenosis, age, or dynamic sagittal imbalance. Future efforts at classification should attempt to incorporate these elements.

References

[1] Schwab F, Dubey A, Gamez L, et al. Adult scoliosis: prevalence, SF-36, and nutritional parameters in an elderly volunteer population. Spine. 2005; 30 (9):1082–1085

[2] Bridwell KH, Lewis SJ, Edwards C, et al. Complications and outcomes of pedicle subtraction osteotomies for fixed sagittal imbalance. Spine. 2003; 28 (18):2093–2101

[3] Puvanesarajah V, Shen FH, Cancienne JM, et al. Risk factors for revision surgery following primary adult spinal deformity surgery in patients 65 years and older. J Neurosurg Spine. 2016; 25(4):486–493

[4] Glassman SD, Dimar JR, II, Carreon LY. Revision rate after adult deformity surgery. Spine Deform. 2015; 3(2):199–203

[5] Kim HJ, Bridwell KH, Lenke LG, et al. Patients with proximal junctional kyphosis requiring revision surgery have higher postoperative lumbar lordosis and larger sagittal balance corrections. Spine. 2014; 39(9):E576–E580

[6] Hart R, McCarthy I, O'Brien M, et al. Identification of decision criteria for revision surgery among patients with proximal junctional failure after surgical treatment of spinal deformity. Spine. 2013; 38(19):E1223–E1227

[7] Cho SK, Bridwell KH, Lenke LG, et al. Major complications in revision adult deformity surgery: risk factors and clinical outcomes with 2- to 7-year follow-up. Spine. 2012; 37(6):489–500

[8] Glassman SD, Bridwell K, Dimar JR, Horton W, Berven S, Schwab F. The impact of positive sagittal balance in adult spinal deformity. Spine. 2005; 30 (18):2024–2029

[9] Glassman SD, Berven S, Bridwell K, Horton W, Dimar JR. Correlation of radiographic parameters and clinical symptoms in adult scoliosis. Spine. 2005; 30 (6):682–688

[10] Youssef JA, Orndorff DO, Patty CA, et al. Current status of adult spinal deformity. Global Spine J. 2013; 3(1):51–62

[11] Savage JW, Patel AA. Fixed sagittal plane imbalance. Global Spine J. 2014; 4 (4):287–296

[12] Taneichi H. Update on pathology and surgical treatment for adult spinal deformity. J Orthop Sci. 2016; 21(2):116–123

[13] Aebi M. The adult scoliosis. Eur Spine J. 2005; 14(10):925–948

[14] Miyakoshi N, Itoi E, Kobayashi M, Kodama H. Impact of postural deformities and spinal mobility on quality of life in postmenopausal osteoporosis. Osteoporos Int. 2003; 14(12):1007–1012

[15] Itoi E. Roentgenographic analysis of posture in spinal osteoporotics. Spine. 1991; 16(7):750–756

[16] Schwab F, Ungar B, Blondel B, et al. Scoliosis Research Society-Schwab adult spinal deformity classification: a validation study. Spine. 2012; 37(12):1077–1082

[17] Milne JS, Lauder IJ. Age effects in kyphosis and lordosis in adults. Ann Hum Biol. 1974; 1(3):327–337

[18] Stagnara P, De Mauroy JC, Dran G, et al. Reciprocal angulation of vertebral bodies in a sagittal plane: approach to references for the evaluation of kyphosis and lordosis. Spine. 1982; 7(4):335–342

[19] Bernhardt M, Bridwell KH. Segmental analysis of the sagittal plane alignment of the normal thoracic and lumbar spines and thoracolumbar junction. Spine. 1989; 14(7):717–721

[20] Takemitsu Y, Harada Y, Iwahara T, Miyamoto M, Miyatake Y. Lumbar degenerative kyphosis. Clinical, radiological and epidemiological studies. Spine. 1988; 13(11):1317–1326

[21] Jackson RP, McManus AC. Radiographic analysis of sagittal plane alignment and balance in standing volunteers and patients with low back pain matched for age, sex, and size. A prospective controlled clinical study. Spine. 1994; 19 (14):1611–1618

[22] Paquet N, Malouin F, Richards CL. Hip-spine movement interaction and muscle activation patterns during sagittal trunk movements in low back pain patients. Spine. 1994; 19(5):596–603

[23] Duval-Beaupère G, Schmidt C, Cosson P. A barycentremetric study of the sagittal shape of spine and pelvis: the conditions required for an economic standing position. Ann Biomed Eng. 1992; 20(4):451–462

[24] Shirazi-Adl A, Parnianpour M. Stabilizing role of moments and pelvic rotation on the human spine in compression. J Biomech Eng. 1996; 118(1):26–31

[25] Jackson RP, Peterson MD, McManus AC, Hales C. Compensatory spinopelvic balance over the hip axis and better reliability in measuring lordosis to the pelvic radius on standing lateral radiographs of adult volunteers and patients. Spine. 1998; 23(16):1750–1767

[26] Legaye J, Duval-Beaupère G, Hecquet J, Marty C. Pelvic incidence: a fundamental pelvic parameter for three-dimensional regulation of spinal sagittal curves. Eur Spine J. 1998; 7(2):99–103

[27] Hanson DS, Bridwell KH, Rhee JM, Lenke LG. Correlation of pelvic incidence with low- and high-grade isthmic spondylolisthesis. Spine. 2002; 27 (18):2026–2029

[28] Jackson RP, Phipps T, Hales C, Surber J. Pelvic lordosis and alignment in spondylolisthesis. Spine. 2003; 28(2):151–160

[29] Labelle H, Roussouly P, Berthonnaud E, et al. Spondylolisthesis, pelvic incidence, and spinopelvic balance: a correlation study. Spine. 2004; 29 (18):2049–2054

[30] Labelle H, Roussouly P, Berthonnaud E, Dimnet J, O'Brien M. The importance of spino-pelvic balance in L5-s1 developmental spondylolisthesis: a review of pertinent radiologic measurements. Spine. 2005; 30(6) Suppl:S27–S34

[31] Boulay C, Tardieu C, Hecquet J, et al. Sagittal alignment of spine and pelvis regulated by pelvic incidence: standard values and prediction of lordosis. Eur Spine J. 2006; 15(4):415–422

[32] O'Brien M, Kuklo T, Blanke K, Lenke L. Spinal Deformity Study Group Radiographic Measurement Manual. Memphis, TN: Medtronic Sofamor Danek; 2005

[33] Vedantam R, Lenke LG, Bridwell KH, Linville DL, Blanke K. The effect of variation in arm position on sagittal spinal alignment. Spine. 2000; 25(17):2204–2209

[34] Roussouly P, Nnadi C. Sagittal plane deformity: an overview of interpretation and management. Eur Spine J. 2010; 19(11):1824–1836

[35] Roussouly P, Gollogly S, Berthonnaud E, Dimnet J. Classification of the normal variation in the sagittal alignment of the human lumbar spine and pelvis in the standing position. Spine. 2005; 30(3):346–353

[36] Schwab F, Lafage V, Patel A, Farcy JP. Sagittal plane considerations and the pelvis in the adult patient. Spine. 2009; 34(17):1828–1833

[37] Van Royen BJ, Toussaint HM, Kingma I, et al. Accuracy of the sagittal vertical axis in a standing lateral radiograph as a measurement of balance in spinal deformities. Eur Spine J. 1998; 7(5):408–412

[38] Obeid I, Boissière L, Yilgor C, et al. Global tilt: a single parameter incorporating spinal and pelvic sagittal parameters and least affected by patient positioning. Eur Spine J. 2016; 25(11):3644–3649

[39] Banno T, Togawa D, Arima H, et al. The cohort study for the determination of reference values for spinopelvic parameters (T1 pelvic angle and global tilt) in elderly volunteers. Eur Spine J. 2016; 25(11):3687–3693

[40] Protopsaltis T, Schwab F, Bronsard N, et al. TheT1 pelvic angle, a novel radiographic measure of global sagittal deformity, accounts for both spinal inclination and pelvic tilt and correlates with health-related quality of life. J Bone Joint Surg Am. 2014; 96(19):1631–1640

[41] Lafage V, Schwab F, Skalli W, et al. Standing balance and sagittal plane spinal deformity: analysis of spinopelvic and gravity line parameters. Spine. 2008; 33(14):1572–1578

[42] Berthonnaud E, Dimnet J, Roussouly P, Labelle H. Analysis of the sagittal balance of the spine and pelvis using shape and orientation parameters. J Spinal Disord Tech. 2005; 18(1):40–47

[43] Dubousset J. Reflections of an orthopaedic surgeon on patient care and research into the condition of scoliosis. J Pediatr Orthop. 2011; 31(1) Suppl: S1–S8

[44] Barrey C, Roussouly P, Perrin G, Le Huec JC. Sagittal balance disorders in severe degenerative spine. Can we identify the compensatory mechanisms? Eur Spine J. 2011; 20 Suppl 5:626–633

[45] Kim KT, Lee SH, Suk KS, Lee JH, Im YJ. Spinal pseudarthrosis in advanced ankylosing spondylitis with sagittal plane deformity: clinical characteristics and outcome analysis. Spine. 2007; 32(15):1641–1647

[46] Joseph SA, Jr, Moreno AP, Brandoff J, Casden AC, Kuflik P, Neuwirth MG. Sagittal plane deformity in the adult patient. J Am Acad Orthop Surg. 2009; 17(6):378–388

[47] Farcy JP, Schwab FJ. Management of flatback and related kyphotic decompensation syndromes. Spine. 1997; 22(20):2452–2457

[48] Lagrone MO, Bradford DS, Moe JH, Lonstein JE, Winter RB, Ogilvie JW. Treatment of symptomatic flatback after spinal fusion. J Bone Joint Surg Am. 1988; 70(4):569–580

[49] Bridwell KH, Lenke LG, Lewis SJ. Treatment of spinal stenosis and fixed sagittal imbalance. Clin Orthop Relat Res. 2001; 384:35–44

[50] Liu S, Schwab F, Smith JS, et al. Likelihood of reaching minimal clinically important difference in adult spinal deformity: a comparison of operative and nonoperative treatment. Ochsner J. 2014; 14(1):67–77

[51] Yoshida G, Boissiere L, Larrieu D, et al. Advantages and disadvantages of adult spinal deformity surgery and its impact on health-related quality of life. Spine. 2017; 42(6):411–419

[52] Schwab F, Dubey A, Pagala M, Gamez L, Farcy JP. Adult scoliosis: a health assessment analysis by SF-36. Spine. 2003; 28(6):602–606

[53] Ames C, Gammal I, Matsumoto M, et al. Geographic and ethnic variations in radiographic disability thresholds: analysis of North American and Japanese operative adult spinal deformity populations. Neurosurgery. 2016; 78 (6):793–801

[54] Berven S, Deviren V, Demir-Deviren S, Hu SS, Bradford DS. Studies in the modified Scoliosis Research Society Outcomes Instrument in adults: validation, reliability, and discriminatory capacity. Spine. 2003; 28(18):2164–2169, discussion 2169

[55] Bridwell KH, Berven S, Glassman S, et al. Is the SRS-22 instrument responsive to change in adult scoliosis patients having primary spinal deformity surgery? Spine. 2007; 32(20):2220–2225

[56] Baldus C, Bridwell KH, Harrast J, et al. Age-gender matched comparison of SRS instrument scores between adult deformity and normal adults: are all SRS domains disease specific? Spine. 2008; 33(20):2214–2218

[57] Pellisé F, Vila-Casademunt A, Ferrer M, et al. Impact on health related quality of life of adult spinal deformity (ASD) compared with other chronic conditions. Eur Spine J. 2015; 24(1):3–11

[58] Schwab F, Patel A, Ungar B, Farcy JP, Lafage V. Adult spinal deformity-postoperative standing imbalance: how much can you tolerate? An overview of key parameters in assessing alignment and planning corrective surgery. Spine. 2010; 35(25):2224–2231

[59] Lowe T, Berven SH, Schwab FJ, Bridwell KH. The SRS classification for adult spinal deformity: building on the King/Moe and Lenke classification systems. Spine. 2006; 31(19) Suppl:S119–S125

[60] Schwab F, Farcy JP, Bridwell K, et al. A clinical impact classification of scoliosis in the adult. Spine. 2006; 31(18):2109–2114

[61] Schwab F, Lafage V, Boyce R, Skalli W, Farcy JP. Gravity line analysis in adult volunteers: age-related correlation with spinal parameters, pelvic parameters, and foot position. Spine. 2006; 31(25):E959–E967

[62] Lafage V, Schwab F, Patel A, Hawkinson N, Farcy JP. Pelvic tilt and truncal inclination: two key radiographic parameters in the setting of adults with spinal deformity. Spine. 2009; 34(17):E599–E606

[63] Rose PS, Bridwell KH, Lenke LG, et al. Role of pelvic incidence, thoracic kyphosis, and patient factors on sagittal plane correction following pedicle subtraction osteotomy. Spine. 2009; 34(8):785–791

[64] Lafage V, Schwab F, Vira S, Patel A, Ungar B, Farcy JP. Spino-pelvic parameters after surgery can be predicted: a preliminary formula and validation of standing alignment. Spine. 2011; 36(13):1037–1045

[65] Terran J, Schwab F, Shaffrey CI, et al. The SRS-Schwab adult spinal deformity classification: assessment and clinical correlations based on a prospective operative and nonoperative cohort. Neurosurgery. 2013; 73(4):559–568

[66] Hallager DW, Hansen LV, Dragsted CR, Peytz N, Gehrchen M, Dahl B. A comprehensive analysis of the SRS-Schwab adult spinal deformity classification and confounding variables: a prospective, non-US cross-sectional study in 292 patients. Spine. 2016; 41(10):E589–E597

[67] Smith JS, Shaffrey CI, Berven S, et al. Operative versus nonoperative treatment of leg pain in adults with scoliosis: a retrospective review of a prospective multicenter database with two-year follow-up. Spine. 2009; 34(16): 1693–1698

[68] Smith JS, Shaffrey CI, Glassman SD, et al. Risk-benefit assessment of surgery for adult scoliosis: an analysis based on patient age. Spine. 2011; 36(10): 817–824

[69] Bridwell KH, Glassman S, Horton W, et al. Does treatment (nonoperative and operative) improve the two-year quality of life in patients with adult symptomatic lumbar scoliosis: a prospective multicenter evidence-based medicine study. Spine. 2009; 34(20):2171–2178

[70] Smith JS, Klineberg E, Schwab F, et al. Change in classification grade by the SRS-Schwab adult spinal deformity classification predicts impact on health-related quality of life measures: prospective analysis of operative and nonoperative treatment. Spine. 2013; 38(19):1663–1671

[71] Ha KY, Jang WH, Kim YH, Park DC. Clinical relevance of the SRS-Schwab classification for degenerative lumbar scoliosis. Spine. 2016; 41(5):E282–E288

[72] Lafage R, Schwab F, Challier V, et al. Defining spino-pelvic alignment thresholds: should operative goals in adult spinal deformity surgery account for age? Spine. 2016; 41(1):62–68

[73] Tonosu J, Takeshita K, Hara N, et al. The normative score and the cut-off value of the Oswestry Disability Index (ODI). Eur Spine J. 2012; 21(8):1596–1602

[74] Nielsen DH, Gehrchen M, Hansen LV, Walbom J, Dahl B. Inter- and intra-rater agreement in assessment of adult spinal deformity using the Scoliosis Research Society-Schwab classification. Spine Deform. 2014; 2(1):40–47

[75] Liu Y, Liu Z, Zhu F, et al. Validation and reliability analysis of the new SRS-Schwab classification for adult spinal deformity. Spine. 2013; 38(11): 902–908

[76] Vialle R, Levassor N, Rillardon L, Templier A, Skalli W, Guigui P. Radiographic analysis of the sagittal alignment and balance of the spine in asymptomatic subjects. J Bone Joint Surg Am. 2005; 87(2):260–267

[77] Le Huec JC, Aunoble S, Philippe L, Nicolas P. Pelvic parameters: origin and significance. Eur Spine J. 2011; 20(Suppl 5):564–571

[78] Mac-Thiong JM, Labelle H, Berthonnaud E, Betz RR, Roussouly P. Sagittal spinopelvic balance in normal children and adolescents. Eur Spine J. 2007; 16 (2):227–234

[79] Mangione P, Gomez D, Senegas J. Study of the course of the incidence angle during growth. Eur Spine J. 1997; 6(3):163–167

[80] Mac-Thiong JM, Berthonnaud E, Dimar JR, II, Betz RR, Labelle H. Sagittal alignment of the spine and pelvis during growth. Spine. 2004; 29(15):1642–1647

[81] Mac-Thiong JM, Roussouly P, Berthonnaud E, Guigui P. Age- and sex-related variations in sagittal sacropelvic morphology and balance in asymptomatic adults. Eur Spine J. 2011; 20 Suppl 5:572–577

[82] Jean L. Influence of age and sagittal balance of the spine on the value of the pelvic incidence. Eur Spine J. 2014; 23(7):1394–1399

[83] Lee JH, Na KH, Kim JH, Jeong HY, Chang DG. Is pelvic incidence a constant, as everyone knows? Changes of pelvic incidence in surgically corrected adult sagittal deformity. Eur Spine J. 2016; 25(11):3707–3714

[84] Arima H, Yamato Y, Hasegawa T, et al. Discrepancy between standing posture and sagittal balance during walking in adult spinal deformity patients. Spine. 2017; 42(1):E25–E30

[85] Shiba Y, Taneichi H, Inami S, Moridaira H, Takeuchi D, Nohara Y. Dynamic global sagittal alignment evaluated by three-dimensional gait analysis in patients with degenerative lumbar kyphoscoliosis. Eur Spine J. 2016; 25 (8):2572–2579

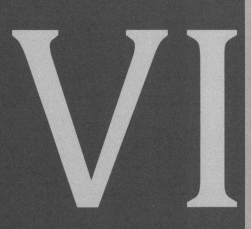

Part VI

Adolescent Idiopathic Scoliosis (AIS)

VI

18 Specificities in Growing Spine

Shahnawaz Haleem and Colin Nnadi

Abstract

Sagittal balance in adults has been the subject of extensive research in the literature. There is very little recorded on the development of sagittal balance in the child. The aim of this chapter is to increase the reader's understanding of processes involved in the evolution of spinal development in children: how these processes differ from the adult population and what childhood conditions impact on the normal sagittal alignment of the immature spine.

Keywords: pediatric sagittal balance, pediatric spinal parameters, pediatric spondylolisthesis, proximal junctional kyphosis (PJK), spinal equilibrium

18.1 Normal Development of Spine

The development of the spine involves longitudinal and axial growth that not only protects the neurological function but also maintains physiological motion. The aim is to have a well-balanced spine that allows achievement of normal everyday activities.

Our early ancestors walked with a bent-hip, bent-knee (BH-BK) gait similar to chimpanzees (▶ Fig. 18.1). This led to a poor upright posture, which in turn meant higher and more costly energy expenditure. This is borne out by the fact that the BH-BK gait throws the center of gravity of the body anterior to the hip joints. This generates an equal and opposite ground reaction force vector with an increased flexion moment arm over the hip joints. These forces need to be counteracted to maintain posture and result in increased energy expenditure.

The "normal" sagittal balance develops from a completely kyphotic spine, which develops into the compensatory lordosis curvature in the cervical and lumbar spine balanced by the

kyphosis in the thoracic spine. This results in placement of the head up over the pelvis.

At birth, the T1-S1 segment measures about 20 cm with a gain in standing height approximately 25 cm during the first year of life and around 12.5 cm during the second year.[1] As mentioned earlier, the spine at this stage is hyperkyphotic with lumbar lordosis (LL) only appearing as the child begins to acquire the upright position initially by sitting (6 to 12 months) and later by a bipedal stance (around one to two years).[2] The thoracic kyphosis (TK) develops to balance the LL as the child grows.[3,4]

The neonatal pelvis has no stance-related locomotion demands as the child is predominantly supine at this stage and the sacrum is vertical.[5] As the child begins to sit up and later stand up, axial weight is transferred to the sacrum leading to its increasing horizontalization.[6,7]

Modern man therefore stands with an upright posture, which means the center of gravity falls between the points of contact with the ground (i.e., the feet). The ground reaction force generated is closer to the hip and knee joints and causes a much smaller flexion moment arm. The energy expenditure of maintaining this posture is much more economical. This progression from the quadrupedal to bipedal posture in humans can be compared to the transition from crawling to walking in the toddler. In both situations, spinopelvic balance is essential for cost-neutral energy expenditure. This is achieved with the development of lordotic curves in the cephalad and caudal regions of the spine and a kyphotic curve in between. Alignment is maintained with adequate muscle tone, diskoligamentous tension, and bony articulation. In the sagittal plane, these segments are interdependent and as a unit articulate with the pelvis and lower limbs to give an equilibrium that maintains an upright posture. In the child, this equilibrium can be disturbed by neurological conditions that affect muscle tone or those that affect alignment such as spondylolisthesis and scoliosis. Iatrogenic causes from treatment with growing rods and their complications is a well-known cause as well.

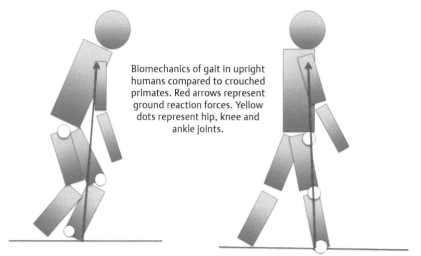

Biomechanics of gait in upright humans compared to crouched primates. Red arrows represent ground reaction forces. Yellow dots represent hip, knee and ankle joints.

Fig. 18.1 Biomechanics of gait. Primate versus modern man.

18.2 Fundamental Parameters in Spinal Alignment

Duval-Beaupère et al described pelvic incidence (PI) as a fundamental pelvic anatomic parameter that is specific and constant for each individual and determines pelvic orientation as well as LL. This principle is somewhat different in the child.[3,8]

As in the adult population, adaptive changes occur in the pelvis and lower limbs in children with sagittal imbalance. Similarly, PI describes the morphology of the pelvis; pelvic tilt (PT) and sacral slope (SS) describe the orientation of the pelvis in relation to the bicoxofemoral axis and the vertical plane. Both PT and SS are positional parameters that change in relation to the orientation of the sacrum. Unlike PI in the adult, in the skeletally immature, PI evolves throughout growth.

Many studies have highlighted the relationship of the spine and pelvis in standing balance in normal adults and children particularly through the effect of LL.[2,4] Schwab et al[9] described the gravitational line to remain fairly constant with age; however, the degree of TK associated with age would shift the plumb line anteriorly with a compensatory retroversion of the pelvis, increasing the PT to keep the gravitational line constant and maintain adequate sagittal balance.

It is thought that there is a trimodal age distribution of sagittal plane deformities. In the teenage years, sagittal plane deformities are usually secondary to Scheuermann's kyphosis. The second group occurs in the 40- to 50-year age range, commonly a result of inflammatory disorders such as ankylosing spondylitis, and the last group is in the over 60 range, where the commonest problem is degenerative arthritis of the spine. The center of gravity line in the standing position lies just in front of the thoracic spine. There is therefore a natural tendency for the upper trunk to move forward but this is counterbalanced by the lordotic lumbar spine. The integrity of the intervertebral disks is important in maintaining this profile. In pathological states, there is collapse of the disk height, which leads to a loss of the normal sagittal curves and a straighter profile that is not biomechanically efficient. This is similarly found in physiological aging of the spine.[10]

Boulay et al[11] found that PI can increase with growth in childhood or adolescence, reaching a constant value in adulthood. Mangione et al[12] showed that PI tended to increase linearly during childhood after the acquisition of walking, but this article did not specifically document the influence of age on PI during adolescence. In another article, Descamps et al[13] showed that PI was relatively stable before 10 years old and then increased significantly during adolescence until reaching its maximum value in adulthood. However, the authors did not evaluate the influence of age on the PI with any correlation studies. In a prospective study, Mac-Thiong et al[14] looked at the sagittal alignment of the spine and pelvis and its change during growth in a normal pediatric population. Lateral standing radiographs in 180 patients were evaluated for TK, LL, SS, PT, and PI. They concluded that PI tended to increase with age from 4 to 18 years. PT and LL increased with age as well but SS was not significantly influenced by age after the onset of walking. There were also no differences between males or females in the study group.

The developing spine with the newly acquired bipedal status and locomotion requires the constant adaptation of the morphology and orientation of the pelvis to align the spine in adequate balance to cope with daily demands. Adequate alignment ensures minimum energy expenditure.[15,16]

Mac-Thiong et al advocated two hypotheses to explain the observed changes in PI. First, the PT seeks to align the center of gravity optimally over the lower limb axis. It does this by keeping the sacral plate behind the hip axis. Because of the increase in body weight during growth and risk of anterior displacement of the center of gravity, the sacral plate is pushed further backward by an increase in PT. Second, with the onset of standing and locomotion, the sacral plate becomes more vertical (i.e., the sacrum becomes more horizontal). This leads to an increase in SS.[14] Geometrically, PI is the sum of SS and PT; hence, any increase in either PT or SS will inevitably lead to an increased PI. Both LL and TK increase with age.[2] LL plays an important role in sagittal balance.[8,17] Adequate lordosis is required to prevent anterior displacement of the center of gravity. The TK balances LL and any changes reflect the evolving status of LL. The development of the respiratory system or thoracic vertebra may also play a role that contradicts the previous hypothesis. This is because of differences observed in TK among patients with adolescent idiopathic curves.[18]

Body mass index has been shown to have a strong correlation with PI and LL.[11] This stems from the remodeling effect on the sacrum, which may continue into the early 20 s.

18.3 Pediatric Spondylolisthesis

The link between pelvic parameters and spondylolisthesis has been well described in the literature.[19,20,21,22] Therefore, it is pertinent that the management of spondylolisthesis requires a clear understanding of spinopelvic parameters in the local and global assessment of balance in the treatment algorithm.

18.4 Causative Factors in the Development of Pediatric Spondylolisthesis

The primary forces acting across the lumbosacral joint include axial loading, forward flexion, and truncal rotation.[23] Sengupta[24] explained that an increased shear force across the lumbosacral disk may explain the association of a large PI and SS with developmental spondylolisthesis, which is a result, primarily, of the loss of the posterior restraint and absence of anterior support allowing the shear forces to propagate the slip. Doming or anterior lipping of the sacral endplate were also noted in patients with high-grade developmental spondylolisthesis.

Spondylolisthesis has a prevalence of about 6% in the general population.[25,26] The prevalence of high-grade spondylolisthesis is unknown. A study by the Spinal Deformity Study Group (SDSG) compared 240 cases with spondylolisthesis to 160 normal, asymptomatic young adults. They found that PI, SS, PT, and LL were significantly greater while TK was significantly lower in the cases with developmental spondylolisthesis when compared to the normal population. They also showed that pelvic anatomy has a direct influence on the development of spondylolisthesis.[22] Shear forces are then generated across the lumbosacral disk in the presence of increased PI and SS in developmental spondylolisthesis.

Table 18.1 SDSG spondylolisthesis classification[25]

Type	Pelvic incidence (°)	Grade
I	<45° (nutcracker type)	Low
II	45°–60°	Low
III	>60°	Low
	Pelvis/spine	
IV	Balanced pelvis	High
V	Retroverted pelvis/balanced spine	High
VI	Retroverted pelvis/unbalanced spine	High

SDSG, Spinal Deformity Study Group.

Historically, the two commonly used classifications were the Wiltse and Meyerding classifications.[27,28] The Wiltse classification is a morphological description of five major types with I (dysplastic) and II (A, stress fracture; B, pars elongation; and C, acute fracture) being commoner in children and adolescents. The Meyerding classification describes slippage of one vertebra relative to another in the form of quadrants. There are five grades with III (50%–75%), IV (75%–100%), and V (>100%) being of most significance in childhood. An all-encompassing classification that incorporates slippage grade, PI, and overall spinopelvic balance has been devised by the SDSG[29,30,31] (▶ Table 18.1).

The SDSG classification describes low-grade slips (1–3) through pelvic PI and high-grade slips (4–6) through PI as well as overall spinopelvic balance. This classification informs decision making about what type of surgery to perform.

18.5 Management of Pediatric Spondylolisthesis

The focus of surgery is to restore spinopelvic balance. Hresko et al,[32] in a study of 133 patients with high-grade slips, defined thresholds beyond which SS and PT values are abnormal. A balanced pelvis in high-grade spondylolisthesis was defined as high PI and SS with low PT, whereas an unbalanced pelvis was defined as that with a low SS and high PT (retroverted pelvis) (▶ Fig. 18.2, ▶ Fig. 18.3). They also have higher lumbosacral kyphosis. The overall spinal balance is defined by the position of the C7 plumb line in relation to the femoral heads. If this line is in front of the femoral heads, the spine is in positive sagittal balance. The presence of an unbalanced pelvis and unbalanced spine require a realignment osteotomy to minimize the lumbosacral shear forces and restore global balance. The L5-S1 slip angle is also gaining prominence as a prognostic indicator. Lundine et al[33] have shown that a slip angle >20° is associated with a worse prognosis in conservatively or surgically treated patients.

The majority of patients with the higher-grade slips will complain of neurological symptoms. The question is how long does the surgeon continue to manage these cases nonoperatively? Long-term outcomes of conservative treatment are

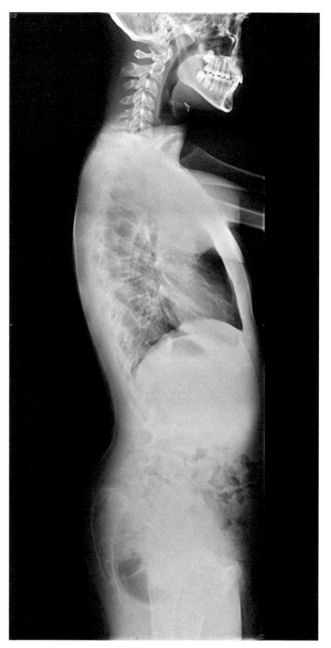

Fig. 18.2 Unbalanced pelvis (retroverted) and balanced spine (C7 plumb line behind hips).

variable with significant pain relief ranging from 10% to 90% of reported cases.[34,35] Bourassa-Moreau et al.[36] concluded that high-grade slips could be treated nonoperatively if there are good baseline quality-of-life scores, a normal neurologic examination, and imaging that remains unchanged over time.

Symptomatic high-grade spondylolisthesis in a growing child will usually require surgical intervention because of the risk of progression. Some children may present with a cauda equina syndrome in which case emergency surgery is necessary. However, neurological symptoms, back pain, and radiculopathy can be seen as relative indications for surgery.

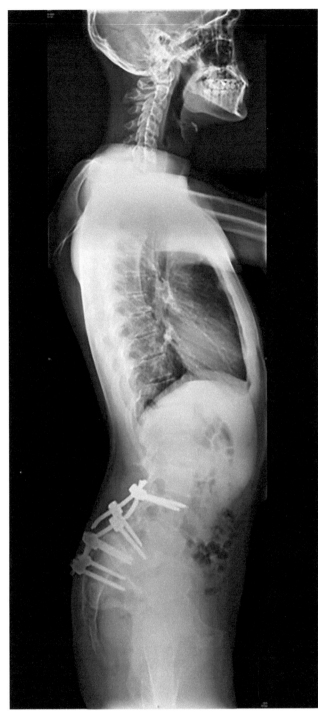

Fig. 18.3 Balanced pelvis (reduced retroversion) and unbalanced spine (C7 plumb line in front of hips).

Noninstrumented fusion techniques have been largely abandoned because of high failure rates.[37] The main controversy with surgery is whether to reduce the deformity or to fix in situ. Reduction is often difficult and associated with complications.[38,39,40,41,42,43,44,45,46,47,48,49]

The goals of surgery are to restore spinopelvic balance, preserve neurological function, improve pain, and achieve a solid fusion. There have been reports of satisfactory outcomes with in situ fusion.[42]

The main concern around reduction techniques is the risk of neurological injury. Recent evidence however does not support this view entirely. Petraco et al[50] showed that the amount of nerve path lengthening rapidly increased from initial reduction of a 100% slip to when it reached the last 25%. Surprisingly, the first half of the reduction led to only 29% of the total nerve strain. Prevalence of nerve root injury is reported as 5%–10% in some series but one suspects the figure may be higher. A Scoliosis Research Society Database query revealed a nerve root deficit rate of 10.2%. One out of nine patients had a permanent deficit and four made a full recovery. Nerve decompression or reduction were not risk factors for a deficit. Osteotomy on the other hand was a risk factor and needs to be taken into consideration when deciding on which surgical procedure to use.[47,51]

A reduction procedure also requires an interbody fusion, which adds to the complexity of the procedure while in situ fusion is limited to posterolateral instrumentation. Anterior column support as provided by interbody fusion does have the advantage of reducing the pseudoarthrosis rate. Reports of 30% pseudoarthrosis rates for instrumented posterolateral fusion, which reduce to less than 10% with anterior column support exist.[52] The main perceived advantage of a reduction is the restoration of spinopelvic balance and minimization of the shear forces across the lumbosacral junction.

The decision to operate also involves deciding on the levels of fusion and whether the pelvis is to be included in the fusion. Studies that involved single-level fusion revealed a 17% nonunion rate in a study of 34 patients and an 11% rate of structural complications prompting the authors to recommend an L4-S1 fusion.[23,46,53] While distal fixation worked well for children and adolescents, involving the pelvis in the fusion proved beneficial for older patients.[54,55]

The use of anterior column support for high-grade slips either with an interbody cage or lumbosacral strut graft has shown to be beneficial because of the reduction in pseudoarthrosis occurrence. These authors postulated that their circumferential fusion technique facilitated correction of local kyphosis and sagittal balance.[56,57] Some authors have also utilized a transsacral interbody fibular or titanium mesh strut (the modified Bohlman technique) successfully to achieve union and reduce kyphosis.[58,59]

18.6 Flat Back Syndrome

The reduction of LL can occur as a result of fusion of the spine with distraction creating a positive sagittal imbalance. This phenomenon is known as iatrogenic flat-back syndrome. This may also include an inability to stand upright and involve back pain.[60]

A loss of lordosis noticed after treatment of thoracolumbar scoliosis has been reported by several authors.[61] Factors that contribute to this condition include preoperative kyphosis in the thoracolumbar spine, growing rod instrumentation, and pseudoarthrosis postoperatively.[62] It has also been noted that a more distal fusion is susceptible to flat-back deformity.[63,64]

18.7 Proximal Junctional Kyphosis (PJK)

A recent meta-analysis showed an overall incidence of PJK in the pediatric and adolescent patients to be 11% (0%–55%).[65] PJK is a radiographic and clinical diagnosis. It is generally picked up earlier on postoperative radiographs and may be symptomatic or asymptomatic. There have been previous radiographic descriptions of PJK but the two most commonly used criteria are those by Glattes et al and Helgeson et al with the latter being the more commonly used.[66,67] The former describes postoperative kyphosis increase at > 15° while the latter uses > 10° as the cutoff.

Risk factors for PJK preoperatively include preexisting thoracic hyperkyphosis while those occurring intraoperatively are ligamentous disruption, facet joint capsule breaches, and the use of pedicle screws in the upper instrumented vertebra. Thoracoplasty may also be a risk factor.[68,69]

The management of PJK depends on the presentation, as there are currently no evidence-based guidelines. A clinical assessment of the neurological status is required with management ranging from observation to surgical correction.

Despite the prevalence of PJK, the radiological appearances do not always correlate with outcome. Successful management relies on an awareness of the risk factors, good sagittal alignment evaluation preoperatively, and good surgical technique.

18.8 Key Points

- Childhood sagittal balance is evolutionary.
- Alignment parameters must be evaluated prior to treatment.
- Important to understand the differences in balanced and unbalanced spine–pelvis relationships for best outcomes in treatment of spondylolisthesis.
- Beware iatrogenic flat-back syndrome and PJK; proper evaluation is needed before treatment.

References

[1] Dimeglio A, Canavese F. The growing spine: how spinal deformities influence normal spine and thoracic cage growth. Eur Spine J. 2012; 21(1):64–70

[2] Voutsinas SA, MacEwen GD. Sagittal profiles of the spine. Clin Orthop Relat Res. 1986; 210:235–242

[3] Legaye J, Duval-Beaupère G, Hecquet J, Marty C. Pelvic incidence: a fundamental pelvic parameter for three-dimensional regulation of spinal sagittal curves. Eur Spine J. 1998; 7(2):99–103

[4] Vaz G, Roussouly P, Berthonnaud E, Dimnet J. Sagittal morphology and equilibrium of pelvis and spine. Eur Spine J. 2002; 11(1):80–87

[5] Yusof NA, Soames RW, Cunningham CA, Black SM. Growth of the human ilium: the anomalous sacroiliac junction. Anat Rec (Hoboken). 2013; 296 (11):1688–1694

[6] Bogduk N, Macintosh JE, Pearcy MJ. A universal model of the lumbar back muscles in the upright position. Spine. 1992; 17(8):897–913

[7] Keen M. Early development and attainment of normal mature gait. J Prosthet Orthot. 1993; 5(2). DOI: 10.1097/00008526–199304000–00004

[8] Duval-Beaupère G, Schmidt C, Cosson P. A barycentremetric study of the sagittal shape of spine and pelvis: the conditions required for an economic standing position. Ann Biomed Eng. 1992; 20(4):451–462

[9] Schwab F, Lafage V, Patel A, Farcy JP. Sagittal plane considerations and the pelvis in the adult patient. Spine. 2009; 34(17):1828–1833

[10] Roussouly P, Nnadi C. Sagittal plane deformity: an overview of interpretation and management. Eur Spine J. 2010; 19(11):1824–1836

[11] Boulay C, Tardieu C, Hecquet J, et al. Sagittal alignment of spine and pelvis regulated by pelvic incidence: standard values and prediction of lordosis. Eur Spine J. 2006; 15(4):415–422

[12] Mangione P, Gomez D, Senegas J. Study of the course of the incidence angle during growth. Eur Spine J. 1997; 6(3):163–167

[13] Descamps H, Commare-Nordmann MC, Marty C, Hecquet J, Duval-Beaupère G. Modification of pelvic angle during the human growth (in French). Biom Hum Anthropol. 1999; 17:59–63

[14] Mac-Thiong JM, Berthonnaud E, Dimar JR, II, Betz RR, Labelle H. Sagittal alignment of the spine and pelvis during growth. Spine. 2004; 29(15):1642–1647

[15] Abitbol MM. Evolution of the lumbosacral angle. Am J Phys Anthropol. 1987; 72(3):361–372

[16] Abitbol MM. Effect of posture and locomotion on energy expenditure. Am J Phys Anthropol. 1988; 77(2):191–199

[17] During J, Goudfrooij H, Keessen W, Beeker TW, Crowe A. Toward standards for posture. Postural characteristics of the lower back system in normal and pathologic conditions. Spine. 1985; 10(1):83–87

[18] Mac-Thiong J-M, Labelle H, Charlebois M, Huot MP, de Guise JA. Sagittal plane analysis of the spine and pelvis in adolescent idiopathic scoliosis according to the coronal curve type. Spine. 2003; 28(13):1404–1409

[19] Labelle H, Roussouly P, Berthonnaud E, Dimnet J, O'Brien M. The importance of spino-pelvic balance in L5-s1 developmental spondylolisthesis: a review of pertinent radiologic measurements. Spine. 2005; 30(6) Suppl:S27–S34

[20] Hanson DS, Bridwell KH, Rhee JM, Lenke LG. Correlation of pelvic incidence with low- and high-grade isthmic spondylolisthesis. Spine. 2002; 27 (18):2026–2029

[21] Rajnics P, Templier A, Skalli W, Lavaste F, Illés T. The association of sagittal spinal and pelvic parameters in asymptomatic persons and patients with isthmic spondylolisthesis. J Spinal Disord Tech. 2002; 15(1):24–30

[22] Labelle H, Roussouly P, Berthonnaud E, et al. Spondylolisthesis, pelvic incidence, and spinopelvic balance: a correlation study. Spine. 2004; 29 (18):2049–2054

[23] Schoenleber SJ, Shufflebarger HL, Shah SA. The assessment and treatment of high-grade lumbosacral spondylolisthesis and spondyloptosis in children and young adults. JBJS Rev. 2015; 3(12):01874474–201512000–00006

[24] Sengupta DK. Spinopelvic balance. JBJS Rev. 2014; 2(8):01874474–201408000–00005

[25] Beutler WJ, Fredrickson BE, Murtland A, Sweeney CA, Grant WD, Baker D. The natural history of spondylolysis and spondylolisthesis: 45-year follow-up evaluation. Spine. 2003; 28(10):1027–1035, discussion 1035

[26] Fredrickson BE, Baker D, McHolick WJ, Yuan HA, Lubicky JP. The natural history of spondylolysis and spondylolisthesis. J Bone Joint Surg Am. 1984; 66 (5):699–707

[27] Wiltse LL, Newman PH, Macnab I. Classification of spondylolisis and spondylolisthesis. Clin Orthop Relat Res. 1976; 117:23–29

[28] Meyerding HW. Spondylolisthesis. Surg Gynecol Obstet. 1932; 54:371–377

[29] Mac-Thiong JM, Labelle H. A proposal for a surgical classification of pediatric lumbosacral spondylolisthesis based on current literature. Eur Spine J. 2006; 15(10):1425–1435

[30] Mac-Thiong JM, Labelle H, Parent S, et al. Reliability and development of a new classification of lumbosacral spondylolisthesis. Scoliosis. 2008; 3:19

[31] Mac-Thiong JM, Duong L, Parent S, et al. Reliability of the Spinal Deformity Study Group classification of lumbosacral spondylolisthesis. Spine. 2012; 37 (2):E95–E102

[32] Hresko MT, Labelle H, Roussouly P, Berthonnaud E. Classification of high-grade spondylolistheses based on pelvic version and spine balance: possible rationale for reduction. Spine. 2007; 32(20):2208–2213

[33] Lundine KM, Lewis SJ, Al-Aubaidi Z, Alman B, Howard AW. Patient outcomes in the operative and nonoperative management of high-grade spondylolisthesis in children. J Pediatr Orthop. 2014; 34(5):483–489

[34] Pizzutillo PD, Hummer CD, III. Nonoperative treatment for painful adolescent spondylolysis or spondylolisthesis. J Pediatr Orthop. 1989; 9(5):538–540

[35] Harris IE, Weinstein SL. Long-term follow-up of patients with grade-III and IV spondylolisthesis. Treatment with and without posterior fusion. J Bone Joint Surg Am. 1987; 69(7):960–969

[36] Bourassa-Moreau É, Mac-Thiong JM, Joncas J, Parent S, Labelle H. Quality of life of patients with high-grade spondylolisthesis: minimum 2-year follow-up after surgical and nonsurgical treatments. Spine. 2013; 13(7):770–774

[37] Lamberg T, Remes V, Helenius I, Schlenzka D, Seitsalo S, Poussa M. Uninstrumented in situ fusion for high-grade childhood and adolescent

isthmic spondylolisthesis: long-term outcome. J Bone Joint Surg Am. 2007; 89(3):512–518

[38] Boachie-Adjei O, Do T, Rawlins BA. Partial lumbosacral kyphosis reduction, decompression, and posterior lumbosacral transfixation in high-grade isthmic spondylolisthesis: clinical and radiographic results in six patients. Spine. 2002; 27(6):E161–E168

[39] Boos N, Marchesi D, Zuber K, Aebi M. Treatment of severe spondylolisthesis by reduction and pedicular fixation. A 4–6-year follow-up study. Spine. 1993; 18(12):1655–1661

[40] Longo UG, Loppini M, Romeo G, Maffulli N, Denaro V. Evidence-based surgical management of spondylolisthesis: reduction or arthrodesis in situ. J Bone Joint Surg Am. 2014; 96(1):53–58

[41] Lonner BS, Song EW, Scharf CL, Yao J. Reduction of high-grade isthmic and dysplastic spondylolisthesis in 5 adolescents. Am J Orthop. 2007; 36(7):367–373

[42] Martiniani M, Lamartina C, Specchia N. "In situ" fusion or reduction in high-grade high dysplastic developmental spondylolisthesis (HDSS). Eur Spine J. 2012; 21 Suppl 1:S134–S140

[43] Molinari RW, Bridwell KH, Lenke LG, Ungacta FF, Riew KD. Complications in the surgical treatment of pediatric high-grade, isthmic dysplastic spondylolisthesis. a comparison of three surgical approaches. Spine. 1999; 24(16):1701–1711

[44] Muschik M, Zippel H, Perka C. Surgical management of severe spondylolisthesis in children and adolescents. Anterior fusion in situ versus anterior spondylodesis with posterior transpedicular instrumentation and reduction. Spine. 1997; 22(17):2036–2042, discussion 2043

[45] Sailhan F, Gollogly S, Roussouly P. The radiographic results and neurologic complications of instrumented reduction and fusion of high-grade spondylolisthesis without decompression of the neural elements: a retrospective review of 44 patients. Spine. 2006; 31(2):161–169, discussion 170

[46] Shufflebarger HL, Geck MJ. High-grade isthmic dysplastic spondylolisthesis: monosegmental surgical treatment. Spine. 2005; 30(6) Suppl:S42–S48

[47] Kasliwal MK, Smith JS, Shaffrey CI, et al. Short-term complications associated with surgery for high-grade spondylolisthesis in adults and pediatric patients: a report from the scoliosis research society morbidity and mortality database. Neurosurgery. 2012; 71(1):109–116

[48] Poussa M, Schlenzka D, Seitsalo S, Ylikoski M, Hurri H, Osterman K. Surgical treatment of severe isthmic spondylolisthesis in adolescents. Reduction or fusion in situ. Spine. 1993; 18(7):894–901

[49] Poussa M, Remes V, Lamberg T, et al. Treatment of severe spondylolisthesis in adolescence with reduction or fusion in situ: long-term clinical, radiologic, and functional outcome. Spine. 2006; 31(5):583–590, discussion 591–592

[50] Petraco DM, Spivak JM, Cappadona JG, Kummer FJ, Neuwirth MG. An anatomic evaluation of L5 nerve stretch in spondylolisthesis reduction. Spine. 1996; 21(10):1133–1138, discussion 1139

[51] Gandhoke GS, Kasliwal MK, Smith JS, et al. A multi-center evaluation of clinical and radiographic outcomes following high-grade spondylolisthesis reduction and fusion. Clin Spine Surg. 2017; 30(4):E363–E369

[52] Dehoux E, Fourati E, Madi K, Reddy B, Segal P. Posterolateral versus interbody fusion in isthmic spondylolisthesis: functional results in 52 cases with a minimum follow-up of 6 years. Acta Orthop Belg. 2004; 70(6):578–582

[53] Lengert R, Charles YP, Walter A, Schuller S, Godet J, Steib JP. Posterior surgery in high-grade spondylolisthesis. Orthop Traumatol Surg Res. 2014; 100 (5):481–484

[54] Kuklo TR, Bridwell KH, Lewis SJ, et al. Minimum 2-year analysis of sacropelvic fixation and L5-S1 fusion using S1 and iliac screws. Spine. 2001; 26 (18):1976–1983

[55] Tsuchiya K, Bridwell KH, Kuklo TR, Lenke LG, Baldus C. Minimum 5-year analysis of L5-S1 fusion using sacropelvic fixation (bilateral S1 and iliac screws) for spinal deformity. Spine. 2006; 31(3):303–308

[56] Molinari RW, Bridwell KH, Lenke LG, Baldus C. Anterior column support in surgery for high-grade, isthmic spondylolisthesis. Clin Orthop Relat Res. 2002; 394:109–120

[57] Mehdian SH, Arun R. A new three-stage spinal shortening procedure for reduction of severe adolescent isthmic spondylolisthesis: a case series with medium- to long-term follow-up. Spine. 2011; 36(11):E705–E711

[58] Sasso RC, Shively KD, Reilly TM. Transvertebral transsacral strut grafting for high-grade isthmic spondylolisthesis L5-S1 with fibular allograft. J Spinal Disord Tech. 2008; 21(5):328–333

[59] Hart RA, Domes CM, Goodwin B, et al. High-grade spondylolisthesis treated using a modified Bohlman technique: results among multiple surgeons. J Neurosurg Spine. 2014; 20(5):523–530

[60] La Grone MO. Loss of lumbar lordosis. A complication of spinal fusion for scoliosis. Orthop Clin North Am. 1988; 19(2):383–393

[61] Moe JH, Denis F. The iatrogenic loss of lumbar lordosis. Orthop Trans. 1977; 1:131

[62] Potter BK, Lenke LG, Kuklo TR. Prevention and management of iatrogenic flatback deformity. J Bone Joint Surg Am. 2004; 86-A(8):1793–1808

[63] Aaro S, Ohlén G. The effect of Harrington instrumentation on the sagittal configuration and mobility of the spine in scoliosis. Spine. 1983; 8(6):570–575

[64] Swank S, Lonstein JE, Moe JH, Winter RB, Bradford DS. Surgical treatment of adult scoliosis. A review of two hundred and twenty-two cases. J Bone Joint Surg Am. 1981; 63(2):268–287

[65] Yan C, Li Y, Yu Z. Prevalence and consequences of the proximal junctional kyphosis after spinal deformity surgery: a meta-analysis. Medicine (Baltimore). 2016; 95(20):e3471

[66] Glattes RC, Bridwell KH, Lenke LG, Kim YJ, Rinella A, Edwards C, II. Proximal junctional kyphosis in adult spinal deformity following long instrumented posterior spinal fusion: incidence, outcomes, and risk factor analysis. Spine. 2005; 30(14):1643–1649

[67] Helgeson MD, Shah SA, Newton PO, et al. Evaluation of proximal junctional kyphosis in adolescent idiopathic scoliosis following pedicle screw, hook, or hybrid instrumentation. Spine. 2010; 35(2):177–181

[68] Kim YJ, Bridwell KH, Lenke LG, Kim J, Cho SK. Proximal junctional kyphosis in adolescent idiopathic scoliosis following segmental posterior spinal instrumentation and fusion: minimum 5-year follow-up. Spine. 2005; 30 (18):2045–2050

[69] Wang J, Zhao Y, Shen B, Wang C, Li M. Risk factor analysis of proximal junctional kyphosis after posterior fusion in patients with idiopathic scoliosis. Injury. 2010; 41(4):415–420

19 Sagittal Balance Incidence on Treatment Strategy in AIS

Stefan Parent

Abstract

Sagittal balance has several implications when treating patients with adolescent idiopathic scoliosis (AIS). Adolescents and young adults have significant mechanisms to compensate for mismatches between spinal and pelvic parameters, which can prevent some of the failures seen following surgery for adult spinal deformities. A basic understanding of the normal spinopelvic sagittal balance and the interactions between these different parameters can lead to better preoperative planning and intraoperative execution to promote a harmonious sagittal balance postoperatively. This chapter will focus on what normal spinopelvic balance is and its influence on the treatment strategy in AIS.

Keywords: adolescent idiopathic scoliosis, pelvic balance, pelvic incidence, spinopelvic parameters

19.1 Introduction

Sagittal balance is an essential component of everyday life. It is the result of complex interactions between the pelvis and the spine but also with the lower extremities. Any alteration between one of these structures can lead to abnormal sagittal balance and have a profound effect on the patient's ability to stand and/or walk for prolonged periods of time. When sagittal balance is preserved, the human body is in a state of minimal energy expenditure.

Adolescent idiopathic scoliosis (AIS) is a three-dimensional deformity of the spine not only affecting the coronal and sagittal plane but also the axial plane. It is this spatial deformity of the spine that creates unbalance in the three planes. Locally, both the intervertebral disk and the vertebral body's shape are affected, contributing to the regional and global deformity. When addressing these deformities surgically, the surgeon must have a good understanding of the impact of the corrective maneuvers and the extent of the instrumentation on the uninstrumented spine. Although surgeons historically focused on the correction in the coronal plane, there has been a renewed interest in the sagittal plane and the impact of different corrective strategies in AIS. From past experience with the Harrington instrumentation, it has become clear that special attention must be given to restore an optimal sagittal balance postoperatively to prevent long-term disability and reoperations.

19.2 Normal Spinopelvic Balance in Children and Adolescents

There are excellent references for sagittal spinopelvic balance in children and adolescents both for normal patients and for patients with AIS.[1,2,3,4] Pelvic incidence (PI) is a pelvic morphometric parameter that increases during adolescent growth and stabilizes in adulthood.[5] PI regulates the relationship between sacral slope (SS) and pelvic tilt (PT), whereby PI = SS + PT.[6] PI is a determinant of lumbar lordosis (LL) and therefore is usually closely related to the lumbar sagittal curve. PI has been shown to be slightly higher in both AIS[7] and adults with idiopathic scoliosis[4] despite the finding that scoliosis deformity is often associated with a hypokyphosis or lordosis of the thoracic segment for thoracic structural curves. The type of curve has not been associated with a change in PI or sagittal balance[7] but the thoracic kyphosis is highly associated with the type of curve. The LL is not influenced by the type of scoliotic deformity but is associated with the pelvic morphology.[7]

Global sagittal balance has also been described in children and adolescents. Different techniques have been proposed to assess global sagittal balance and C7 is generally used as a reference point to represent where the spine is in space relatively to the pelvis. These global measurements typically will encompass a larger number of parameters such as sacropelvic parameters, thoracic kyphosis and LL. One such parameter is based on the distance between the C7 plumb line and the anterosuperior corner of S1. This measurement was found to evolve between adolescents and adults with a progressive displacement of C7 over the pelvis denoting a form of modification in the sagittal curvatures with growth.[8,9]

Linear parameters are, however, subject to measurement error if using uncalibrated radiographs. Descriptive angular parameters have been introduced to overcome these limitations. The spinosacral angle is an angle subtended by the upper sacral endplate and the line from the center of C7 vertebral body to the center of the upper sacral endplate, as described by Roussouly et al.[10] The spinal tilt (ST) angle is subtended by the horizontal line and the line from the center of the C7 vertebral body to the center of the upper sacral endplate. A value greater than 90° indicates that the center of the C7 vertebral body is behind the center of the upper sacral endplate, while for values less than 90°, the center of the C7 vertebral body is in front of the center of the upper sacral endplate. Spinopelvic tilt (SPT) is an angle subtended by the horizontal line and the line from the center of the C7 vertebral body to the hip axis. A value greater than 90° indicates that the center of the C7 vertebral body is behind the hip axis, while for values less than 90°, the center of the C7 vertebral body is in front of the center of the hip axis.

Finally, a classification has been proposed that does not use an angular or linear measurement but is based on the relative position of the C7 plumb line to both the sacrum and vertical axis.[11] This provides a simple and intuitive understanding of the position of the spine relative to the sacrum and hips. Six types are proposed, three where the center of the upper endplate of the sacrum lies in front of the hip axis and three where it lies behind the hip axis. Types 3 and 6 represent the situation where C7 is in front of both the center of the upper endplate of the sacrum and the hip axis.[11] This classification could be used to identify patients at higher risk of developing degenerative changes later in their adult life. ▶ Fig. 19.1 shows the six types as described by Mac-Thiong et al.[11] The classification

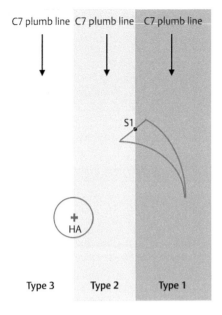

C7 plumb line C7 plumb line C7 plumb line

S1

+ HA

Type 3 Type 2 Type 1

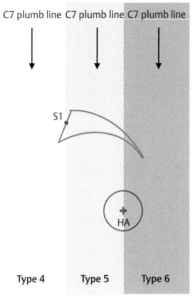

C7 plumb line C7 plumb line C7 plumb line

S1

+ HA

Type 4 Type 5 Type 6

Fig. 19.1 Determination of the global balance type (types 1–6) from the position of C7 plumb line relative to the center of upper sacral endplate of S1 (S1) and to the hip axis (HA). Types 1–3 correspond to cases when HA lies in front of S1, whereas types 4–6 are present when HA is behind S1.

determines global balance without relying on angular parameters. An evaluation of 646 children and adolescents has provided normative data for these types. A C7 plumb line in front of the hip axis and in front of the sacrum (types 3 and 6) is not necessarily associated with spinal pathology with 22% of asymptomatic patients having this configuration. The large variation in asymptomatic patients may reflect the complex interaction in patients' shape, muscle tone, and spine morphology to obtain an upright stable posture.

19.3 How the Spine Reacts to Surgical Correction in Adolescent Idiopathic Scoliosis

Adolescents and young adults are particularly resilient to postural imbalance and will be able to accommodate for imperfect sagittal realignment through different mechanisms. Such mechanisms include pelvic retroversion and, as further imbalance occurs through degenerative changes, further pelvic retroversion, knee flexion and forward trunk displacement (▶ Fig. 19.2). Fortunately, this process usually happens over a long period of time and is more common in adult spinal deformities than in AIS. In adult spinal deformities, the focus is to restore sagittal balance to prevent proximal junctional issues and to minimize sagittal and coronal imbalance. The focus in recent years has been much more on restoring the sagittal alignment than on pure coronal correction, thereby creating a state of least energy expenditure. The long-term goal of AIS surgery is to prevent progression of the scoliotic deformity. This should also include the prevention of distal and proximal junctional issues as well as sagittal balance issues.

When surgical correction of a specific deformity is performed, there are typically two distinct mechanisms involved to produce the resultant sagittal alignment. First, there is an imposed correction that is highly dependent on the surgical maneuver and the instrumentation that will impose a fixed sagittal profile in the instrumented segment. The second mechanism is the reactive changes observed in the uninstrumented segment of the spine both above and below the instrumentation. A delicate balance between imposing too much correction in the instrumented segment and the extent of the fusion can limit the spontaneous adjustment usually observed following spinal arthrodesis.

19.4 Treatment Strategies and Implications for Adolescent Idiopathic Scoliosis Surgery

The preoperative evaluation of a patient should start on the preoperative visit by assessing the patient's posture. Careful evaluation of the lower extremities, including flexion contractures and skeletal rotational deformities (e.g., increased femoral anteversion), should be carefully evaluated. The evaluation should include the patient's sitting and standing posture as well as an evaluation of gait to elicit any compensatory mechanisms involved in activities of daily living. The focus of the evaluation should then be turned to the patient's spinal deformity. An assessment of the thoracic hypokyphosis (or lordosis) and the LL should be performed. Taking the patient through different flexion and extension motions to determine whether the patient's spine is flexible or stiff, and lateral bendings and traction maneuvers (either standing or supine), can also help in determining whether the deformity is relatively flexible or may be difficult to treat. All these preoperative assessments will complement any static imaging studies that will be ordered prior to surgery.

Preoperative imaging should include posteroanterior and lateral standing long radiographs. These images should ideally include the proximal femurs to determine PI and the proximal femoral angle. Nowadays, there are new imaging modalities allowing for full-body standing radiographs, which can be useful in the preoperative assessment. For patients with right thoracic curves presenting increased thoracic kyphosis and

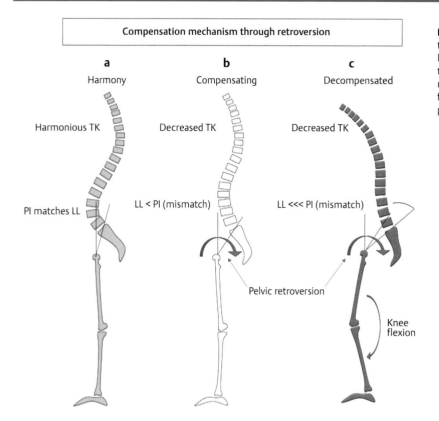

Compensation mechanism through retroversion

a
Harmony

Harmonious TK

PI matches LL

b
Compensating

Decreased TK

LL < PI (mismatch)

c
Decompensated

Decreased TK

LL <<< PI (mismatch)

Pelvic retroversion

Knee flexion

Fig. 19.2 (a-c) Compensation mechanism through retroversion: as lumbar lordosis (LL) is lost, the pelvis is retroverted to accommodate the pelvic incidence (PI) versus LL mismatch. As retroversion is maximized and, in the face of further lordosis loss or increased thoracic kyphosis (TK), knee flexion occurs.

thoracic rotation, preoperative magnetic resonance imaging (MRI) should be used to rule out any neural axis anomalies.[12] Routine use of preoperative MRI is otherwise not mandatory.

The preoperative evaluation should then proceed with an evaluation of the pelvic morphology. Pelvic indices, including PI, SS, and PT should all be measured. LL and thoracic kyphosis can then be measured. The exact lordosis and kyphosis measurement may be poorly evaluated because of the rotational deformity present in AIS. Newton et al[13] have reported on the differences between 2D measured kyphosis versus 3D measured kyphosis from 3D reconstructions of the spine. They found a mean difference of 11° between the 3D derotated kyphosis and the 2D measured kyphosis. This difference was also more important as vertebral rotation increased thereby creating a false impression of preserved kyphosis in larger more rotated curves. The summation of local kyphosis obtained in 3D by derotating each spinal segment can only be obtained by mathematically rearranging the spinal segments and observing them in 3D (▶ Fig. 19.3).

PI and sagittal balance should then influence the corrective strategy to be used for a specific patient.[2,14] Patients with higher than normal PI will need a higher lordosis either through a combination of increased segmental lordosis in the uninstrumented portion of the spine or by additional lordosis in the instrumented segment of the lumbar spine. Typically, for a patient with a high PI, the patient can create lordosis by tilting the pelvis forward and increasing the segmental lordosis under the instrumentation. It is thus important to leave as many free segments distally for the spine to compensate or to create more

lordosis into the instrumented segments. For patients with a smaller value of PI, care should be taken to avoid hyperlordosis creating, in turn, a posterior shift of the fusion mass putting the proximal and distal junctions at risk of failure.[15]

Once the pelvic morphology has been recognized, attention should be turned toward the thoracic segment. If the patient is normokyphotic, the surgical strategy should emphasize careful positioning to avoid extension of the T5-T12 segment and proper rod contouring, including overcontouring the concave rod to promote kyphosis generation and/or maintenance. Derotation maneuvers, especially directed at vertebral derotation either direct or en bloc, should be performed by avoiding pushing down on the convex side of the thorax. These maneuvers have been shown to generate hypokyphosis when the center of rotation was around the concave rod as opposed to the center of the vertebral axis.[16] By using careful corrective maneuvers and appropriate rod contouring techniques, significant correction with restoration of sagittal balance is possible (▶ Fig. 19.4).

For patients with thoracic hypokyphosis or thoracic lordosis, the surgical strategy may need to be tailored to the amount of correction needed. Thoracic kyphosis can be generated either by lengthening the posterior portion of the spine or by shortening the anterior portion of the spine. Although initially described to correct kyphotic deformities, the Ponte osteotomy has become an intrinsic part of the treatment of spinal deformities.[17] By releasing the posterior elements, it produces marked increased flexibility in extension, flexion, and rotation. It does not require a separate anterior procedure and can

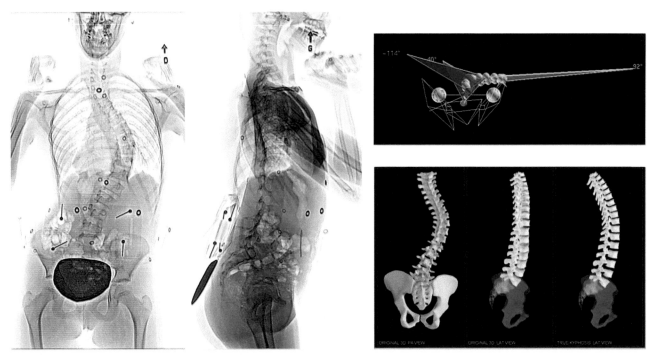

Fig. 19.3 Posteroanterior and lateral images of a patient with significant thoracic lordosis in a Lenke 1A pattern. The 3D reconstruction shows the significant thoracic lordosis on the segmentally derotated 3D reconstruction (third reconstruction, bottom right). The Da Vinci view (top view right) shows the main thoracic curve to be projected forward in front of the hip axis (green triangle).

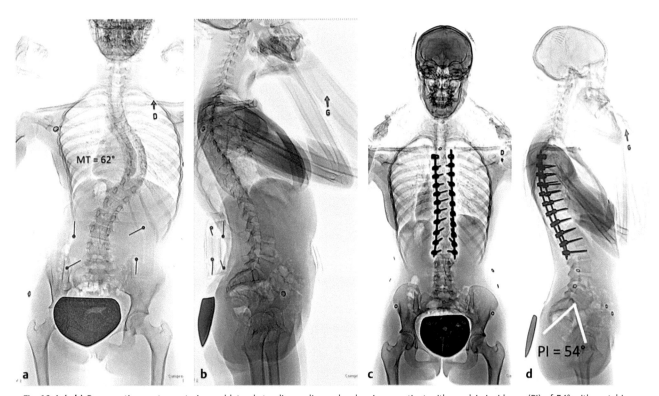

Fig. 19.4 (a,b) Preoperative posteroanterior and lateral standing radiographs showing a patient with a pelvic incidence (PI) of 54° with matching lordosis and normokyphosis. **(c,d)** The surgical strategy was to restore segmental thoracic kyphosis with rod differential contouring and direct vertebral derotation maneuvers. The correction in the sagittal plane was coupled to the correction in the coronal plane, creating a very satisfactory result postoperatively. MT, Main thoracic.

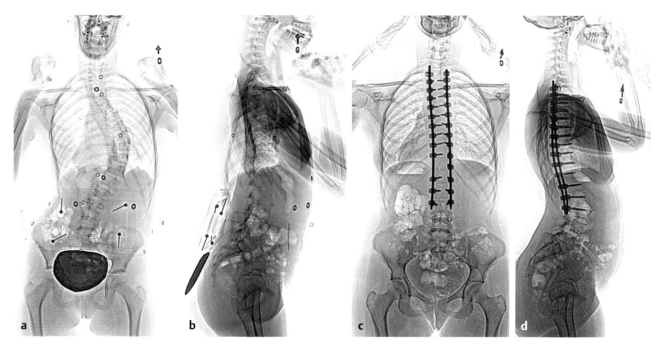

Fig. 19.5 (a,b) Same patient as ▶ Fig. 19.3. Significant thoracic lordosis despite a pelvic incidence (PI) of 58°. The patient's deformity was considered to be relatively stiff on physical exam and progressed rapidly in the 6 months prior to surgery. **(c,d)** Surgical strategy included an anterior thoracoscopic release between T8 and T12 followed by posterior instrumentation from T2 to L3 and multiple Ponte osteotomies between T6 and L2. Correction was achieved by translation instead of rod derotation to help pull the spine back toward the rods. Thoracic kyphosis improved to 20° postop with a significant decrease in cervical kyphosis.

produce adequate segmental correction and produce kyphosis segmentally. Care must, however, be taken when lengthening the posterior column as this may also stretch the spinal cord. Careful monitoring during this portion of the correction is of utmost importance. As the osteotomy site opens, care must be taken to avoid inadvertent trauma to the spinal cord.

In the face of significant thoracic lordosis (as illustrated by the segmental thoracic lordosis; ▶ Fig. 19.3, ▶ Fig. 19.5), the surgeon may elect to proceed with an anterior release thereby creating kyphosis by shortening the anterior part of the spine. This anterior release can be performed through an open thoracotomy or, more commonly, through a video-assisted thoracoscopy. This allows for removal of the intervertebral disk, release of the anterior longitudinal ligament, and bone grafting. Nonstructural bone graft is usually preferred, and care is taken not to overfill the resected disk space to avoid limiting kyphosis generation. Once the release is completed, the patient is then positioned prone and the thoracic pad is placed so as to maximize kyphosis generation with positioning. Posterior instrumentation then proceeds with the addition of Ponte osteotomies to generate as much kyphosis as possible (▶ Fig. 19.5).

For patients with lower PI, different facts must be considered when planning the surgical correction. Patients with lower PI do not need as much lordosis to create sagittal balance and may tolerate hypokyphosis much better than patients with a higher PI. Care should be taken to avoid aggressive lordosis generation in the instrumented portion of the lumbar spine to avoid posterior displacement of the fusion mass that could, in turn, increase the stresses both distally or proximally putting the spine at risk of junctional failure. Transition from the thoracic region to the lumbar region should be done progressively with lordosis creation concentrated in the distal segments (▶ Fig. 19.6).

19.5 Conclusion

Spinopelvic and global sagittal balance are important factors to consider both in the preoperative assessment and in the intraoperative treatment strategies to optimize the postoperative outcome. Restoration of near-normal sagittal balance should decrease the risk of long-term junctional issues and hopefully preserve motion distally and proximally to the instrumented segment. Surgeons need to have a solid understanding of the implications of sagittal balance and weigh the benefits of sagittal plane restoration against the risk of perturbing this state of harmony for a perfectly aligned spine in the coronal plane.

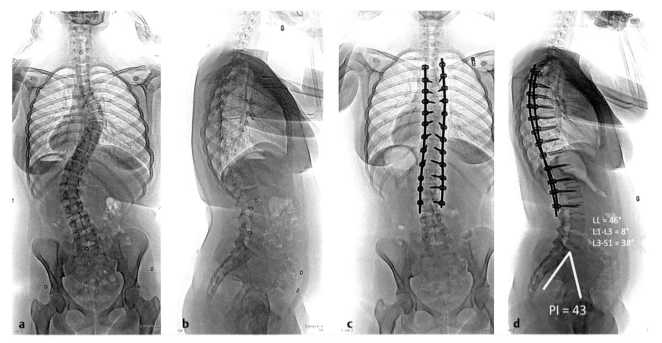

Fig. 19.6 (a,b) patient with a lower pelvic incidence (PI) and double major curve pattern. Surgical strategy was aimed at preventing posterior displacement of the instrumented segment to prevent junctional issues. **(c,d)** Total lumbar lordosis (LL) was 46° postop for a PI of 43°. Most of the lordosis was in the last three segments with 38° between L3 and S1. The instrumented segment accounted for only 8°, creating a smooth transition between the thoracic kyphosis and LL.

References

[1] Mac-Thiong J-M, Labelle H, Berthonnaud E, Betz RR, Roussouly P. Sagittal spinopelvic balance in normal children and adolescents. Eur Spine J. 2007; 16 (2):227–234

[2] Tanguay F, Mac-Thiong J-M, de Guise JA, Labelle H. Relation between the sagittal pelvic and lumbar spine geometries following surgical correction of adolescent idiopathic scoliosis. Eur Spine J. 2007; 16(4):531–536

[3] Mac-Thiong J-M, Labelle H, Roussouly P. Pediatric sagittal alignment. Eur Spine J. 2011; 20 Suppl 5:586–590

[4] Roussouly P, Labelle H, Rouissi J, Bodin A. Pre- and post-operative sagittal balance in idiopathic scoliosis: a comparison over the ages of two cohorts of 132 adolescents and 52 adults. Eur Spine J. 2013; 22 Suppl 2:S203–S215

[5] Marty C, Boisaubert B, Descamps H, et al. The sagittal anatomy of the sacrum among young adults, infants, and spondylolisthesis patients. Eur Spine J. 2002; 11(2):119–125

[6] Legaye J, Duval-Beaupère G, Hecquet J, Marty C. Pelvic incidence: a fundamental pelvic parameter for three-dimensional regulation of spinal sagittal curves. Eur Spine J. 1998; 7(2):99–103

[7] Mac-Thiong J-M, Labelle H, Charlebois M, Huot M-P, de Guise JA. Sagittal plane analysis of the spine and pelvis in adolescent idiopathic scoliosis according to the coronal curve type. Spine. 2003; 28(13):1404–1409

[8] Vedantam R, Lenke LG, Keeney JA, Bridwell KH. Comparison of standing sagittal spinal alignment in asymptomatic adolescents and adults. Spine. 1998; 23 (2):211–215

[9] Cil A, Yazici M, Uzumcugil A, et al. The evolution of sagittal segmental alignment of the spine during childhood. Spine. 2005; 30(1):93–100

[10] Roussouly P, Gollogly S, Noseda O, Berthonnaud E, Dimnet J. The vertical projection of the sum of the ground reactive forces of a standing patient is not the same as the C7 plumb line: a radiographic study of the sagittal alignment of 153 asymptomatic volunteers. Spine. 2006; 31(11):E320–E325

[11] Mac-Thiong J-M, Roussouly P, Berthonnaud E, Guigui P. Sagittal parameters of global spinal balance: normative values from a prospective cohort of seven hundred nine Caucasian asymptomatic adults. Spine. 2010; 35(22):E1193–E1198

[12] Richards BS, Sucato DJ, Johnston CE, et al. Right thoracic curves in presumed adolescent idiopathic scoliosis: which clinical and radiographic findings correlate with a preoperative abnormal magnetic resonance image? Spine. 2010; 35(20):1855–1860

[13] Newton PO, Fujimori T, Doan J, Reighard FG, Bastrom TP, Misaghi A. Defining the "three-dimensional sagittal plane" in thoracic adolescent idiopathic scoliosis. J Bone Joint Surg Am. 2015; 97(20):1694–1701

[14] Ilharreborde B. Sagittal balance and idiopathic scoliosis: does final sagittal alignment influence outcomes, degeneration rate or failure rate? Eur Spine J. 2018; 27 Suppl 1:48–58

[15] Vidal C, Mazda K, Ilharreborde B. Sagittal spino-pelvic adjustment in severe Lenke 1 hypokyphotic adolescent idiopathic scoliosis patients. Eur Spine J. 2016; 25(10):3162–3169

[16] Martino J, Aubin C-E, Labelle H, Wang X, Parent S. Biomechanical analysis of vertebral derotation techniques for the surgical correction of thoracic scoliosis. A numerical study through case simulations and a sensitivity analysis. Spine. 2013; 38(2):E73–E83

[17] Ponte A, Orlando G, Siccardi GL. The true Ponte osteotomy: by the one who developed it. Spine Deform. 2018; 6(1):2–11

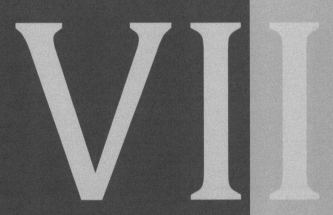

Part VII

Adult Scoliosis (AS)

VII

20 From Pathological to Normal Shapes in Adult Scoliosis

Pierre Roussouly and Amer Sebaaly

Abstract

Treatment of adult spinal deformity remains a surgical dilemma for most of spinal surgeons and even spinal deformity surgeons. The most important aspect of spinal surgery is to restore the spinal balance. Once a surgeon has accepted the importance of restoring good sagittal balance, he must answer several questions before embarking on the surgical journey. What is the compensatory mechanism used in this patient for restoring its sagittal balance? What was his or her normal profile before having the degenerative changes? What is the best surgical strategy to achieve complication-free outcomes? What techniques does the surgeon have in his armamentarium to achieve his surgical goals? What are the expected outcomes of this surgery? This chapter will review a proposed algorithm for the treatment of adult spinal deformity with a rapid review of the possible techniques.

Keywords: Adult spinal deformity, spinal osteotomy, Roussouly classification

20.1 Introduction

Recognizing sagittal imbalance in adult spinal deformity is of primary importance as restoring the patient's horizontal gaze is important not only for less energy expenditure but also for normal social interaction.[1] To achieve optimum outcomes when treating these pathologies, a good understanding of the principles of sagittal balance is needed as well as a good understanding of the compensatory mechanism employed by the patient to maintain a horizontal gaze.[2] One cannot stress enough the importance of these mechanisms as failure to identify them could lead to mediocre surgical results. In fact, Kumar et al[3] found, in 2001, that even short posterior fusion has a great risk of adjacent segment disease (more than 50%) if the fusion is done in an unbalanced state, while the risk of this complication is lowered by more than 20-fold if the fusion is done in a perfectly balanced state.

Once a surgeon has accepted the importance of restoring good sagittal balance, they must answer several questions before embarking on the surgical journey. What is the compensatory mechanism used in this patient for restoring its sagittal balance? What was his or her normal profile before having the degenerative changes? What is the best surgical strategy to achieve an outcome with minimal complications? What techniques does the surgeon have in his armamentarium to achieve his surgical goals? What are the expected outcomes of this surgery?

Based on angles reciprocity, American authors demonstrated that a good correlation between the pelvic incidence (PI) and the lumbar lordosis (LL) T12-S1 may be a basic requirement to obtain a good clinical result by using control with health-related quality of life (HRQoL).[4,5] For a period of time, this theory was becoming a "credo," with alternating good and bad results, mainly proximal junctional kyphosis (PJK). Even if many

attempts at an explanation have been made, it seems that the intrinsic spinal shape was not well understood until now. Based on the normal sagittal shapes and their possible pathological evolution, we would like to propose treatment options for restoring the pelvic shape evaluated by PI.

20.2 From Normal to Pathological: Classification of Pathological Shapes of the Aging Spine

As presented in Chapter 6 in this book, Roussouly et al evaluated the spinal shapes in an asymptomatic population.[6] The authors defined four types of normal spinal shapes and they recently updated their classification to include a fifth type[7] (▶ Fig. 20.1). Recognizing normal sagittal profiles is important as it may help the surgeon to identify its degenerative evolution. Thus, every pathological sagittal shape could and should have come from one of the five described shapes depending on the PI.

The first phenomenon of local degeneration is the disk height loss with subsequent imbalance as a result of local kyphosis. As the compensation end point is having an upward gait and horizontal tilt of the head for a normal sight, several mechanisms for spinal compensation are observed as shown by the study of Berthonnaud et al.[8] If the spine is flexible, there is an increased extension of the flexible spine above and/or below this local kyphosis with contraction of the posterior spinal muscles, which lifts the trunk vertically, requiring painful abnormal effort from the spinal muscles to prevent falling forward with increased pressure on the posterior facets (▶ Fig. 20.2). If the spine is rigid, with progressive kyphosis, the gravity line moves forward and the pelvis rotates backward (retroversion), inducing a decrease in the sacral slope (SS) and increase of pelvic tilt (PT).[2] Hyperextension of the hips follows, which is limited by the extension reserve (generally 10°) and, finally, a flexion of the knees in severe cases, controlled by the quadriceps.[2]

It is fundamental to recognize both mechanisms. They have different clinical expressions and may be divided into local compensation and global unbalance. The first one (extension above and below the flexion accident) induces local compensations in the shape of the spine to restore a new alignment allowing slight global adaptations. It could be, for instance, an L3-L4 hyperextension above an insufficient lordotic L4-S1 arthrodesis, or a flattening of thoracic spine above a hypo-lordotic lumbar fusion. However, these local compensations are painful, both by local hyperextensive stress on the posterior facets, creating sometimes, at its maximum, a retrolisthesis, and by muscle contracture to maintain an abnormal local positioning as thoracic hypokyphosis. These patients are difficult to diagnose because they may have pain and discomfort without global unbalance, but, nonetheless, they have balance troubles.

The second mechanism is the well-known classical unbalance: loss of lordosis and/or hyperkyphosis, where

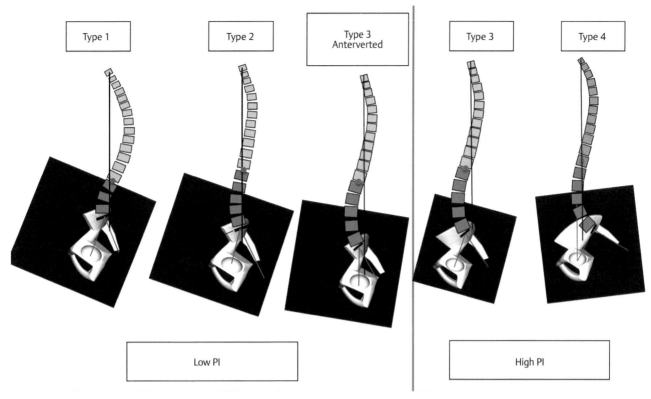

Fig. 20.1 The modified Roussouly classification.[7] Normal human spines could be divided into five different shapes according to sacral slope (SS) and pelvic incidence (PI). Types 1 and 2 have small SS and PI with the former having a small SL and a long thoracic kyphosis (TK), whereas the latter have a straight spine. Anteverted type 3 have small PI but high SS and low pelvic tilt (PT). Type 3 has high PI and medium range SS, whereas type 4 has very high PI and SS.

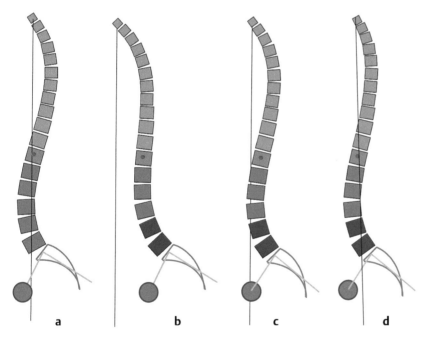

Fig. 20.2 Drawing showing the mechanisms of compensation of the spine and the pelvis following a kyphosing event. Normal alignment **(a)**. Degenerative changes occur in the lower lumbar levels (navy blue inducing anterior displacement of the plumb line **(b)**. Two compensations occur: retroversion of the pelvis (increasing pelvic tilt [PT] and decreasing sacral slope [SS]) **(c)**, and a decrease of the kyphosis in the mobile segments (decrease in thoracic kyphosis) **(d)**.

compensation mechanisms are unable to balance the system, overpassed or, because of rigidity, retroverted pelvis, and forward displacement of the C7 plumb line (C7PL). This mechanism of pelvic retroversion is linked to PI value by the relation: PI = PT + SS. The higher the PI, the higher the ability of PT to increase. This mechanism has a double effect: horizontal positioning of SS and backward positioning of the whole spine regarding the femoral heads (FHs). This phenomenon is limited by the hip reserve of extension.[9] Maintaining this position is not economical and may induce muscle contractures (gluteus and hamstrings). Even if the balance seems controlled in a standing position, when walking, the expression of forward unbalance is stronger as a result of hip positioning in gait during a posterior step. When the spine is rigid, the forward unbalance provides discomfort but little pain.

Based on this, and on the Barrey ratio (BR), in a first attempt of classification, Le Huec proposed to divide sagittal spinal balance into three categories (▶ Fig. 20.3)[10]:

- Type A or normal spinal balance: characterized by global balance of the trunk measured BR < 100% (C7PL behind or just in front of the sacral plateau) and normal 10° < PT < 25°. Lower limbs are completely extended in the standing position.
- Type B or compensated balance: global balance of the trunk is still normal, BR is less than 100% (C7PL behind FH), but the pelvis is retroverted (PT > 25°). The lower limbs show extension of the hips (femur straight) and the knees are in full extension.
- Type C or decompensated balance: global balance of the trunk shows a positive C7PL, with a value that falls generally in front of the FHs (BR > 100%), and the pelvis shows a PT in retroversion. In the lower limbs, there is extension of the hips (pelvic retroversion) and flexion of the knees. Hip extension is overpassed.
- A fourth type could be added by describing the association of a lumbar hyperlordosis and an anteverted pelvis (PT > 5°). Hips are in normal position or in slight flexion and knees may be in recurvatum. There is frequently a compensation in thoracic hypokyphosis. This is a frequent finding in anteverted type 3 spines (▶ Fig. 20.4).

It is important to differentiate sagittal balance or compensated balance. It was found that posterior fusion in a compensated balanced position was associated with increased adjacent segment disease compared to fusion patients in a balanced position.[3]

Even though this classification is simplistic, one could not plan a surgical strategy based on this classification and no attempt was made to classify sagittal imbalance beyond this primitive reasoning. In fact, many attempts have been made to classify degenerative spine diseases, like the degenerative spondylolisthesis classification[11,12] or adult deformity (Schwab-Scoliosis Research Society [SRS] classification).[13] The Schwab-SRS classification defines four types of basic deformities: T for thoracic scoliosis, D for double scoliosis, L for lumbar scoliosis, and S for sagittal deformity without coronal deformity. Added to the basic deformity are three modifiers: PT, PI-LL, and sagittal vertical axis (SVA) (▶ Fig. 20.5). All the parameters used in these classifications are positional parameters without any attempt to analyze the shape of the spine and its pathological evolution. In addtion, HRQoL scores and mechanical complications (PJK, nonunion, etc.) were correlated to some local parameters (PI-LL) or overall parameters (T1 pelvic angle, global tilt) without taking into consideration the shape of the degenerative spine.

Recently, we have proposed a classification and degenerative evolution of the aging spine based on the initial Roussouly classification and the compensatory mechanisms to local kyphosis (▶ Fig. 20.6, ▶ Fig. 20.7, ▶ Fig. 20.8, ▶ Fig. 20.9). This study was done by analyzing a cohort of 331 nonoperated degenerative spines to identify possible degenerative evolution of normal

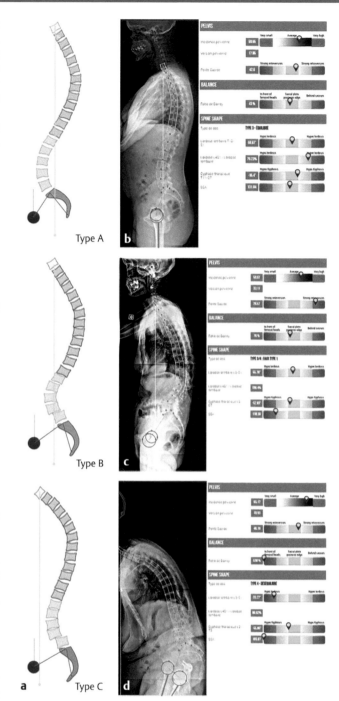

Fig. 20.3 Sagittal imbalance could be divided into three clinical scenarios **(a)**. Type A is a balanced spine with Barrey ratio (BR) < 100% and a pelvic tilt (PT) corresponding to pelvic incidence (PI) **(b)**. Type B is a compensated balanced spine where the compensation of the sagittal imbalance begets normal BR (< 100%) with the caveat of having higher than normal PT **(c)**. Type C is an unbalanced spine where all compensatory mechanisms are lost **(d)**. SSA, Spinosacral angle.

shapes.[14] To make this classification easier to understand, it is divided into 11 types clustered into four categories (▶ Table 20.1):

- Classical types: the described types 1 to 4 of the initial Roussouly classification (see Chapter 6).

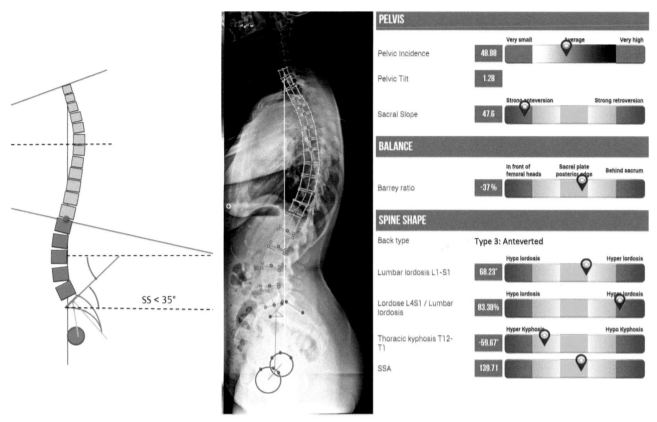

Fig. 20.4 Anteverted type 3 spines have the same characteristics of type 3 spines but with pelvic tilt (PT) < 5°. The pelvic incidence (PI) has a low value. SS, Sacral slope.

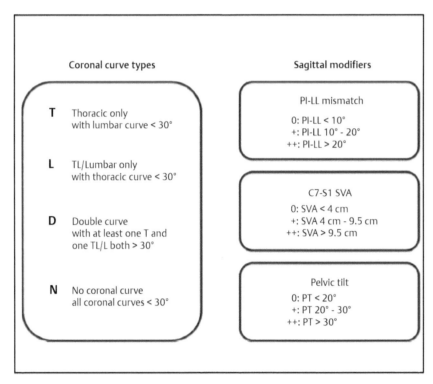

Fig. 20.5 The Scoliosis Research Society (SRS)-Schwab classification of adult deformity with four main classes and three modifiers (sagittal vertical axis [SVA], pelvic incidence [PI]-lumbar lordosis [LL], and pelvic tilt [PT]).

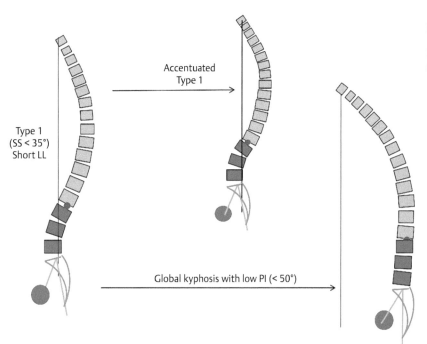

Fig. 20.6 Possible degenerative evolution of type 1 into accentuated type 1 and then global kyphosis with low pelvic incidence (PI). SS, Sacral slope; LL, lumbar lordosis.

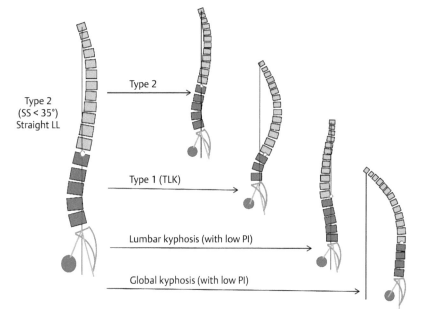

Fig. 20.7 Possible degenerative evolution of type 2 into type 1, type 2, or global or lumbar kyphosis (with low pelvic incidence [PI]). SS, Sacral slope; LL, lumbar lordosis; TLK, thoracolumbar kyphosis.

- Anteverted types 3 and 4: these types have, respectively, the same characteristics of the classical types 3 and 4 (medium and high SS) but with a low PT (PT ≤ 5°) (see Chapter 6).
- Retroverted (or false) types: these types arise from the four classical types with a pelvic retroversion. False types 2 and 3 have, respectively, the same characteristics of the classical types according to the SS and LL shape, but they have a high PT (PT ≥ 25). False type 2 with thoracic kyphosis (TK) has a low SS, straight LL, high PI, and high TK.

- Kyphotic types: when all compensatory mechanisms are consumed, kyphosis occurs. It can be divided into two subtypes according to the possibility of compensation in the thoracic spine:
  ○ Lumbar kyphosis shape: characterized by lumbar kyphosis with a hypokyphotic thoracic compensation curve (BR < 100%).
  ○ Global kyphosis shape: characterized by lumbar kyphosis without a hypokyphotic thoracic compensation curve (and thus an unbalanced spine, BR ≥ 100%).

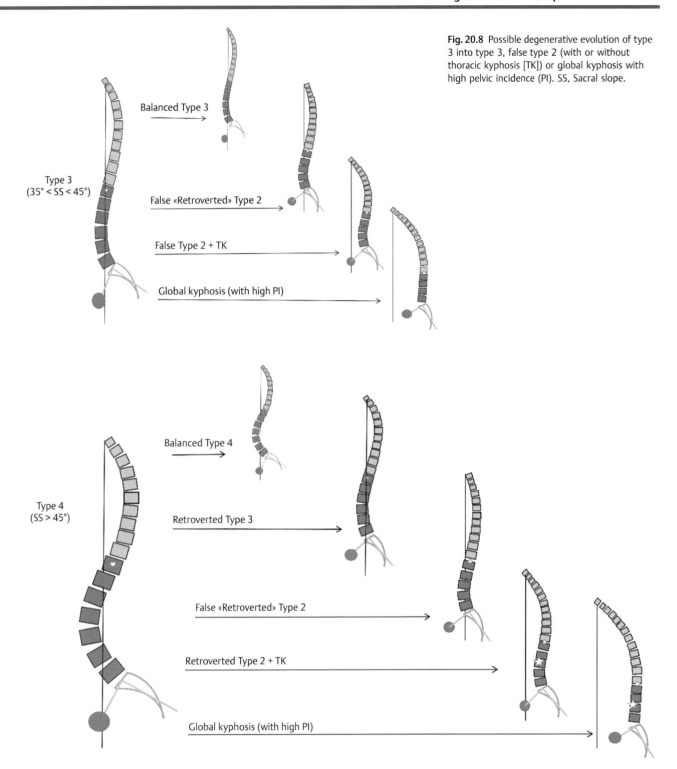

Fig. 20.8 Possible degenerative evolution of type 3 into type 3, false type 2 (with or without thoracic kyphosis [TK]) or global kyphosis with high pelvic incidence (PI). SS, Sacral slope.

Fig. 20.9 Possible degenerative evolution of type 4. SS, Sacral slope; TK, thoracic kyphosis; PI, pelvic incidence.

Table 20.1 Different types of degenerative types according to the classification of Roussouly of degenerative spinal diseases and their incidence in our cohort

	Spinal shape type	Incidence
Classical subtypes	Type 1	15.4%
	Type 2	13.9%
	Type 3	19.0%
	Type 4	23.6%
Anteverted	Type 3 Ant	1.2%
	Type 4 Ant	0.3%
Retroverted	Retrov T1	0%
	Retrov T2	13.9%
	Retrov T2 + TK	1.8%
	Retrov T3	5.1%
	Retrov T4	0%
Kyphosis	Global kyphosis	2.7%
	Lumbar kyphosis	3.3%

To simply understand this classification of spinal degenerative evolution, one must bear in mind the appropriate compensatory mechanism for local kyphosis: hyperlordosis of the adjacent mobile spine and/or retroversion of the pelvis. Considering these facts, this description of the sagittal alignment of the degenerative human spine is created by adding kyphosis to the four classical types, depending on PI.

20.2.1 For Low Pelvic Incidence (< 50°), No Retroversion, or Slightly Retroverted Pelvis

- When type 1 spine degenerates, compensation is done below in the lumbar spine by increasing the lordosis on a short segment (accentuating the type 1). On the other hand, when compensation mechanisms are inefficient, LL disappears, giving rise to a "global kyphosis" type with a very small PI (▶ Fig. 20.6).
- Type 2 spines also have little range of compensation (▶ Fig. 20.7). Depending on the level where kyphosis occurs:
  ○ At the thoracic level without altering the type 2 lordosis (type 2 + TK).
  ○ At the thoracolumbar level, generating a type 1 spine (thoracolumbar kyphosis).
  ○ At the lumbar level, generating "lumbar kyphosis" type (if the thoracic spine could compensate with a hypokyphosis).
  ○ "Global kyphosis type" (with a low PI), or lumbar spine lordosis disappears.

20.2.2 For High Pelvic Incidence (50°), Retroverted Pelvis

In types 3 and 4 spines, the initial shape may remain the same. Degenerative changes occur on posterior facets with facet arthritis as a result of the posterior hyperpressure

(see Chapter 9). This may be the initial step for a degenerative spondylolisthesis when the facet stability fails. When a degenerative loss of lordosis occurs, pelvic retroversion is the rule with decreasing SS (▶ Fig. 20.8, ▶ Fig. 20.9). A type 4 may change in type 3 with increasing retroversion, generating a false type 3, then a type 3 may change in type 2. As it is a type 2 with a retroverted pelvis (as it is called):

- It is a false type 2 if there is a compensation in the thoracic area by flattening the kyphosis.
- It is a false type 2 + TK if the TK is not altered.

The last step is the total loss of lordosis with a global kyphosis and widely retroverted pelvis generally with knee flexion.

One should bear in mind the absence of retroverted or false type 1 as type 1 has a very low PI and a very low maneuver margin to compensate for pelvis retroversion. One more type that was not found was the retroverted type 4 as it shares the same characteristics with type 3 spines.

This description of a degenerative spine could help the surgeon identify the initial spinal type and help identify the best surgical strategy to optimize surgical results. PI remains the only signature of the initial type and its recognition is required for surgical treatment. Low PI originates from types 1 or 2, whereas high PI originates from types 3 or 4.

20.3 Techniques for Reduction of Fixed Sagittal Imbalance

Rigid spinal deformities require great surgical ability but most importantly thorough preoperative preparation. One could never stress enough the importance of surgical planning for treating adult spinal deformity whether it involves posterior approaches, anterior approaches, or both. In fact, a recent study has shown that 23% of deformity corrective surgery does not reach the desired goals even if performed by experts.[4]

The oldest and most primitive technique in surgical planning of adult deformities is using tracing paper. It involves replicating the deformity on tracing paper and simulating various scenarios for osteotomies. With the advent of technology, computer software became routine for measurement of spinal parameters as well as for surgical planning. Two software packages have been excessively used in adult spinal deformity: KEOPS spine and Surgimap. While the latter offers the opportunity to measure the sagittal balance parameters and to plan surgical strategy (osteotomy, cages, etc.), the former adds the ability to store the data online as well as to serve as a surgeon's database, including physical exam and HRQoL scores. KEOPS has been found to be a reliable tool for measurement of coronal and sagittal parameters in adult deformity with nearly excellent inter- and intraobserver reliability.[15] On the other hand, Surgimap was found to have a slightly lower reliability for measuring sagittal parameters,[5] but offers the possibility of exact prediction of the postoperative alignment after major corrective surgery of adult deformity.[16] Regardless of the method used for planning the surgery, it should always abide by the rules stated in the next section.

When planning corrective surgery for adult spinal deformity, surgeons can look into their armamentarium of surgical techniques. They can be divided into posterior corrective techniques (posterior osteotomies) or anterior release first techniques.

20.3.1 Posterior First Techniques

Posterior surgeries for treating spinal pathology are the most frequently used approach and the best known to spinal surgeons.[17] Posterior spinal osteotomies have been popularized since the first description of spinal osteotomies by Smith-Petersen in 1945.[18] The main strategy and the extent of fixation is detailed in the next section. Posterior correction parametrium could be divided into three main categories: the posterior column osteotomies, the three-column osteotomies, and the posterior vertebral column resection. Diebo et al[19] then subdivided the osteotomies into two types each having a total of six types of posterior osteotomies. One should bear in mind that a three-column osteotomy is a posterior column osteotomy with some added, more complex steps with increasing complexity.

20.3.2 Anterior First Techniques

Since the publication of the International Spine Study Group (ISSG) report on adult deformity complications (with more than 100% complication rate!),[20] the attention has shifted toward an anterior first correction of the deformity. The first techniques used to reduce deformities by an anterior approach with instrumentation were the Dwyer, and then the ventral derotation spondylodese (VDS). Besides the aggressive thoracolumbar approach, insufficient sagittal correction was the main feature of those techniques. The use of a more rigid rod improved this problem, but the former remains an obstacle for routinely using these procedures. More recently, the use of dedicated interbody cages placed by the minimally invasive spine surgery (MISS) technique (extreme lateral interbody fusion [XLIF], and more recently oblique lumbar interbody fusion [OLIF]) has improved the approach morbidity, with a high possibility of frontal and coronal reduction. In addtion, the access to the L5-S1 disk has become more popular using an oblique approach.[21] This prompted the idea of restoring the disk height inducing simultaneous deformity correction and indirect neurological decompression.

Recent studies have shown the same corrective power of a single-level pedicle subtraction osteotomy (PSO) and anterior corrective surgery in the setting of adult spinal deformity.[22] The minimally invasive surgery (MIS) ISSG group has recently showed that using these approaches reduces construct length, reoperation rates, blood loss, and length of stay without affecting clinical and radiographic outcomes when compared to open procedures. The main limitation of anterior first approaches is its inability to perform high correction rates and to address the posterior facet osteoarthritis. For that reason, the MIS ISSG committee recommended the use of these minimally invasive techniques for the correction of small (SVA < 6 cm), flexible, and compensated balanced deformities (▶ Fig. 20.10).[23]

20.4 From Pathology to Normal Shapes: Strategy for Reduction of Fixed Sagittal Balance

Based on the SRS classification, the aim of sagittal correction is based on LL versus PI correlation as if there was a linear relation between LL and PI, with the idea that LL increases with PI. Even if, roughly, this relation is acceptable, it does not include TK and the reciprocity between LL and TK as, for example, in Roussouly's type 1 where LL is higher than the expected value correlated with a low PI. On the other hand, we have seen in a

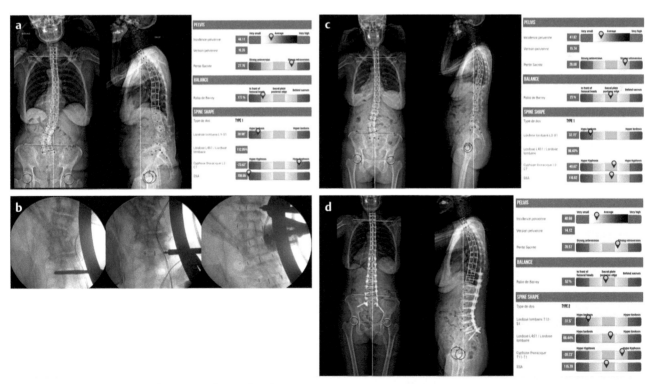

Fig. 20.10 Case 1. See Section 20.5.1. SSA, Spinosacral angle.

previous chapter that, for the same value of LL, the repartition of extension between the upper and lower arc of lordosis is of great importance in the TK organization.

Before proposing our algorithm for surgical management of adult deformity based on the above proposed classification, some basic rules for management should be laid down. First, there is a tendency to use different surgical goals between genders. In fact, males tolerate better undercorrection than females, probably because of a better posterior musculature. Second, when the spine is not rigid, Smith-Petersen osteotomy (SPO) or polysegmental osteotomy (PO) are preferred over PSO since they yield the same results with fewer complications.[24]

The most important aspect of surgical strategy (▶ Fig. 20.11, ▶ Fig. 20.12) in the correction of adult deformity is to avoid undercorrection as well as overcorrection, which could lead to several early complications (see below). According to PI, the aim of the sagittal reduction is to maintain the present shape, to restore a shape that respects the pelvis shape (PI).

20.4.1 When Pelvic Incidence Is Small (< 50°) (▶ Fig. 20.11)

- Type 1 shapes[25]:
  - To maintain type 1 shape in the reduction is a good option mainly in the absence of scoliosis.
  - To turn it into a type 2 by reducing the thoracolumbar kyphosis may be a good option in the case of associated thoracolumbar scoliosis.
  - It is imperative to avoid a too long lordosis inducing an anteverted type 3, which is always a bad option.[26]
- Type 2 shapes:
  - Maintain the same type 2. It is generally not necessary to address the thoracic spine. There is low risk of PJK if low lordosis values are maintained with appropriate space available for lung.

- Type 2 with TK:
  - To maintain the type 2 shape, it is necessary to reduce the TK. That could be very hazardous in the older patient population. We recommend turning the patient's spine into a type 1 spine with a longer Scheuermann's kyphosis and a short distal lumbosacral lordosis. It is always preferable to integrate the thoracic spine in the construction.
  - In any case, too much lordosis would result in an anteverted type 3, which cannot be a good option.[26]
- Lumbar kyphosis:
  - Restoration of lordosis by a posterior approach needs generally a small L4 PSO because of the rigidity of the lumbar spine.
  - Reduction of lordosis by anterior first interbody cages (OLIF) could be a good option for opening the disk spaces and restoring the lordosis.[27]

20.4.2 When Pelvic Incidence Is High (50°)

- Degenerative changes with persistent type 3 or 4 spines:
  - The main objective of spinal correction is to maintain the same spinal shape.
  - If the spine is well balanced with an adapted SK, it is not necessary to address the whole spine.
- Decreasing lordosis without thoracic compensation (false type 2 with TK), and retroverted pelvis (PT > 25°):
  - It is necessary to increase the lordosis, with either a global release (posterior column osteotomies) if the spine is still flexible or an L4 PSO when the spine is rigid.
  - As there is no compensation at the thoracic level, it is possible not to extend the fusion to the upper thoracic area.
- Decreasing lordosis with a double compensation, thoracic hypokyphosis, and retroverted pelvis (false type 2):

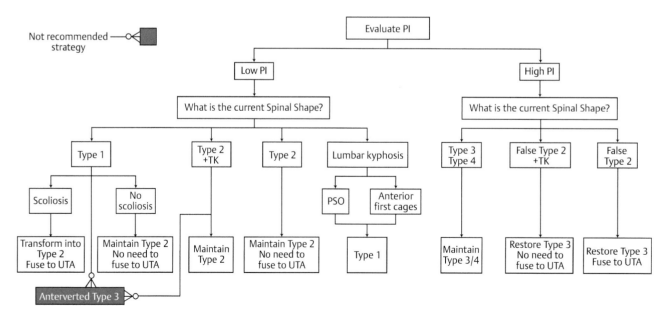

Fig. 20.11 Algorithm for treating fixed spinal deformity. PI, Pelvic incidence; PSO, pedicle subtraction osteotomy; TK, thoracic kyphosis; UTA: upper thoracic area.

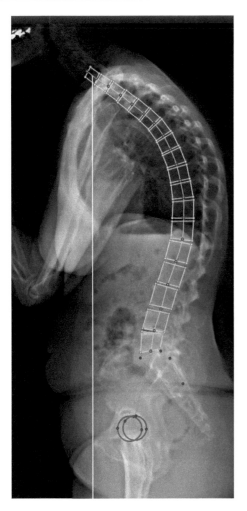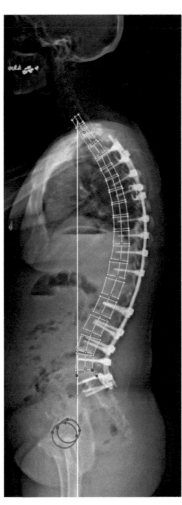

Fig. 20.12 Case 2. See Section 20.5.2.

○ When the lordosis is restored, the thoracic spine always flexes forward as the thoracic spine will always find its original shape.
  – If the fusion stops at T10, there is an increased risk of junctional failure. It may be necessary to extend the fusion to T2 or T3 depending on SK.
  – If the fusion extends to the proximal thoracic area, it is difficult to predict the precise need of kyphosis restoration. If this SK restoration is insufficient, there is an increased risk of cervicothoracic PJK with a risk of proximal instrumentation loosening.
○ When restoring the lordosis, it is necessary to respect the shape of lordosis. The bigger angle of lordosis must be given distally between L4 and S1. If the lordosis is extended too proximally, up to T12-L1, it reduces the place for TK and increases the risk of upper PJK. Too long and too strong lordosis is not a good option (see Section 8).

20.5 Case Examples

20.5.1 Case 1

A 48-year-old female presented with increasing low lumbar pain and with an increasing sensation of bending forward. She had an Oswestry disability index of 48. Full spine X-rays (▶ Fig. 20.10) show a low PI with a type 1 spine and a relatively straight thoracic spine as well as a lumbar scoliosis of 36° (▶ Fig. 20.10a). It is possible that this patient will maintain the type 1 or transform into a type 2 with scoliosis reduction according to the proposed treatment algorithm (▶ Fig. 20.11). She was operated on with anterior reduction of her kyphoscoliosis using the OLIF approach from L1 to S1 (▶ Fig. 20.10b). After this first procedure, there was a partial reduction of the scoliosis (to 24°) and of the sagittal balance (▶ Fig. 20.10c). One week later, she was operated on with posterior instrumentation and reduction. Postoperative full spine X-rays showed a well-balanced type 2 and reduction of the lumbar scoliosis to 13° (▶ Fig. 20.10d).

20.5.2 Case 2

A 62-year-old woman presented with increasing low back pain. Full spine X-rays showed a type 2 spine with TK. According to the treatment algorithm, maintaining type 2 or transformation to a type 1 are both options with an instrumentation of the thoracic spine with partial reduction of the scoliosis (▶ Fig. 20.12).

20.5.3 Case 3

Full spine X-rays showing a flat back with upper TK (▶ Fig. 20.13). There is an increased PT and a PI of 57°. This

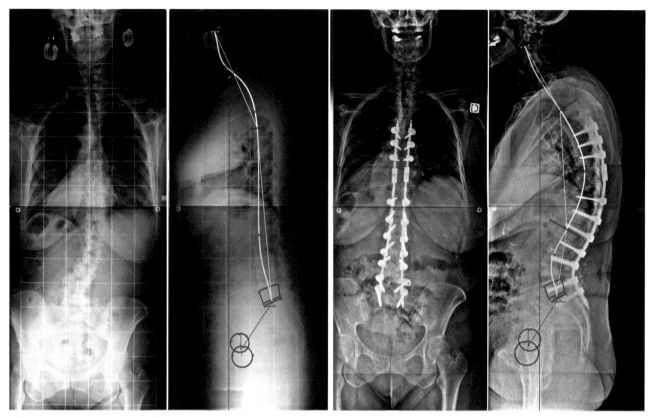

Fig. 20.13 Case 3. See Section 20.5.3.

renders the patient in a false type 2 with TK. The only option is to restore a type 3. This was done with a PSO at the L4 level and fusion to the upper thoracic spine.

20.6 Conclusion

Because of age and mechanical stresses, degeneration induces local and global changes on the spine affecting intervertebral disks and posterior facets. Recognition of initial normal shapes and the stress they may induce on each intervertebral segment allows a prediction of degeneration localization and its effect on shape changing. Linked to its almost constant value in adult life, PI is a true signature of the sagittal status of each person and allows a characterization of the most probable "ideal balanced shape." If angle correlation is of great importance in treatment evaluation, the curves shape identification, associated length, and curve repartition is needed to avoid misalignments and bad curve evolution with PJK.

References

[1] Roussouly P, Nnadi C. Sagittal plane deformity: an overview of interpretation and management. Eur Spine J. 2010; 19(11):1824–1836

[2] Barrey C, Roussouly P, Perrin G, Le Huec JC. Sagittal balance disorders in severe degenerative spine. Can we identify the compensatory mechanisms? Eur Spine J. 2011; 20 Suppl 5:626–633

[3] Kumar MN, Baklanov A, Chopin D. Correlation between sagittal plane changes and adjacent segment degeneration following lumbar spine fusion. Eur Spine J. 2001; 10(4):314–319

[4] Schwab FJ, Patel A, Shaffrey CI, et al. Sagittal realignment failures following pedicle subtraction osteotomy surgery: are we doing enough? Clinical article. J Neurosurg Spine. 2012; 16(6):539–546

[5] Lafage R, Ferrero E, Henry JK, et al. Validation of a new computer-assisted tool to measure spino-pelvic parameters. Spine J. 2015; 15(12):2493–2502

[6] Roussouly P, Gollogly S, Berthonnaud E, Dimnet J. Classification of the normal variation in the sagittal alignment of the human lumbar spine and pelvis in the standing position. Spine. 2005; 30(3):346–353

[7] Laouissat F, Sebaaly A, Gehrchen M, Roussouly P. Classification of normal sagittal spine alignment: refounding the Roussouly classification. Eur Spine J. 2018; 27(8):2002–2011

[8] Berthonnaud E, Dimnet J, Roussouly P, Labelle H. Analysis of the sagittal balance of the spine and pelvis using shape and orientation parameters. J Spinal Disord Tech. 2005; 18(1):40–47

[9] Hovorka I, Rousseau P, Bronsard N, et al. Extension reserve of the hip in relation to the spine: comparative study of two radiographic methods. Rev Chir Orthop Repar Appar Mot. 2008; 94(8):771–776

[10] Le Huec JC, Charosky S, Barrey C, Rigal J, Aunoble S. Sagittal imbalance cascade for simple degenerative spine and consequences: algorithm of decision for appropriate treatment. Eur Spine J. 2011; 20 Suppl 5:699–703

[11] Kepler CK, Hilibrand AS, Sayadipour A, et al. Clinical and radiographic degenerative spondylolisthesis (CARDS) classification. Spine J. 2015; 15(8):1804–1811

[12] Gille O, Challier V, Parent H, et al. Degenerative lumbar spondylolisthesis: cohort of 670 patients, and proposal of a new classification. Orthop Traumatol Surg Res. 2014; 100(6) Suppl:S311–S315

[13] Schwab F, Ungar B, Blondel B, et al. Scoliosis Research Society-Schwab adult spinal deformity classification: a validation study. Spine. 2012; 37(12):1077–1082

[14] Sebaaly A, Grobost P, Mallam L, Roussouly P. Description of the sagittal alignment of the degenerative human spine. Eur Spine J. 2018; 27(2):489–496

[15] Maillot C, Ferrero E, Fort D, Heyberger C, Le Huec JC. Reproducibility and repeatability of a new computerized software for sagittal spinopelvic and scoliosis curvature radiologic measurements: Keops. Eur Spine J. 2015; 24(7):1574–1581

[16] Langella F, Villafañe JH, Damilano M, et al. Predictive accuracy of Surgimap surgical planning for sagittal imbalance: a cohort study. Spine. 2017; 42(22): E1297–E1304

[17] Polly DW, Jr, Chou D, Sembrano JN, Ledonio CG, Tomita K. An analysis of decision making and treatment in thoracolumbar metastases. Spine. 2009; 34 (22) Suppl:S118–S127

[18] Smith-Petersen MN, Larson CB, Aufranc OE. Osteotomy of the spine for correction of flexion deformity in rheumatoid arthritis. Clin Orthop Relat Res. 1969; 66(66):6–9

[19] Diebo B, Liu S, Lafage V, Schwab F. Osteotomies in the treatment of spinal deformities: indications, classification, and surgical planning. Eur J Orthop Surg Traumatol. 2014; 24 Suppl 1:S11–S20

[20] Smith JS, Klineberg E, Lafage V, et al. Prospective multicenter assessment of perioperative and minimum 2-year postoperative complication rates associated with adult spinal deformity surgery. J Neurosurg Spine. 2016; 25(1): 1–14

[21] Zairi F, Sunna TP, Westwick HJ, et al. Mini-open oblique lumbar interbody fusion (OLIF) approach for multi-level discectomy and fusion involving L5-S1: preliminary experience. Orthop Traumatol Surg Res. 2017; 103(2):295–299

[22] Mundis GM, Jr, Turner JD, Kabirian N, et al. Anterior column realignment has similar results to pedicle subtraction osteotomy in treating adults with sagittal plane deformity. World Neurosurg. 2017; 105:249–256

[23] Mummaneni PV, Shaffrey CI, Lenke LG, et al. The minimally invasive spinal deformity surgery algorithm: a reproducible rational framework for decision making in minimally invasive spinal deformity surgery. Neurosurg Focus. 2014; 36(5):E6

[24] Cho K-J, Bridwell KH, Lenke LG, Berra A, Baldus C. Comparison of Smith-Petersen versus pedicle subtraction osteotomy for the correction of fixed sagittal imbalance. Spine. 2005; 30(18):2030–2037, discussion 2038

[25] Scemama C, Laouissat F, Abelin-Genevois K, Roussouly P. Surgical treatment of thoraco-lumbar kyphosis (TLK) associated with low pelvic incidence. Eur Spine J. 2017; 26(8):2146–2152

[26] Ferrero E, Vira S, Ames CP, et al. Analysis of an unexplored group of sagittal deformity patients: low pelvic tilt despite positive sagittal malalignment. Eur Spine J. 2016; 25(11):3568–3576

[27] Ohtori S, Mannoji C, Orita S, et al. Mini-open anterior retroperitoneal lumbar interbody fusion: oblique lateral interbody fusion for degenerated lumbar spinal kyphoscoliosis. Asian Spine J. 2015; 9(4):565–572

21 Sagittal Balance Treatment Strategy in a Posterior Approach

Fethi Laouissat and Pierre Roussouly

Abstract

The purpose of this chapter is to show how to manage a spinal surgery for degenerative or deformity issues by a posterior approach to restore an adequate sagittal alignment and balance of the spine.

Keywords: deformity reduction, monoaxial screws, monoplanar screws, reduction strategy, rod contouring, Roussouly classification, sagittal balance, spinal alignment

21.1 Introduction and Controversies

Sagittal balance has become an increasingly important matter for spine surgeons when dealing with spinal degenerative or deformity conditions. All spine surgeons agree on the fact that painstaking preoperative planning must be established before entering the operating theater because "failing to plan is planning to fail."

However, despite the fact that tactical and technical basic skills are well known throughout the spine surgeon community, strategy and philosophy of sagittal spinal alignment are still controversial. Questions surrounding some crucial points regarding the relationship between spine curvature and pelvis are still discussed.

It is well recognized that pelvic incidence (PI) is a constant parameter that determines the shape of the pelvis. Pelvic rotation around the hip axis permits adaptation of the sacral plateau by retroversion or anteversion. This adaptation is framed by a geometrical relation: PI = SS + PT (SS, sacral slope; PT, pelvic tilt)[1] (▶ Fig. 21.1).

To guide surgical planning, a widespread parameter relating PI and lumbar lordosis (LL) (measured between L1 and S1) has been proposed to enable a patient-specific approach to treatment goals by quantifying the mismatch between pelvic morphology and lumbar curve.[2] The threshold identified as a spinopelvic sagittal alignment goal was PI-LL < 10°. However, the PI-LL mismatch appears to be a "one size fits all" theory, as well as the Schwab-SRS classification cut-offs.[3]

On the other hand, Roussouly et al[4] investigated sagittal spinal shapes in asymptomatic populations and defined four sagittal types of lumbar curvatures. The Roussouly classification was refined by Laouissat et al[5] by integrating a fifth type of sagittal shape, which held the anteverted pelvis concept. The difference between the two concepts is fundamental. The "PI-LL mismatch" approach appears to be mathematical; it gives only an "ideal" global angle of lordosis without an instruction about curvature repartition. The L1-S1 definition of LL is another paradigm that treats all kinds of lordotic shapes in the same manner: "one size fits all."

Introduction of lordosis shape variation according to PI by Roussouly et al[4] emphasizes not only angle relationships but also lordosis curve organization and distribution of LL and thoracic kyphosis. Based on this concept, sagittal balance treatment tends to restore better balance parameters such as PT and C7PL and, therefore, aims to restore the shape most approaching normal shape according to PI. In pathology, the fundamental reference is the pelvic shape regarding the PI value (high- or low-grade PI), which is, as a constant shape parameter, the only signature of the previous spinal shape (before degenerative changes).

We may roughly divide pelvic shapes into two classes: low PI (< 50°) and high PI (> 50°). For low PI, it is necessary to restore type 1 or 2 shapes, and for high PI, type 3 or 4 shapes (▶ Fig. 21.2).

This said, the authors of this chapter aim to give to the reader some technical notes and points of view based on their experience in a comprehensive manner to help spine surgeons set up their preop planning.

21.2 Reduction Technique by Posterior Approach

21.2.1 Evaluation of the Length of Fusion

Short Fusion (One or Two Levels)

This option is efficient mainly when unbalance may be linked to painful compensation as a result of a local spinal disease (instability, stenosis). However, for a fixed or structural deformity, short fusion is insufficient for balance restoration.

PI = PT + SS

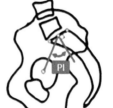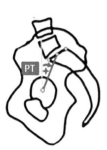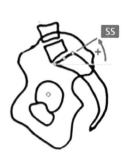

Fig. 21.1 Sacropelvic parameters: pelvic incidence (PI), pelvic tilt (PT), and sacral slope (SS).

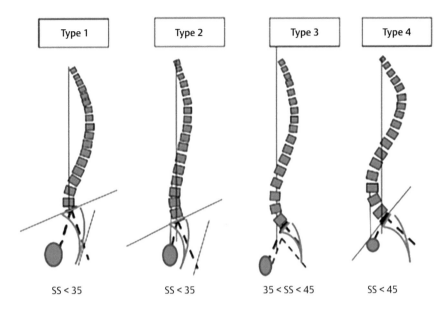

Fig. 21.2 Subdivision of the sagittal spinal curvatures according to the Roussouly classification. SS, Sacral slope.

Long Fusion (More than Three Levels)

Proximal instrumented level: this is probably the most controversial issue and the most difficult decision. There are three major levels: L2, T10, and T2–T4. The most problematic is the longer fusion to the upper thoracic spine. It is generally imposed by a severe thoracic kyphosis that needs to be controlled by the extended fusion.

Distal instrumented level "fuse or not to the sacrum?": There is a lot of controversy surrounding fusion to L5 or to the sacrum/pelvis. Fusion to the sacrum is technically demanding. It needs a multifocal fixation for long constructs with several screws in various anatomic positions: sacral plate, sacral alar, iliac, sacroiliac.[6,7,8,9,10,11] These extensions of instrumentation are at a high risk of pseudarthrosis.[12] To enhance fusion, circumferential or "360°" fusions and instrumentations have proved to yield good to excellent results both clinically and biomechanically.[13,14] An associated L5–S1 cage with anterior fusion is needed if disk height exceeds 6 mm. Fusion to L5 is technically easier but less efficient on balance restoration. In the case of suboptimal alignment of the fused spine above L5 as a distal instrumented vertebra, compensation may occur on the free L5–S1 level, mainly with painful local extension. The initial compensation mechanism starts at the L5–S1 level by bending backward the fused spine to avoid forward C7 tilt. Therefore, local stress forces are focused on L5–S1 facets and posterior elements. On long-term follow-up, diskal degenerative evolution may induce a loss of disk height and an anterior imbalance by L5–S1 flexion (kyphosis) or L5–S1 degenerative spondylolisthesis. Revision with disk height restitution is difficult and, generally, a pedicle subtraction osteotomy (PSO) must be used.

21.2.2 Evaluation of Spine Flexibility

Release strategy depends on the flexibility status of the deformed spine. Preoperative radiological means allow this evaluation. Stress films plus computed tomography (CT) scans are generally sufficient. A CT scan combines a stress film effect, because of the supine position, and intervertebral fusion evaluation. Different stages of fusion may be as follows:

- Normal intervertebral status: the level is free of degenerative effect.
- Degenerative rigidity: but neither the disk nor the facets are fused and a deep posterior release (total articular process resection plus interlaminar release) is sufficient for mobilization.
- Total posterior fusion but disk space is free: indication for Smith-Petersen osteotomy (SPO).
- Total anterior fusion by disk ossification associated to posterior fusion: indication for PSO. These techniques are well described in Chapter 23. We want to insist on asymmetrical osteotomies, which are very useful in rigid kyphoscoliosis cases, allowing the correction of both deformities.

Remark

The level of PSO is of great importance for the reduction strategy. Some authors[15] emphasized the L3 level because of better accessibility and reduction of neurological troubles. But recent studies have demonstrated the relation between height of the apex of lordosis and proximal junctional kyphosis (PJK) occurrence.[16] We have seen previously that it is necessary to restitute the inferior arch of lordosis and to concentrate the correction of lordosis on L4 or L5. If an L4 PSO procedure is already well known, L5 PSO[17] is less common and has a bad reputation mainly because of the higher risk of neurological complications. To avoid these, we propose a modified L5 PSO, which performs only a proximal hemipediculectomy that preserves the foramens of L5–S1 and avoids an L5 root trapping when closing the osteotomy. The best indication for such an L5 PSO is a fixed sagittal imbalance in a very high PI that imposes a restoration of a very high SS with a very curved lordosis.

21.2.3 Screws Placement and Mechanics

Following principles of modern instrumentation, pedicle screws are widely used anchors because of their strong fixation in the bone. They are connected to the rods either directly with tulips or by means of a connector. There is an advantage to superpose the screw direction with the vertebra anatomy. Positioning the screw with regard to the rod contour, the corresponding vertebra, follows the same orientation. On the contrary, if two screws inserted in both pedicles of one vertebra are in divergent directions, other than the vertebral plane and axis, it will be impossible to correlate the screw direction with the vertebra orientation. We recommend a perfect position of each screw in each pedicle in symmetry regarding the vertebral sagittal plane and parallel to the upper plateau (▶ Fig. 21.3).

21.2.4 Rod Contouring

This is probably the most demanding stage. Planning the sagittal correction of a deformed spine is the key point of spinal surgery. We have seen that there are two main objectives based on angle and shape correction of the respective spinal curvatures: lordosis and kyphosis. The main tool for surgery reduction is the rod contouring. At the beginning of spinal instrumentation, rods were poorly or not bent, and the effect on the lumbar spine was the loss of lordosis that led to a "flat back." In the 1990s, the literature described this iatrogenic complication.[18] More recently, a prescription of lordosis restitution based on LL versus PI reciprocity conducted on very bent rods with long lordosis length has been mentioned as the cause of PJK.[19] This said, it appears that "quantitative" angle restoration is necessary but not sufficient. We propose a strategy of restitution of "normal" shapes according to PI following Roussouly's classification. We know that the main area to restitute lordosis is L4-L5-S1, the lower angle of lordosis being equal to SS. Furthermore, the rods have to be bent with a maximum of angle from S1 to L4, and poorly or not bent at the level of the spine above. According to Roussouly's classification, we propose the following method of rod bending (▶ Fig. 21.4):

- Type 1: Rods are strongly bent distally to restore the short acute distal lordosis, then immediately at the L3 level begin

Symmetrical positioning of the screws

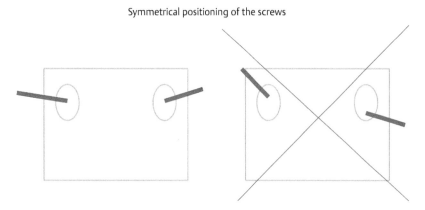

Achieve a screw positioning parallel to the upper plateau

Fig. 21.3 Pedicle screw positioning superposed to vertebral anatomy.

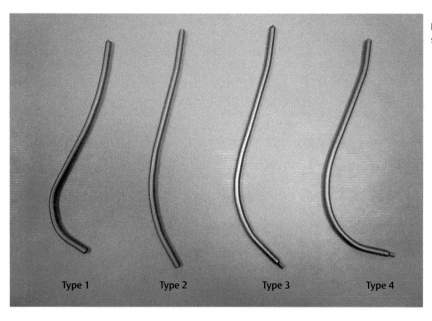

Type 1   Type 2   Type 3   Type 4

Fig. 21.4 Rods bending according to the four sagittal types of Roussouly classification.

kyphosis bending to correspond to the thoracolumbar kyphosis specific of type 1. Occasionally, a type 2 with thoracic kyphosis may be turned into type 1 by type 1 rod contouring.

- Type 2: Same distal shape with less angle (<35°) in distal lordosis; then the rods stay straight without lordosis curvature.
- Type 3: Same distal shape with more angle (between 35° and 45°), then the rods stay straight or very poorly bent. The kyphosis inflection begins at T11-T10.
- Type 4: Increasing distal lordosis (>45°), then slightly bent until the T12 and kyphosis inflection is at T11-T10.

Whatever the situation, a correcting rod shape has to remain close to the pathological situation. It is not appropriate to use an overly drastic strategy and to reduce excessively. When the patient is under anesthesia in a prone position, the deformity is always partially reduced and the gap to a reduced situation is generally very short.[20] This is important for thoracic kyphosis reduction; there is always a tendency to overly flatten the kyphosis using poorly bent rods. Therefore, rods have to be bent close to the initial thoracic shape with a slight correction. (But the rod aspect always seems overbent when radiological control shows a "good" correction.)

21.2.5 Spine Approximation and Implant Connection

This is the time of reduction (▶ Fig. 21.5, ▶ Fig. 21.6). During this time, the spine has to reach the rods and follow their shape. Ideally, in deformities, the rods bent adequately according to the desired sagittal shape are positioned in the sagittal patient plane to be straight in front (scoliosis reduction) and curved in the sagittal plane (sagittal reduction). Instrumentation for spinal arthrodesis offers two main types of connection: direct tulip systems and connector or translation systems, and two possibilities of liberty: polyaxial (there is a 2D mobility between the rod and the connection system) and monoaxial (there is no mobility between rod and connection). In polyaxial systems, the connection appears easy, but once the locking nut is tight, the screw is stabilized randomly regarding the rod.

Moreover, the use of a polyaxial connection leads to a limited range of reduction because of the poor relation between vertebral position and rod orientation. The ability of reduction of a polyaxial system is limited and has to be reserved for short instrumentation especially in a percutaneous approach.

When looking for a deformity reduction, a monoaxial connection must be preferred. The use of monoaxial screws in spinal deformity corrections has been routine for decades, because monoaxial screws provide greater rotational correction, correction of thoracic torsion, and correction of thoracic symmetry than multiaxial screws.[21,22] When dealing with traumatic conditions, monoaxial screws provide more stability than multiaxial screws.[23] We think that these concepts prevail for sagittal restoration of spinal lordosis in degenerative conditions and adult spinal deformity. With monoaxial screws, once the nut is tightened, the screw is fixed perpendicular to the rod. When the rod is curved after being bent, the final screw orientation is perpendicular to the curve tangent. The screw positioning into the vertebral pedicle is more demanding and, as described earlier, must follow the vertebral axis to represent the 3D vertebral orientation. With a monoaxial connection, when final screws are perpendicular to the rods (▶ Fig. 21.7), the final vertebral position follows the rod curvature exactly. There are generally some degrees of freedom before the complete nut tightening that allows a tilt between screw and rod. By compression or distraction, it is possible to bring the screw into its ideal position perpendicular to the rod. This action combined with a very curved rod allows the restitution of very acute and distal lordosis, especially in the type 1 shape.

Monoaxial or monoplanar screws have proved their biomechanical superiority compared to multiaxial screws regarding the failure of the screw–head interface in multiaxial screws.[24] In a practical way, the polyaxial screw-head shift could cause a loss of segmental lordosis, even more for multilevel pedicle instrumentation. Sequential losses of segmental lordosis in multilevel pedicle instrumentation using multiaxial screw results in a suboptimal restoration of postoperative LL and implementation of pelvic compensation mechanisms (pelvic retroversion), worsening clinical results.

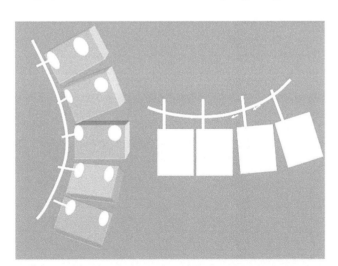

Fig. 21.5 Deformity reduction maneuver: The rod is connected to the monoaxial screws. The nuts are loose. Frontal plane is on the left. Sagittal plane is on the right.

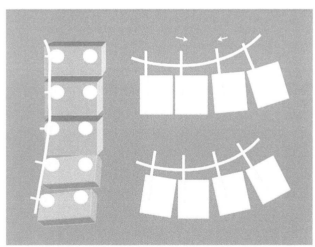

Fig. 21.6 Finished reduction maneuver: The rod is connected to the monoaxial screws. The nuts are tightened and segmental compression is applied. Frontal plane is on the left. Sagittal plane is on the right.

21.3 Spine Fusion and Stabilization

Anterior support with structural interbody cages or bone grafts is required to restore the height of disks preoperatively collapsed, or to maintain disk height. Our strategy proposes a staged surgery:

During the first surgery the spine is approached posteriorly, allowing fundamental actions for spinal deformities treatment

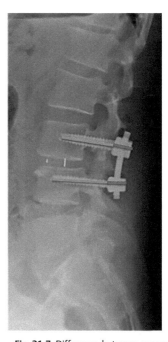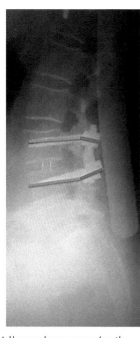

Fig. 21.7 Difference between monoaxial/monoplanar screws (on the left) and polyaxial screws (on the right). Monoaxial/monoplanar screws provide screw head positioning perpendicular to the rods.

such as: release, decompression and osteotomies if necessary, instrumentation, reduction and stabilization, and posterior grafting.

The second surgery (3 to 4 weeks later) permits an anterior support and grafting for the anterior column through a retroperitoneal approach: anterior lumbar interbody fusion (ALIF) or oblique lateral interbody fusion (OLIF).[25] Minimally invasive ALIF or OLIF offer minimal blood loss, shorter operative times, and less postoperative painkiller consumption because of less postop pain.

▶ Fig. 21.8 shows an example of pre- and postoperative sagittal balance analysis realized with KEOPS software (Optispine, Lyon, France) for a 63-year-old man who suffered from multilevel diskopathies, L3-L4 degenerative spondylolisthesis, and canal stenosis. The patient presented with a degenerative flat back in the framework of an average PI (50°) and a sagittal imbalance with a retroverted pelvis. The first surgery was an L2-sacrum posterior spinal fusion, L3-L4 and L4-L5 SPO. Correction of the sagittal imbalance was obtained postoperatively and the patient stood with less PT than preoperatively.

Three weeks later, the patient underwent a second procedure for anterior column support via a minimally invasive OLIF approach.[25] If we compare OLIF and transforaminal lumbar interbody fusion (TLIF) procedures, we can observe that OLIF is associated with less bleeding, less operative times, and less neurological damage and infection. Also, OLIF offers better preparation of the disk space, greater disk excision, and larger cartilage removal of the vertebral plateau. Moreover, reduction of segmental kyphosis or disk collapse occurs during the first surgery, before the positioning of the anterior support.

Some exceptions have to be highlighted regarding the benefits offered by TLIF, such as greater frontal correction especially for oblique takeoff of L5 and frontal deformity correction of the lumbosacral area,[26] and patients who cannot handle two surgeries for any reason.

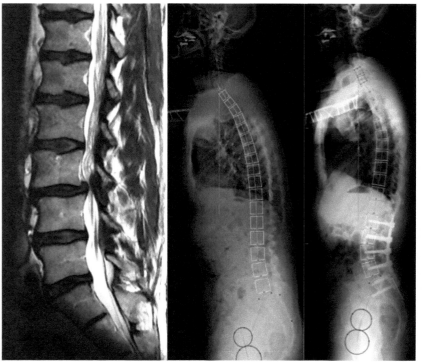

Fig. 21.8 Multilevel diskopathies, L3-L4 degenerative spondylolisthesis, and canal stenosis in a 63-year-old male. Magnetic resonance image on the left, preop in the middle, postop sagittal alignment analysis on the right. The patient runs an L2-sacrum posterior spinal fusion (PSF), L3-L4 and L4-L5 Smith-Petersen osteotomies, then an L3-L4 and L4-L5 oblique lateral interbody fusion (OLIF) procedure.

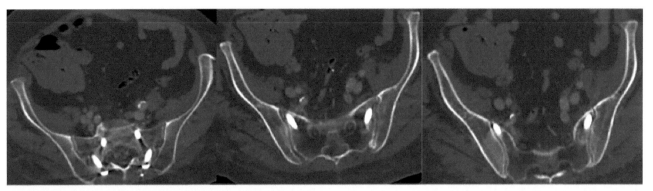

Fig. 21.9 Computed tomography scan showing an S2 alar screw trajectory.

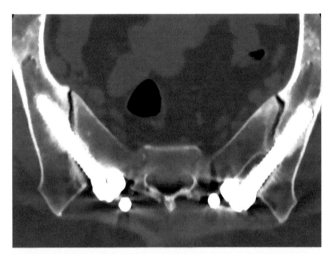

Fig. 21.10 Computed tomography (CT) scan showing an S2 alar-Iliac screw placement.

21.4 Sacropelvic Fixation

Strong pelvic fixation plays an essential role in achieving solid fusion in the lumbosacral junction.[7] Historically, several techniques have emerged and found their indications and specificities for each pathology.[7] Recently, there is a trend to use fewer iliac screws because of their possible complications (extensive subfascial dissection, implant prominence).[27] Local and regional anatomy of the sacrum and pelvis offers other points of anchorage,[28] and a four-screws strategy is preferred rather than S1 screws only for long instrumentations extended to the sacrum.

Our preference is the S2 alar screw inserted through the sacral plate. This technique offers solid anchorage to the sacrum without affecting the sacroiliac joint[9] (▶ Fig. 21.9). However, the S2 alar screwing technique can be demanding because of the small corridor offered by the local sacral anatomy to the surgeon. Therefore, the S2 alar-iliac (S2AI) technique can be a good alternative (▶ Fig. 21.10).

The S2AI technique is gaining more popularity among spine surgeons in adult deformities and neuromuscular scoliosis when fusion to the sacrum has been chosen.[6,8,10,11,29]

References

[1] Legaye J, Duval-Beaupère G, Hecquet J, Marty C. Pelvic incidence: a fundamental pelvic parameter for three-dimensional regulation of spinal sagittal curves. Eur Spine J. 1998; 7(2):99–103

[2] Diebo BG, Varghese JJ, Lafage R, Schwab FJ, Lafage V. Sagittal alignment of the spine: what do you need to know? Clin Neurol Neurosurg. 2015; 139:295–301

[3] Schwab F, Ungar B, Blondel B, et al. Scoliosis Research Society-Schwab adult spinal deformity classification: a validation study. Spine. 2012; 37(12):1077–1082

[4] Roussouly P, Gollogly S, Berthonnaud E, Dimnet J. Classification of the normal variation in the sagittal alignment of the human lumbar spine and pelvis in the standing position. Spine. 2005; 30(3):346–353

[5] Laouissat F, Sebaaly A, Gehrchen M, Roussouly P. Classification of normal sagittal spine alignment: refounding the Roussouly classification. Eur Spine J. 2018; 27(8):2002–2011

[6] Burns CB, Dua K, Trasolini NA, Komatsu DE, Barsi JM. Biomechanical comparison of spinopelvic fixation constructs: iliac screw versus S2-alar-iliac screw. Spine Deform. 2016; 4(1):10–15

[7] Jain A, Hassanzadeh H, Strike SA, Menga EN, Sponseller PD, Kebaish KM. Pelvic fixation in adult and pediatric spine surgery: historical perspective, indications, and techniques: AAOS exhibit selection. J Bone Joint Surg Am. 2015; 97(18):1521–1528

[8] Lombardi JM, Shillingford JN, Lenke LG, Lehman RA. Sacropelvic fixation: when, why, how? Neurosurg Clin N Am. 2018; 29(3):389–397

[9] Nottmeier EW, Pirris SM, Balseiro S, Fenton D. Three-dimensional image-guided placement of S2 alar screws to adjunct or salvage lumbosacral fixation. Spine J. 2010; 10(7):595–601

[10] Shillingford JN, Laratta JL, Tan LA, et al. The free-hand technique for S2-alar-iliac screw placement: a safe and effective method for sacropelvic fixation in adult spinal deformity. J Bone Joint Surg Am. 2018; 100(4):334–342

[11] Smith EJ, Kyhos J, Dolitsky R, Yu W, O'Brien J. S2 alar iliac fixation in long segment constructs, a two- to five-year follow-up. Spine Deform. 2018; 6(1):72–78

[12] How NE, Street JT, Dvorak MF, et al. Pseudarthrosis in adult and pediatric spinal deformity surgery: a systematic review of the literature and meta-analysis of incidence, characteristics, and risk factors. Neurosurg Rev. 2018. DOI: 1 0.1007/s10143-018-0951-3

[13] Cunningham BW, Polly DW, Jr. The use of interbody cage devices for spinal deformity: a biomechanical perspective. Clin Orthop Relat Res. 2002; 394:73–83

[14] Kim YJ, Bridwell KH, Lenke LG, Rhim S, Cheh G. Pseudarthrosis in long adult spinal deformity instrumentation and fusion to the sacrum: prevalence and risk factor analysis of 144 cases. Spine. 2006; 31(20):2329–2336

[15] Ferrero E, Liabaud B, Henry JK, et al. Sagittal alignment and complications following lumbar 3-column osteotomy: does the level of resection matter? J Neurosurg Spine. 2017; 27(5):560–569

[16] Endo K, Suzuki H, Nishimura H, Tanaka H, Shishido T, Yamamoto K. Characteristics of sagittal spino-pelvic alignment in Japanese young adults. Asian Spine J. 2014; 8(5):599–604

[17] Alzakri A, Boissière L, Cawley DT, et al. L5 pedicle subtraction osteotomy: indication, surgical technique and specificities. Eur Spine J. 2018; 27(3): 644–651

[18] Wiggins GC, Ondra SL, Shaffrey CI. Management of iatrogenic flat-back syndrome. Neurosurg Focus. 2003; 15(3):E8

[19] Sebaaly A, Riouallon G, Obeid I, et al. Proximal junctional kyphosis in adult scoliosis: comparison of four radiological predictor models. Eur Spine J. 2018; 27(3):613–621

[20] Yasuda T, Hasegawa T, Yamato Y, et al. Effect of position on lumbar lordosis in patients with adult spinal deformity. J Neurosurg Spine. 2018:1–5

[21] Kuklo TR, Potter BK, Polly DW, Jr, Lenke LG. Monaxial versus multiaxial thoracic pedicle screws in the correction of adolescent idiopathic scoliosis. Spine. 2005; 30(18):2113–2120

[22] Lonner BS, Auerbach JD, Boachie-Adjei O, Shah SA, Hosogane N, Newton PO. Treatment of thoracic scoliosis: are monoaxial thoracic pedicle screws the best form of fixation for correction? Spine. 2009; 34(8):845–851

[23] Wang H, Li C, Liu T, Zhao WD, Zhou Y. Biomechanical efficacy of monoaxial or polyaxial pedicle screw and additional screw insertion at the level of fracture, in lumbar burst fracture: an experimental study. Indian J Orthop. 2012; 46 (4):395–401

[24] Schroerlucke SR, Steklov N, Mundis GM, Jr, Marino JF, Akbarnia BA, Eastlack RK. How does a novel monoplanar pedicle screw perform biomechanically relative to monoaxial and polyaxial designs? Clin Orthop Relat Res. 2014; 472 (9):2826–2832

[25] Silvestre C, Mac-Thiong JM, Hilmi R, Roussouly P. Complications and morbidities of mini-open anterior retroperitoneal lumbar interbody fusion: oblique lumbar interbody fusion in 179 patients. Asian Spine J. 2012; 6(2):89–97

[26] Dorward IG, Lenke LG, Bridwell KH, et al. Transforaminal versus anterior lumbar interbody fusion in long deformity constructs: a matched cohort analysis. Spine. 2013; 38(12):E755–E762

[27] Kuklo TR, Bridwell KH, Lewis SJ, et al. Minimum 2-year analysis of sacropelvic fixation and L5-S1 fusion using S1 and iliac screws. Spine. 2001; 26 (18):1976–1983

[28] Wagner D, Kamer L, Sawaguchi T, et al. Morphometry of the sacrum and its implication on trans-sacral corridors using a computed tomography data-based three-dimensional statistical model. Spine J. 2017; 17(8):1141–1147

[29] Lin JD, Tan LA, Wei C, et al. The posterior superior iliac spine and sacral laminar slope: key anatomical landmarks for freehand S2-alar-iliac screw placement. J Neurosurg Spine. 2018; 29(4):429–434

22 Adult Scoliosis Treatment with an Anterior Approach

Anthony M. DiGiorgio, Mohanad Alazzeh, and Praveen V. Mummaneni

Abstract

Surgical techniques accessing the anterior column of the spine continue to evolve. These techniques show utility in correction of spinal deformity. Each technique has its unique advantages and disadvantages. This chapter covers the anterior, lateral transpsoas and pre-psoas approaches. These provide useful tools in treating sagittal imbalance and lumbar-pelvic mismatch. The versatile deformity correction surgeon may be familiar with all. Additionally, interbody cage types and biologics are reviewed, thus giving an overview of the multitude of technologies available to the spinal deformity surgeon.

Keywords: spinal deformity correction, anterior lumbar interbody fusion, lateral transpsoas lumbar interbody fusion, lateral prepsoas lumbar interbody fusion, interbody cage, spine biologics

22.1 Introduction

Adult degenerative scoliosis is becoming increasingly prevalent as the population ages.[1] If conservative measures fail, surgical correction is considered. Outcomes are best if sagittal balance and lumbar-pelvic mismatch are normalized.[2] A combination of techniques, including osteotomies and interbody graft placements, are employed to achieve this correction. Recently, some surgeons have employed anterior lumbar interbody fusion (ALIF) and minimally invasive surgery (MIS) posterior approaches as a treatment option.

22.2 Approaches

22.2.1 Anterior Approach

Lumbar spine pathologies have been addressed via an anterior approach for decades.[3] The transperitoneal and retroperitoneal ALIF are widely used techniques for degenerative disk disease as well as deformity correction.

The anterior approach to the lumbar spine has many advantages. A large graft can be inserted, as there is access to the entirety of the anterior disk space. This allows for restoration of disk height and lordosis, as well as providing a large fusion surface. Releasing the anterior longitudinal ligament, which is required to access the disk, also assists with deformity correction. The amount of lordosis gained from a single interbody fusion alone is typically between 4° and 10°.[4,5,6] The disk height restoration has the added benefit of indirectly decompressing the neural foramen, increasing foraminal height by up to 18%.[7]

The Food and Drug Administration (FDA) approved the use of bone morphogenic protein (BMP) in ALIF. The large fusion surface provided by the ALIF, along with the use of BMP, can give fusion rates greater than 90% at 12 months.[8] Combining this approach with posterior decompressions and fusions can give dramatic deformity corrections and improved patient-reported outcomes.[9]

Both the transperitoneal and retroperitoneal approaches may involve mobilizing major vasculature. This may necessitate the use of an approach surgeon. The L5-S1 disk can typically be accessed in the bifurcation of the iliac veins. Above L5-S1, the vena cava and aorta will likely have to be mobilized laterally. Care must be taken to avoid tearing the iliolumbar vein on the left when exposing L4-L5, as it can retract and cause significant bleeding. While vascular injuries are rare with this approach, they are a possibility and the patient must be counseled about the risks.[10] Manipulation and prolonged retraction of these vessels can also lead to an increased deep vein thrombosis rate.[10,11] The use of neuromonitoring and pulse oximetry on the foot can alert the operating team to intraoperative ischemia from vessel retraction.

Abdominal surgery carries a higher risk of postoperative ileus. This complicates pain management as it can be aggravated by opioid analgesics. Patients' diets should be advanced slowly after this procedure. Even more serious is acute colonic pseudo-obstruction, which occurs after manipulation of the sacral plexus and disrupts colonic autonomic function. This uncommon condition can lead to cecal perforation. This can be treated by bowel rest, nasogastric suctioning, enemas, neostigmine, and, if needed, colonoscopic decompression.[11]

Injury to the superior hypogastric plexus can cause retrograde ejaculation in male patients. The rates have been reported from 1% to 45%.[8,12] These rates may be increased with BMP usage and laparoscopic approaches.[12,13,14] Other complications can include abdominal hernia, wound infection, ureter injury, retroperitoneal hematoma, and lymphocele.[5,15]

▶ Fig. 22.1 demonstrates an example of a 77-year-old female who presented with low back pain and was found to have degenerative scoliosis and spondylolisthesis. She underwent an anterior retroperitoneal approach, and she had 8° cages placed at L2-L3 and L3-L4, a 15° cage placed at L4-L5, and a 20° cage placed at L5-S1. BMP was used for fusion. The cages were secured with anterior screw fixation, and she had posterior instrumentation via an MIS approach using intraoperative computed tomography (CT) and navigation. She also had MIS laminoforaminotomies at L1-L2, L2-L3, and L4-L5.

22.2.2 Transpsoas Lateral Approach

The transpsoas lateral technique provides access to the lumbar disk space without many of the complications associated with the anterior procedure. By dissecting through the psoas muscle, the lateral lumbar spine can be accessed. This allows for interbody grafts to be inserted that span the apophyseal ring.

This procedure is done from the lateral position in a completely retroperitoneal trajectory. The approach is perpendicular to the spine and patient positioning is key to ensure this angle. If fluoroscopy is to be used, the patient must be positioned in a true lateral position. This helps ensure perpendicular trajectories, decreases the chances that anterior structures will be injured, and provides clear fluoroscopic guidance. Navigation can also be used for this approach, which decreases the amount of radiation exposure.

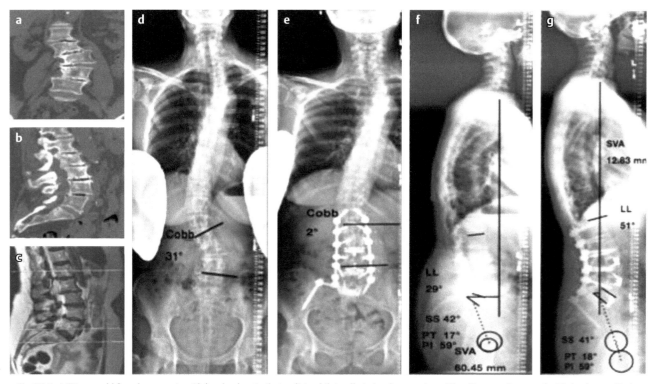

Fig. 22.1 A 77-year-old female presents with low back pain that radiates bilaterally to her lower extremities. She was diagnosed with lumbar scoliosis, stenosis, and spondylisthesis. A four-level anterior lumbar interbody fusion at the L2-L3, L3-L4, L4-L5, and L5-S1 levels was performed. Panel **(a)** shows a preop coronal computed tomography (CT) scan, and **(b)** a preop sagittal CT scan. **(c)** Preop L5-S1 sagittal magnetic resonance imaging cut. Panel **(d)** shows the preop, and **(e)** the postop anteroposterior 36-inch cassette X-rays, with a reduction of the coronal Cobb angle from 31° to 1°. **(f,g)** Lateral cassette X-rays with a reduction in sagittal vertical axis (SVA) from 60.45 mm to 12.83 mm.

If L4-L5 is to be fused, standing radiographs must be examined preoperatively as iliac crest height will determine accessibility. If the iliac crest height is above the disk space, another approach should be considered, as it may be difficult to access the disk space.

Another benefit to the lateral approach is correction of coronal deformity. Approaching from the concavity of the curve allows for asymmetric disk degeneration to be addressed. Upward of 20° of coronal correction are reported in the literature with the use of a lateral approach.[16]

Whereas coronal correction is achieved with the lateral approach, it may not have the same benefit as the anterior approach with respect to lordosis.[17] This is because the approach does not routinely release the anterior longitudinal ligament, as the ALIF does. However, if anterior column release is added to the lateral approach, better lumbar lordosis (LL) correction can be achieved as well.[18,19]

Härtl et al showed a lower overall complication rate with lateral approaches in a meta-analysis comparing it to the ALIF. However, the transpsoas lateral approach did have a higher rate of neurologic complications.[10] This is because of the various nerves that run superficial to or within the psoas muscle, the most commonly injured or stretched being the femoral or genitofemoral nerves.

Injuries to these nerves can lead to anterolateral thigh/groin pain and numbness or hip flexor/quadriceps weakness. These nerves lie in the posterior third of the plexus and can be avoided either with triggered electromyography monitoring or by dissecting them under direct visualization.[20] Even with these

techniques, thigh numbness can occur in up to 40% of patients and weakness in up to 55%.[21] A meta-analysis by Joseph et al[22] showed a 9.4% transient and 2.5% permanent deficit with the transpsoas lateral approach, along with a 27.1% rate of sensory deficits.

Other complications secondary to this approach include injuries to the retroperitoneal structures. While the lateral approach has fewer incidents of this than the anterior approach, injuries to the great vessels and even abdominal viscera are still possible.[23,24] Distortions of the anatomy as a result of the degenerative scoliosis can increase the chances of this.[25] Pseudohernia is also a possible complication.[26]

▶ Fig. 22.2 demonstrates an example of deformity correction via the lateral approach. The patient presented with degenerative scoliosis and lumbar stenosis, and underwent an L2-L3, L3-L4, and L4-L5 lateral retroperitoneal exposure and interbody fusion. Neuromonitoring was used. The patient underwent a minimally invasive posterior instrumentation as a separate procedure.

22.2.3 Prepsoas Oblique Lateral Approach

The prepsoas MIS access to the lumbar spine is one of the more recently described approaches, first described by Mayer in 1997.[27] This technique offers the benefits of the lateral approach with a lower rate of complications associated with dissecting through the psoas, notably thigh numbness and weakness.

The procedure is performed in much the same manner as the transpsoas lateral. The patient is positioned laterally, but the

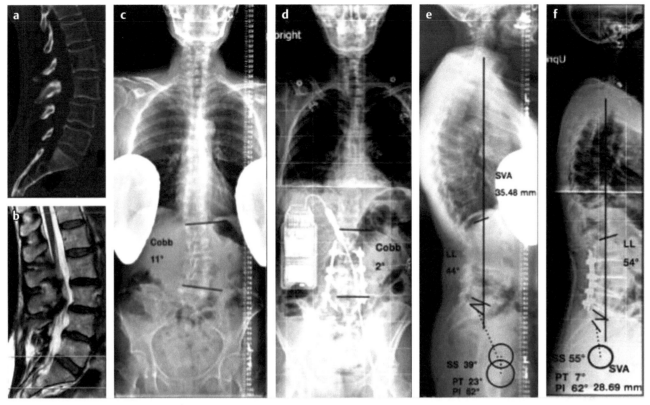

Fig. 22.2 A 69-year-old female presents with lumbar scoliosis and stenosis. She complained of back and radicular pain. After conservative measures failed, surgery was discussed. An L2-L3, L3-L4, and L4-L5 left-sided retroperitoneal exposure, interbody diskectomies, and interbody arthrodesis and fusion with a lateral lumbar interbody fusion cage at L2-L3, L3-L4, and L4-L5 was performed. Panel **(a)** shows a preop coronal sagittal computed tomography scan, and **(b)** is a preop L5-S1 sagittal magnetic resonance imaging cut. Panel **(c)** shows the preop anteroposterior 36-inch cassette X-rays with a coronal Cobb angle of 11°. **(d)** The postop anteroposterior 36-inch cassette X-rays showing a coronal Cobb of 2°. **(e)** Pre- and **(f)** postop lateral 36-inch cassette X-rays with the sagittal balance improved from 35.48 mm to 28.69 mm after surgery.

incision is anterolateral and only the left side can be accessed. This means that coronal deformities that are concave to the right are ill-suited for this approach. Staying retroperitoneal, the lumbar spine can be accessed in the narrow corridor between the psoas muscle and the vena cava. This approach also has the benefit of easier access to L4-L5 with a high riding iliac crest. L5-S1 can also be accessed, but usually requires an approach surgeon; and even with this, the rate of vascular injury approaches 10%.[28]

Similar to the lateral technique, the prepsoas approach allows inserting a large, lordotic graft. Although direct comparisons are not available, limited literature on this approach shows improvement of lumbar spine alignment variables.[29]

A drawback to the prepsoas technique is that the oblique trajectory can be disorienting. Whereas the anterior and transpsoas lateral approaches allow a perpendicular angle to the spinal column, the oblique approach does not. The use of navigation can help offset this.[30,31]

Complications with the prepsoas approach are similar to those from both the ALIF and transpsoas lateral approaches. Although the psoas is not violated, working around it can still lead to paresis or a psoas hematoma. Groin numbness and paresthesias have also been reported. Ileus, major vascular injury, peritoneal laceration, sympathetic chain injury, and incisional hernia can all occur as well.[32]

▶ Fig. 22.3 demonstrates an example of a 55-year-old female presenting with degenerative scoliosis and lumbar stenosis. She underwent a retroperitoneal, prepsoas approach to the lumbar spine for interbody fusions at L1-L2, L2-L3, L3-L4, and L4-L5. Intraoperative CT scan and navigation were also used, as well as neuromonitoring. She underwent staged minimally invasive posterior instrumentation as well.

22.3 Instrumentation

22.3.1 Hyperlordotic Cages

The introduction of hyperlordotic cages has advanced the ability of surgeons to perform deformity correction with the anterior and lateral approaches. These cages have large angles, 20°–30°, to restore LL and correct pelvic incidence (PI)-LL mismatch.

From an anterior approach, the restoration of lordosis using these cages can be dramatic. Saville et al[33] found that using a 30° ALIF cage gave, on average, 29° of LL and a 20° cage averaged 19° of LL. Thus, the radiographic changes in lordosis nearly matched the angle of the cage. However, there was some settling in follow-up, and the patients lost 4.5° on average.

Early results with the lateral approach and hyperlordotic cages were not as remarkable. The taller cages tended to settle

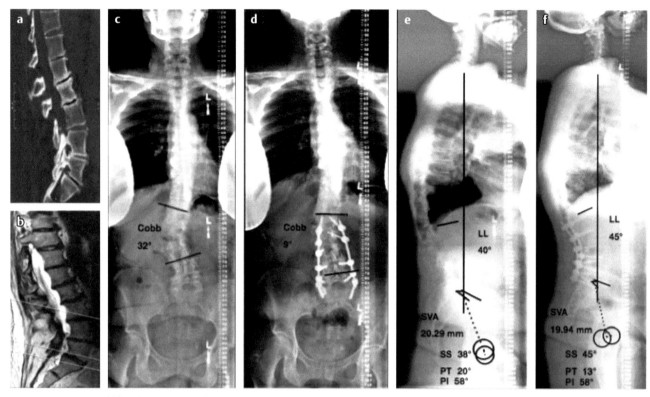

Fig. 22.3 A 55-year-old female presents with low back pain located in the lumbosacral region, with radiation into the left buttock and posterior thigh. She was diagnosed with adult scoliosis and degenerative lumbar spine pathology. After conservative treatment failed, a minimally invasive oblique lateral approach to the left-sided spine with lateral interbody fusion at L1-L2, L2–3, L3-L4, and L4-L5 was performed. Panel **(a)** shows a preop sagittal computed tomography scan with bony deformities and endplate sclerosis with severe disk degeneration. **(b)** Preop L5-S1 sagittal magnetic resonance imaging cut. Panel **(c)** shows pre- and **(d)** postop anteroposterior 36-inch cassette X-rays with a coronal Cobb angle reduction of 23°. **(e,f)** Pre- and postop lateral 36-inch cassette X-rays that show that sagittal balance was maintained after surgery.

and radiographic changes in lordosis did not come close to matching the cage angles.[34,35] However, with release of the anterior longitudinal ligament, Uribe et al found that laterally inserted hyperlordotic cages can substantially increase LL in a 3D model.[36] A recent study by Leveque et al[37] shows that a lateral hyperlordotic cage restored LL equivalent to that of a posterior subtraction osteotomy, but with less blood loss.

22.3.2 Cage Composition

There is a wide variety of interbody cages on the market. The three most common compositions of anterior and lateral cages are polyethylethyl ketone (PEEK), titanium, and titanium-coated PEEK.

PEEK has many advantages over titanium. It is radiolucent, making postoperative imaging (both CT and magnetic resonance imaging) easier to interpret. Additionally, the rigidity of titanium makes endplate damage and subsidence more likely than with PEEK. PEEK cages with an autograft have shown fusion rates of greater than 95% when used in an ALIF approach.[38] However, PEEK is inert when it comes to bony growth, while titanium can be osteoconductive. This has led to the adoption of titanium-coated PEEK cages, which have shown good fusion and low subsidence rates.[39,40]

Advances in 3D printing technology have led to the creation of printed titanium cages. This allows the manufacturer to create cages with pores that are the theoretically optimum size

to stimulate osteoblast proliferation. These have been shown to provide good osseointegration, but literature describing the new technology is limited. There are no direct comparison studies among all the different types of implants and the lumbar fusion guidelines do not give preference to any one type over another.[41]

22.4 Biologics

22.4.1 Bone Morphogenic Protein

Recombinant BMP (rhBMP-2) received FDA approval for use in single-level ALIF procedures in 2002. Despite this limited application, its use has become widespread as an "off-label" adjunct in many spine procedures. There have been many studies on its use in other interbody approaches and posterolateral fusions as well.[42,43]

The joint American Association of Neurological Surgeons and Congress of Neurological Surgeons guidelines on lumbar fusions suggested some options on the use of rhBMP-2. It can be considered as an alternative to iliac crest autograft in both anterior and posterior interbody fusions as well as posterolateral fusions. However, the evidence for these recommendations is grade B and C.[44]

There are a few studies in the literature evaluating rhBMP-2 for use in deformity. Annis et al[45] found a 97% fusion rate at L5-S1 (the most common pseudoarthrosis location) when using rhBMP-2 at that level in long deformity corrections. Kim et al[46] found a significantly better fusion rate in thoracolumbar deformity correction surgeries when rhBMP-2 was used over iliac crest autograft.

One benefit of rhBMP-2 is the reduction of donor site morbidity from harvesting iliac crest autografts. However, rhBMP-2 does have potential complications and patients should be counseled on its use prior to surgery. It can cause heterotopic bone formation, osteolysis, radiculitis, and postoperative seromas.[47,48] Some literature also shows a higher rate of retrograde ejaculation after the use of rhBMP-2 in ALIF procedures.[14]

22.4.2 Demineralized Bone Matrix

Demineralized bone matrix (DBM) has been shown to have osteoinductive properties. There are various studies showing it to be an effective substitute for iliac crest autografts in single-level lumbar fusions.[49,50] However, there is no literature assessing its use in deformity surgery.

22.5 Conclusion

Anterior, transpsoas lateral, and prepsoas oblique lateral approaches are used for the treatment of adult scoliosis. The surgical goal is a reduction of the LL-PI mismatch and normalization of the sagittal balance. The different approaches have their advantages and disadvantages.

Because of the unique advantages each technique offers, the versatile deformity surgeon may be proficient in all. The ALIF offers a large graft and maximal lordosis correction, while the lateral approaches offer better coronal correction (▶ Table 22.1).

Preoperative planning includes choosing the most suitable approach as well as understanding the instrumentation to be used. Newer instrumentation has advanced the techniques and improved outcomes of deformity correction. Hyperlordotic cages as well as their composition are important advancements that aid in surgery when appropriately selected. BMP and DBM are often used in deformity surgery as patients over the age of 70 often have osteopenia. All of these techniques, instrumentation, and biologics are used to treat the growing incidence of adult degenerative scoliosis.[1]

Table 22.1 Complications: ALIF versus transpsoas versus ACR versus prepsoas

Complication	ALIF[5,10,12,15]	Transpsoas	Transpsoas with ACR[10, 21,22,23,24,26]	Prepsoas[30]
Ileus	+ +	+	+	+ +
Vascular injury	+	+	+ +	+
Neurologic injury	+	+ +	+ +	+
Hip flexor weakness	+	+ +	+ +	+

ALIF, Anterior lumbar interbody fusion; ACR, anterior column release.

References

[1] O'Lynnger TM, Zuckerman SL, Morone PJ, Dewan MC, Vasquez-Castellanos RA, Cheng JS. Trends for spine surgery for the elderly: implications for access to healthcare in North America. Neurosurgery. 2015; 77 Suppl 4:S136–S141

[2] Than KD, Park P, Fu KM, et al. Clinical and radiographic parameters associated with best versus worst clinical outcomes in minimally invasive spinal deformity surgery. J Neurosurg Spine. 2016; 25(1):21–25

[3] Lane JD, Jr, Moore ES, Jr. Transperitoneal approach to the intervertebral disc in the lumbar area. Ann Surg. 1948; 127(3):537–551

[4] Hsieh MK, Chen LH, Niu CC, Fu TS, Lai PL, Chen WJ. Combined anterior lumbar interbody fusion and instrumented posterolateral fusion for degenerative lumbar scoliosis: indication and surgical outcomes. BMC Surg. 2015; 15:26

[5] Flouzat-Lachaniette CH, Ratte L, Poignard A, et al. Minimally invasive anterior lumbar interbody fusion for adult degenerative scoliosis with 1 or 2 dislocated levels. J Neurosurg Spine. 2015; 23(6):739–746

[6] Watkins RG, IV, Hanna R, Chang D, Watkins RG, III. Sagittal alignment after lumbar interbody fusion: comparing anterior, lateral, and transforaminal approaches. J Spinal Disord Tech. 2014; 27(5):253–256

[7] Hsieh PC, Koski TR, O'Shaughnessy BA, et al. Anterior lumbar interbody fusion in comparison with transforaminal lumbar interbody fusion: implications for the restoration of foraminal height, local disc angle, lumbar lordosis, and sagittal balance. J Neurosurg Spine. 2007; 7(4):379–386

[8] Malham GM, Parker RM, Ellis NJ, Blecher CM, Chow FY, Claydon MH. Anterior lumbar interbody fusion using recombinant human bone morphogenetic protein-2: a prospective study of complications. J Neurosurg Spine. 2014; 21(6):851–860

[9] Dorward IG, Lenke LG, Bridwell KH, et al. Transforaminal versus anterior lumbar interbody fusion in long deformity constructs: a matched cohort analysis. Spine. 2013; 38(12):E755–E762

[10] Härtl R, Joeris A, McGuire RA. Comparison of the safety outcomes between two surgical approaches for anterior lumbar fusion surgery: anterior lumbar interbody fusion (ALIF) and extreme lateral interbody fusion (ELIF). Eur Spine J. 2016; 25(5):1484–1521

[11] Than KD, Wang AC, Rahman SU, et al. Complication avoidance and management in anterior lumbar interbody fusion. Neurosurg Focus. 2011; 31(4):E6

[12] Comer GC, Smith MW, Hurwitz EL, Mitsunaga KA, Kessler R, Carragee EJ. Retrograde ejaculation after anterior lumbar interbody fusion with and without bone morphogenetic protein-2 augmentation: a 10-year cohort controlled study. Spine J. 2012; 12(10):881–890

[13] Kaiser MG, Haid RW, Jr, Subach BR, Miller JS, Smith CD, Rodts GE, Jr. Comparison of the mini-open versus laparoscopic approach for anterior lumbar interbody fusion: a retrospective review. Neurosurgery. 2002; 51(1): 97–103, discussion 103–105

[14] Carragee EJ, Mitsunaga KA, Hurwitz EL, Scuderi GJ. Retrograde ejaculation after anterior lumbar interbody fusion using rhBMP-2: a cohort controlled study. Spine J. 2011; 11(6):511–516

[15] Mobbs RJ, Phan K, Daly D, Rao PJ, Lennox A. Approach-related complications of anterior lumbar interbody fusion: results of a combined spine and vascular surgical team. Global Spine J. 2016; 6(2):147–154

[16] Wang MY, Mummaneni PV. Minimally invasive surgery for thoracolumbar spinal deformity: initial clinical experience with clinical and radiographic outcomes. Neurosurg Focus. 2010; 28(3):E9

[17] Anand N, Baron EM, Khandehroo B, Kahwaty S. Long-term 2- to 5-year clinical and functional outcomes of minimally invasive surgery for adult scoliosis. Spine. 2013; 38(18):1566–1575

[18] Turner JD, Akbarnia BA, Eastlack RK, et al. Radiographic outcomes of anterior column realignment for adult sagittal plane deformity: a multicenter analysis. Eur Spine J. 2015; 24 Suppl 3:427–432

[19] Manwaring JC, Bach K, Ahmadian AA, Deukmedjian AR, Smith DA, Uribe JS. Management of sagittal balance in adult spinal deformity with minimally invasive anterolateral lumbar interbody fusion: a preliminary radiographic study. J Neurosurg Spine. 2014; 20(5):515–522

[20] Tender GC, Serban D. Genitofemoral nerve protection during the lateral retroperitoneal transpsoas approach. Neurosurgery. 2013; 73(2) Suppl:ons192–ons196, discussion ons196–ons197

[21] Dahdaleh NS, Smith ZA, Snyder LA, Graham RB, Fessler RG, Koski TR. Lateral transpsoas lumbar interbody fusion: outcomes and deformity correction. Neurosurg Clin N Am. 2014; 25(2):353–360

[22] Joseph JR, Smith BW, La Marca F, Park P. Comparison of complication rates of minimally invasive transforaminal lumbar interbody fusion and lateral lumbar interbody fusion: a systematic review of the literature. Neurosurg Focus. 2015; 39(4):E4

[23] Vasiliadis HS, Teuscher R, Kleinschmidt M, Marrè S, Heini P. Temporary liver and stomach necrosis after lateral approach for interbody fusion and deformity correction of lumbar spine: report of two cases and review of the literature. Eur Spine J. 2016; 25 Suppl 1:257–266

[24] Assina R, Majmundar NJ, Herschman Y, Heary RF. First report of major vascular injury due to lateral transpsoas approach leading to fatality. J Neurosurg Spine. 2014; 21(5):794–798

[25] Regev GJ, Chen L, Dhawan M, Lee YP, Garfin SR, Kim CW. Morphometric analysis of the ventral nerve roots and retroperitoneal vessels with respect to the minimally invasive lateral approach in normal and deformed spines. Spine. 2009; 34(12):1330–1335

[26] Galan TV, Mohan V, Klineberg EO, Gupta MC, Roberto RF, Ellwitz JP. Case report: incisional hernia as a complication of extreme lateral interbody fusion. Spine J. 2012; 12(4):e1–e6

[27] Mayer HM. A new microsurgical technique for minimally invasive anterior lumbar interbody fusion. Spine. 1997; 22(6):691–699, discussion 700

[28] Molinares DM, Davis TT, Fung DA. Retroperitoneal oblique corridor to the L2–S1 intervertebral discs: an MRI study. J Neurosurg Spine. 2016; 24(2):248–255

[29] Ohtori S, Mannoji C, Orita S, et al. Mini-open anterior retroperitoneal lumbar interbody fusion: oblique lateral interbody fusion for degenerated lumbar spinal kyphoscoliosis. Asian Spine J. 2015; 9(4):565–572

[30] DiGiorgio AM, Edwards CS, Virk MS, Mummaneni PV, Chou D. Stereotactic navigation for the prepsoas oblique lateral interbody fusion: technical note and case series. Neurosurg Focus. 2017; 43(2):E14

[31] DiGiorgio AM, Edwards CS, Virk MS, Chou D. Lateral prepsoas (oblique) approach nuances. Neurosurg Clin N Am. 2018; 29(3):419–426

[32] Silvestre C, Mac-Thiong JM, Hilmi R, Roussouly P. Complications and morbidities of mini-open anterior retroperitoneal lumbar interbody fusion: oblique lumbar interbody fusion in 179 patients. Asian Spine J. 2012; 6(2):89–97

[33] Saville PA, Kadam AB, Smith HE, Arlet V. Anterior hyperlordotic cages: early experience and radiographic results. J Neurosurg Spine. 2016; 25(6):713–719

[34] Uribe JS, Smith DA, Dakwar E, et al. Lordosis restoration after anterior longitudinal ligament release and placement of lateral hyperlordotic interbody cages during the minimally invasive lateral transpsoas approach: a radiographic study in cadavers. J Neurosurg Spine. 2012; 17(5):476–485

[35] Tohmeh AG, Khorsand D, Watson B, Zielinski X. Radiographical and clinical evaluation of extreme lateral interbody fusion: effects of cage size and instrumentation type with a minimum of 1-year follow-up. Spine. 2014; 39(26):E1582–E1591

[36] Uribe JS, Harris JE, Beckman JM, Turner AW, Mundis GM, Akbarnia BA. Finite element analysis of lordosis restoration with anterior longitudinal ligament release and lateral hyperlordotic cage placement. Eur Spine J. 2015; 24 Suppl 3:420–426

[37] Leveque JC, Yanamadala V, Buchlak QD, Sethi RK. Correction of severe spinopelvic mismatch: decreased blood loss with lateral hyperlordotic interbody grafts as compared with pedicle subtraction osteotomy. Neurosurg Focus. 2017; 43(2):E15

[38] Ni J, Zheng Y, Liu N, et al. Radiological evaluation of anterior lumbar fusion using PEEK cages with adjacent vertebral autograft in spinal deformity long fusion surgeries. Eur Spine J. 2015; 24(4):791–799

[39] Rao PJ, Pelletier MH, Walsh WR, Mobbs RJ. Spine interbody implants: material selection and modification, functionalization and bioactivation of surfaces to improve osseointegration. Orthop Surg. 2014; 6(2):81–89

[40] Sclafani JA, Bergen SR, Staples M, Liang K, Raiszadeh R. Arthrodesis rate and patient reported outcomes after anterior lumbar interbody fusion utilizing a plasma-sprayed titanium coated PEEK interbody implant: a retrospective, observational analysis. Int J Spine Surg. 2017; 11:4

[41] Mummaneni PV, Dhall SS, Eck JC, et al. Guideline update for the performance of fusion procedures for degenerative disease of the lumbar spine. Part 11: interbody techniques for lumbar fusion. J Neurosurg Spine. 2014; 21(1):67–74

[42] Glassman SD, Carreon L, Djurasovic M, et al. Posterolateral lumbar spine fusion with INFUSE bone graft. Spine J. 2007; 7(1):44–49

[43] Mummaneni PV, Pan J, Haid RW, Rodts GE. Contribution of recombinant human bone morphogenetic protein-2 to the rapid creation of interbody fusion when used in transforaminal lumbar interbody fusion: a preliminary report. Invited submission from the Joint Section Meeting on Disorders of the Spine and Peripheral Nerves, March 2004. J Neurosurg Spine. 2004; 1(1):19–23

[44] Kaiser MG, Groff MW, Watters WC, III, et al. Guideline update for the performance of fusion procedures for degenerative disease of the lumbar spine. Part 16: bone graft extenders and substitutes as an adjunct for lumbar fusion. J Neurosurg Spine. 2014; 21(1):106–132

[45] Annis P, Brodke DS, Spiker WR, Daubs MD, Lawrence BD. The fate of L5-S1 with low-dose BMP-2 and pelvic fixation, with or without interbody fusion, in adult deformity surgery. Spine. 2015; 40(11):E634–E639

[46] Kim HJ, Buchowski JM, Zebala LP, Dickson DD, Koester L, Bridwell KH. RhBMP-2 is superior to iliac crest bone graft for long fusions to the sacrum in adult spinal deformity: 4- to 14-year follow-up. Spine. 2013; 38(14):1209–1215

[47] Rihn JA, Makda J, Hong J, et al. The use of RhBMP-2 in single-level transforaminal lumbar interbody fusion: a clinical and radiographic analysis. Eur Spine J. 2009; 18(11):1629–1636

[48] Garrett MP, Kakarla UK, Porter RW, Sonntag VK. Formation of painful seroma and edema after the use of recombinant human bone morphogenetic protein-2 in posterolateral lumbar spine fusions. Neurosurgery. 2010; 66(6):1044–1049, discussion 1049

[49] Schizas C, Triantafyllopoulos D, Kosmopoulos V, Tzinieris N, Stafylas K. Posterolateral lumbar spine fusion using a novel demineralized bone matrix: a controlled case pilot study. Arch Orthop Trauma Surg. 2008; 128(6):621–625

[50] Cammisa FP, Jr, Lowery G, Garfin SR, et al. Two-year fusion rate equivalency between Grafton DBM gel and autograft in posterolateral spine fusion: a prospective controlled trial employing a side-by-side comparison in the same patient. Spine. 2004; 29(6):660–666

23 Techniques for Spine Osteotomies and Clinical Applications

Ibrahim Obeid and Derek T. Cawley

Abstract

Achieving a satisfactory outcome in surgery mostly involves making the correct diagnosis, performing the appropriate procedure, and on a patient suited to the surgical process. Nowhere is this truer than in the adult spinal deformity patient. Conventional modes of diagnosis include focused spine-specific questionnaires and examinations, clinical photography, static, dynamic and alignment radiographs, magnetic resonance imaging, combined computed tomography and scintigraphy, and their associated software programs, which have armed us with an extraordinary insight into spinal pathoanatomy. The evolution in instrumentation is even more impressive, tempting us to perform even more challenging operations, as outlined below. Yet our patients have simple requests: to have less pain, to have better daily function, and to appear more "normal." We must match our objectives with their expectations.

Keywords: adult spinal deformity, ankylosing spondylitis, degenerative, osteotomy, rigid, sagittal balance, scoliosis, vertebral column

23.1 Introduction

Life is a kyphogenic process affected mostly by the invariable onset of degenerative disk disease. Severe spinal kyphotic deformity occurs exclusively or collectively from additional conditions, including inflammatory (for example, ankylosing spondylitis), metabolic (osteoporotic fractures), congenital (failure of adjacent anterior vertebral endplate segmentation), traumatic, postinfectious (collapsed spondylodiskitis), iatrogenic (postcervicothoracic laminectomy), tumoral or neurodegenerative conditions expressed as "bent-spine syndrome," or camptocormia (Parkinson's disease, among many others). In the presence of severe kyphosis, the body may compensate through intraspinal or extraspinal measures to remain upright within its "cone of economy." Alternatively, the body requires a support (crutch or walking frame) or the body may undergo corrective surgery to achieve this. Crucially, in addition to functional requirements, patients have other key objectives including pain relief and cosmesis. Surgery should be planned to the extent that it follows a well-thought-out plan to the point that its execution requires minimal intraoperative thinking. Predictably, following the same steps makes intraoperative teamwork more effective.

23.2 Imaging of Spinal Deformity

Whereas radiographs provide the assessment of alignment, it is worth taking a photograph of the patient pre- and postoperatively to document the changes in posture, particularly if more than one operation is justified. From this, two angles are relevant. The whole-body kyphosis tilt angle (▶ Fig. 23.1) is used, with the apex set at the posterior spine at the level of the umbilicus and the angle subtended from the external auditory meatus to the apex to the lateral femoral condyle.[1] Second, decompensation of cervical sagittal balance can be represented as an increase in the chin-brow vertical angle (CBVA) (▶ Fig. 23.2),[2] the angle between that of the face and the vertical, a reliable clinical measure of horizontal gaze. This angle reflects activities of daily living and quality of life.

Standard radiographs of the spine and pelvis form both diagnostic and planning information when considering surgery. When considering surgery, it is critical to know whether there are a normal number of lumbar vertebrae and ribs. Hyperextension views are useful to highlight any residual intradiskal mobility. They are best taken in the supine position with a cushion under the apex of the rigidity. If one were reliant on fluoroscopy intraoperatively, preoperative radiographs are helpful to identify the vertebral anatomy because pedicle

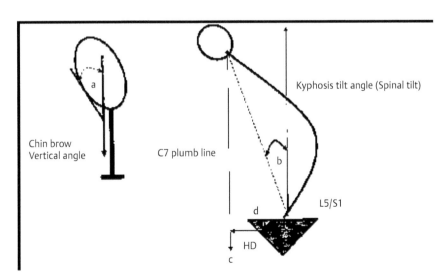

Fig. 23.1 (a) Chin-brow vertical angle, (b) kyphosis tilt angle, (c) C7 plumb line (sagittal vertical axis), (d) horizontal distance (HD) of displaced sagittal vertical axis from reference point on sacral endplate[1] (courtesy of Pierre Roussouly).

Kyphosis tilt angle (Spinal tilt)

Chin brow Vertical angle

C7 plumb line

b

L5/S1

d

HD

c

a

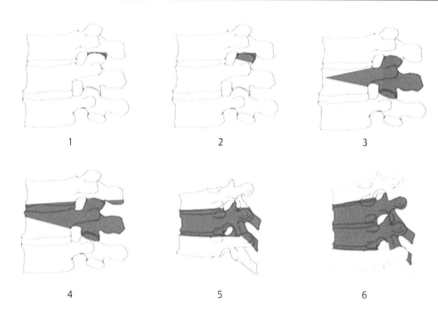

Fig. 23.2 The comprehensive anatomical spinal osteotomy classification as per Schwab.[2]

outlines, for example, may be difficult to visualize on fluoroscopy. EOS imaging or erect full-spine radiographs are used to assess sagittal and coronal spinal balance. The position of the femurs must be included to add this to alignment calculations.

The traditional technique for planning osteotomy involves the printing of the radiograph on paper, drawing and cutting along the osteotomy lines, and manually adjusting the image to approximate the required correction. The digital manipulation of erect full-spine radiographs with software programs such as Spineview (Paris, France) or Surgimap (New York, NY) are conventionally used in planning surgical correction. Correction should be planned at the apex of the deformity as it best approximates the normal anatomy and avoids persistence of postoperative compensatory mechanisms.[3] The software programs are particularly helpful where multiple osteotomies are likely. For example, they can demonstrate whether more than one osteotomy is required and which type. Whichever method is employed should be clearly presented to the patient to ensure that they receive sufficient information.

Computed tomography (CT) invariably yields the best osseous analysis, which is helpful to identify bone quality, pedicle morphology, previous fusion attempts, and integrity of posterior elements. A pseudarthrosis from an old fracture, hypermobile degenerative disk, or previous instrumentation will not have traversing trabeculae but corticated appositional surfaces. Lytic margins are also evident around loose screws/interbody devices or implant breakage. Preoperative CT also provides insight and simulation for what to expect on intraoperative CT. It is helpful to use software (e.g., OsiriX) to reconstruct digitally an axial profile of each vertebra, which can then be displayed as a set of images/prints to be referenced during the case. This exercise mandates thinking about pedicle screw insertion beforehand and then uses this aide-memoire during the "easy" part of the case.

Magnetic resonance imaging is valuable for cord compression but may be difficult because of the deformity. Patients are often uncomfortable within the scanner and may move. The spine may be some distance from the coil thus inhibiting optimal visualization. Consider positioning in lateral decubitus where possible.

23.3 Perioperative Management

If hip arthritis is present, it is worth treating before any spinal deformity correction. As hip arthritis is commonly present with ankylosing spondylitis (AS), hip arthroplasty will aid secondary spinal compensation and help patient positioning if operating on the spine at a later point. The acetabulum is more vertical and anteverted, and reconstruction is best guided by pelvis positioning and not the operating table. A large femoral head may help reduce the risk of anterior dislocations after total hip arthroplasty. By contrast, degenerative knee flexion contractures with AS may help secondary compensation to maintain sagittal balance.

Multidisciplinary input is important regarding aligning the patient's treatment preferences and coordinating cessation of medical therapy. Smokers should be strongly urged to quit. A full anesthetic work-up is required preoperatively to identify AS-associated comorbidities such as right bundle branch block, aortic valve insufficiency, anemia, respiratory compromise from decreased diaphragmatic excursion and restrictive lung disease, aortitis, and so on. Preoperative evaluation of the cervical spine is essential. As the atlanto-occipital joint is the last to fuse, it may be unstable, and thus planning for video-assisted intubation is safest.

Preoperative planning may be a routine process in spine centers where this surgery takes place regularly, but it is always worth ensuring that ancillary services are adequately briefed, including anesthetics, nursing, rehabilitation, and so forth. One has the luxury of time preoperatively so that unexpected intraoperative events are minimized. For example, it is not ideal to discover during the surgery that the L2 left pedicle is malformed or that some material is missing in the operating theater. Developing a predictable pattern makes it easier for the staff, particularly the theater nursing team and surgical assistants (who will benefit more from the learning experience).

Spinal cord monitoring is advisable for these cases, including transcranial motor-evoked potentials, somatosensory-evoked potentials, and free-running electromyography (EMG) of the lower extremities. Evoked EMGs with pedicle screw stimulation is an additional safety measure for checking the proximity of pedicle screws to nearby nerve roots.

Prone positioning the patient is required in most cases with the aid of four padded supports—one under each of the anterior superior iliac spines and one supporting either side of the upper chest. The lower supports must not inhibit blood return from the lower extremities and allow the abdomen to hang unopposed. Thus, they are best placed slightly more distally. The upper supports must be distal enough not to compress the brachial plexus. Given the deformities in AS, it is possible that the head will lie below the level of the chest, and slight head-up positioning or supplementary higher thoracic bolsters may help this.

23.4 Osteotomy

Meticulously ensure that the size and limits of the deformity are analyzed and measured preoperatively, then one can plan what osteotomy is required and at what level(s). The apex of the deformity is the most appropriate level to plan correction as this will best approximate the normal anatomy. The anatomic Schwab classification of spinal osteotomy provides a broad guide for the type of osteotomy needed in most spinal deformities, all of which have been reported in the treatment of AS deformity (▶ Fig. 23.2). Each grade has several described modifications, thus creating significant correctional overlap and, thus, a specific classification is not possible. However, the principle is to release the posterior column and/or the anterior column to allow correction of the deformity; then reconstruction is made by instrumentation with or without anterior column reconstruction. Globally, spinal osteotomies can be divided into posterior column osteotomies and three-column osteotomies (3COs).

Historically, the osteotomy for treatment of AS deformity was a Smith-Petersen osteotomy (SPO), with a resection of the posterior elements, including spinous process, laminae and facets, manual three-point pressure on the spine to complete an audible rupture of the anterior longitudinal ligament (ALL), and application of a molded plaster jacket. This was typically performed in the lumbar spine and could, in theory, achieve corrections of up to 90° but was associated with aortic and gastrointestinal rupture.[4,5] Thus, SPO, in its original format, is not used currently and, when referred to, is understood to mean a chevron or Ponte osteotomy, or at multiple levels, a polysegmental wedge osteotomy.

Grade 1 osteotomy involves inferior facetectomy and joint capsulectomy and is performed with most simple lumbar fusions. It provides minimal correction (5°) at each level but is more effective when combined with the insertion of an anteriorly placed interbody cage to increase the anterior opening angle.

Grade 2 osteotomy requires resection of both inferior and superior facets of the articulation at a given spinal segment, with the ligamentum flavum and potentially the lamina, or the spinous processes. This is an opening wedge osteotomy, also known as the Ponte procedure, requiring anterior column mobility. As most disks are ossified in AS, anterior opening occurs with disruption of the ALL or osteoclasis of the endplate. Mobilizing a rigid anterior column can lead to vascular and neurological sequelae; thus, one should be cautious with older patients displaying atheromatous plaques on preoperative imaging. The resection of multiple facets, along with resection of the spinous processes, involves a substantial amount of bone and ligament resection to afford deformity correction. Given that these osteotomies do not violate the pedicles, pedicle screws can be inserted into the osteotomized levels. Cage insertion may correct the spine more than the same procedure performed at the same level on a flat spine because the number of degrees that will change the affected level from kyphotic to neutral will be added to the usual 8°–10° achieved with this technique.[6]

Grade 3 osteotomy includes grades 1 and 2 resections along with a pedicle subtraction osteotomy (PSO), a closing wedge-shaped transpedicular resection extending into the posterior and middle portion of the vertebral body, achieving up to 40° correction. This posterior-only approach is the "workhorse" of correctional procedures for most severe deformities. Some metanalyses have shown that PSO is the osteotomy of choice for sagittal deformities in AS,[7,8] but others have shown equivalence of correction for both Ponte osteotomy and PSO.[9] Ponte osteotomies are technically easier, less bleeding and shorter than PSO, but aortic rupture and related death, albeit rare, during correction are reported during Ponte osteotomies and should be taken into consideration for decision-making. If there is a solid anterior fusion and immobility, then this greatly inhibits correction. PSO is considered more appropriate for more acute kyphotic deformities. PSOs are usually performed at the L3 or L4 level to correct the lack of lumbar lordosis. An L3 osteotomy is technically easier to perform because of its location, and L3 osteotomies can provide a substantial correction. As two-thirds of lumbar lordosis occur between L4 and S1, L3 PSO thus moves the lordotic apex proximally, which may increase the incidence of proximal junctional kyphosis (PJK). L4 PSO achieves a more anatomical correction.

Grade 4 osteotomy includes a transpedicular bivertebrae wedge osteotomy and diskectomy so that the more oblique caudal aspect opposes the relatively transverse inferior endplate of the cephalad vertebra. A limited amount of posterior translation occurs as the cephalad vertebra approximates the inferior aspect of the caudal vertebra. Given the smaller vertebral height and access to the disk, this has greater application at the lumbosacral junction. Therefore, advantages include a greater correction up to 50° and a decreased risk of pseudarthrosis by eliminating the disk above and allowing direct bone-to-bone contact between the osteotomized vertebra and the vertebra above. The location of the pedicle in the thoracic spine is high relative to the vertebral body and very close to the disk. Thus, when the thoracic pedicle is removed, the disk above is immediately involved.[10]

Grade 5 osteotomy is otherwise known as a vertebral column resection (VCR) or vertebral column decancellation (VCD), including the vertebral body and both adjacent disks. It requires anterior column support. Although VCR is the most potent form of single-level osteotomy, it carries a high risk, is very complex, and, in terms of deformity correction, is for a narrow set of indications. One should avoid excessive spinal shortening in the thoracic spine to avoid spinal cord kinking. This can be performed through a combined anterior/posterior or all-posterior approach. The sharper and more angular the kyphosis, the easier the VCR is through an all-posterior approach.

Grade 6 osteotomy involves the removal of more than one vertebra, indicated for short-wedged or flat vertebral deformities. In cases of severe rotation, anterior instrumentation is possible through a posterior approach.

Surgical management of the deformity may also include treatment of posttraumatic pseudarthrosis with AS. As mentioned, hyperextension radiographs will outline this. Between T11 and L1, 77% of pseudarthroses will occur, but they have been described from T9 to L3.[11] Mild neurological dysfunction is common. Both grades 2 (Ponte osteotomy) and 3 (PSO) are described treatments for these, with corrections of 38° to 45°, respectively.[12,13] After PSO, supplemental anterior fusion is sometimes necessary to support the anterior and middle column in a second stage if there is a bone defect at the osteotomy site.[9,14] Chang et al[13], with a series of 30 pseudarthrosis cases fixed with Ponte osteotomy from the posterior only, suggests that the superior fusion capacity of AS, the rigid fixation, and the improved biomechanical environment with decreased shearing and distraction forces, together contributed to achieving solid fusion. Consideration for anterior column support must include the diaphragmatic detachment associated with anterior thoracolumbar surgery, which may not be ideal in older or compromised patients. The osteoclasis required to perform a Ponte osteotomy is already present in an AS pseudarthrosis, thus lowering the potential for vascular injury. If a pseudarthrosis exists, it should be taken advantage of for deformity correction in addition to a PSO at a nonadjacent level.

Normally, the deformities are corrected from caudal (mostly lumbar), where they are more powerful, to cephalad (mostly cervicothoracic). Severe "chin-on-pubis" deformities have been described, and their severity mandated working in a staged fashion starting with bilateral staged hip resectional arthroplasty, then C6 PSO, T11T12 VCR, and L3 PSO, then bilateral total hip arthroplasty.[15]

As most AS deformities include both lumbar-based and cervicothoracic-based deformities, it is, therefore, logical to perform multiple staged procedures to address this—either at single or multiple outings—depending on intraoperative tolerance and likely correction gained (► Fig. 23.3, ► Fig. 23.4). Even within the lumbar and thoracolumbar spine, multiple osteotomies may be indicated. ► Fig. 23.4 demonstrates the placement of instrumentation from iliac crests to T9 with PSO at L4. The patient was assessed in anticipation of a second PSO, which was carried out at L1. It is possible that a second PSO may not have been necessary and by extending the instrumentation to T9 on the first surgery was still relevant—not adding significant additional morbidity to an already stiff spine. Two-level PSO is better than aiming to achieve greater than 60° with a one-level PSO.[16] The advantages of this include a more harmonious correction, better global balance, less focal cord manipulation, and less force on the pedicle screws. T12 and L3 are the apical vertebrae of global thoracolumbar kyphosis and the normal lumbar lordosis in AS, respectively. Staged L4 then L1 PSOs are demonstrated in ► Fig. 23.3. Higher corrections (>45°) at one level may increase the risk of excessive dural buckling, curving, or even kinking at the apex of the deformity. Fragile patients with severe deformity should be considered for staged procedures if this decreases the complexity of the surgery and the risk for the patient including blood loss and medical complications.

Restoration of lumbar lordosis affects alignment of the cervical region.[17] The C7 slope becomes more horizontal after lumbar PSO. This affects intracervical adjustment if the neck is flexible, as proximal (C0-C2) and distal (C2-C7) lordosis

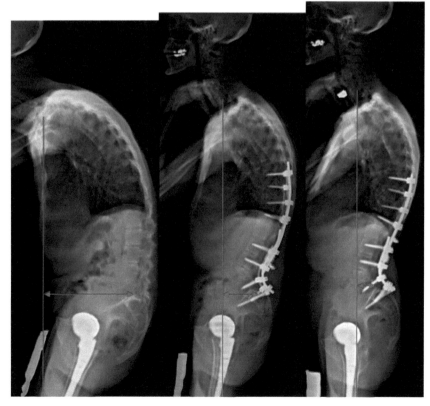

Fig. 23.3 Sagittal profile radiographs of a 45-year-old male patient with ankylosing spondylitis (hip prosthesis in situ), preoperative, post-L4 pedicle subtraction osteotomy (PSO) with instrumentation extending to T9, and post-L1 PSO. Vertical line from C7 indicating the sagittal vertebral axis, which decreases in size after both L4 and L1 PSO.

reciprocate each other to optimize horizontal sight.[18] The CBVA will also improve after more caudal corrective surgery and, as mentioned, reliably demonstrates the requirement for a cervicothoracic osteotomy (▶ Fig. 23.5).

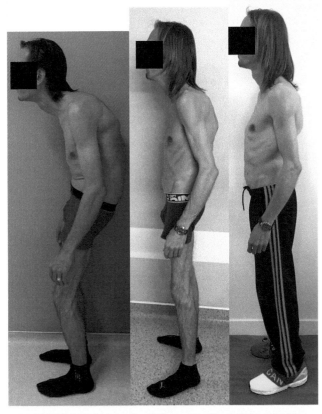

Fig. 23.4 Clinical photographs of the same patient who received two adjacent pedicle subtraction osteotomies. Both the correction of spinal alignment and the loss of secondary compensation measures are evident.

23.5 Surgical Treatment

In this section, we will describe the surgical approaches taken at our institution, most of which have been described in the literature. Posterior approaches to the spine for deformity correction are usually midline and extensive, from three levels above to three levels below the osteotomy site. This can be guided by preoperative on-table imaging, but the anatomic intraoperative level assessment is best done by using anatomical landmarks, including the sacrum and ribs (having counted preoperatively), checking in both directions. The spine is exposed subperiosteally, going laterally to the transverse processes in the lumbar spine and the costotransverse junction in the thoracic spine. When exposing the sacrum, the S1 foramen can bleed if perforated and dissection can be performed slightly superficial to the bone. Lumbar procedures or more caudal are helped by the insertion of Steinmann pins inserted at the posterior aspects of the iliac crests to aid in skin retraction. The prominent ends are cut and protected with a plastic cap. For lumbar spinal osteotomies, fixation to the sacrum is most frequently needed, with iliac screws for an optimal distal fixation.

Hemostasis should be aggressively pursued at this stage accompanied by interval washouts and adjustment of self-retainers. While proceeding with bilateral muscle releases, capsulectomies, and inferior facet resections, the spine will gain increased flexibility, and one can evaluate how much correction is achieved with each step, thus only performing the required amount. The spinous processes are left intact at the three most cephalad levels and the caudal level to preserve ligamentous stability at the ends of the construct.

Spinous process preservation at the cephalad and caudal ends also serve to hold the navigation reference arc for intraoperative CT if required, which is best placed at the cephalad end, communicating with the navigation. Whereas pedicle screws are inserted mostly using a freehand technique, proximal thoracic and cervical pedicles tend to be more difficult in the presence of severe kyphosis. Thus, accuracy is improved with navigation. Navigation is also beneficial during this

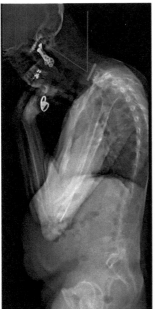
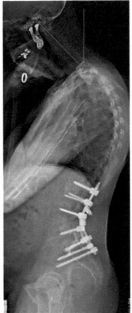
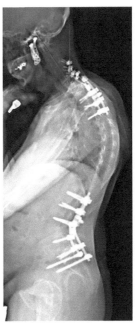

Fig. 23.5 A 52-year-old man with severe global kyphosis secondary to ankylosing spondylitis. Stage 2 site pedicle subtraction osteotomies (PSOs) were performed on L4 and C7. C7 slope decreases after L3 PSO, and external auditory meatus tilt decreases after L3 PSO and C7 PSO.

procedure for placing implants in old fusion masses or abnormal osseous morphology and for identifying the limit of the depth of bone resection during the osteotomy procedure. Areas of greater relative mobility are at greater risk of navigation inaccuracies, particularly at the cervicothoracic junction.

23.5.1 Lumbar Osteotomy

To perform a lumbar osteotomy, both transverse processes of the concerned vertebra are cut at their bases using an osteotome to expose the lateral wall of the vertebra. A Cobb elevator is than placed on the lateral wall of the vertebra, preferentially subperiosteally or at least under the segmental vessels to retract the lateral soft tissues as far as the anterolateral quadrant. An oxidized cellulose polymer mesh (e.g., Surgicel) is left in place to maintain a safe distance between the bone and the soft tissues. This is repeated on the other side. The lateral wall control presents many advantages: it is mostly undisturbed by previous surgeries, it enables control of the segmental vessels laterally, and the dura is not exposed during this technically demanding procedure.

Two complete foraminotomies, both cephalad and caudal to the pedicles on both sides, are made. Having preoperatively planned the resection dimensions, mark out and complete the laminectomy of the concerned level, with partial laminectomies of the levels just above and below, thus exposing the pedicles. Both pedicles are then removed exposing the posterior wall of the vertebra, and the nerve roots above and below are identified. Two osteotomes are then placed above and below each pedicle separated by the distance defined in preoperative planning, which may differ between the right and left sides in the case of an asymmetrical PSO. Cancellous bone is removed in a wedge fashion from posterior to anterior on both sides, leaving a 5 mm thickness of the anterior wall to maintain stability. The medial part of the posterior wall is finally removed with an up-angled pituitary rongeur. The central canal is decompressed, particularly at the cephalad aspect, before closing the osteotomy site to ensure that there will be adequate space. Cobalt chrome rods of 6 mm are used at this institution for the caudal segment. If a lumbar-based coronal deformity occurs, then the working rod is best applied to the convex side. The rod is contoured and applied to the caudal pedicle screws. A domino connector is applied to the end of the rod. This is because the load is spread over all proximal and distal screws while performing the compression at the level of the osteotomy site. The cephalad rod is measured, contoured, and then inserted into the domino (as opposed to the cephalad screws).

For the correction technique, the cephalad rod is then lowered into the cephalad screws as the osteotomy is closed (cantilever bending). The osteotomy is further closed by compression with the use of the domino. The reduction is assessed during surgery and may be completed by other correction techniques, including compression, distraction, or in situ bending if necessary. The bone-on-bone contact at the osteotomy site should be checked, and in the case of a remaining gap, it should be filled with autologous bone graft. The dural sac should be carefully checked for kinking and the foramen for any compression. The contralateral rod is placed and secured, and both rods are then completely locked. Two further satellite rods are applied to span the osteotomy site, for example from L1-L2 to L5-S1 with open side-connecting dominoes. A Capener gouge is used to delaminate exposed laminae, a burr is used to decorticate exposed facets, and prepared graft is placed to cover the maximum surface. Local vancomycin powder (2 g) is used on top of the graft, and fascia and a deep drain are left to prevent epidural hematoma.[19]

23.5.2 Cervicothoracic/Thoracic Osteotomy

For upper thoracic or cervicothoracic procedures, before positioning prone, the patient's head is attached to a Mayfield frame, which is attached to the table after turning the patient. The kyphosis warrants positioning considerations, including, if necessary, placing the thoracic bolsters slightly more distally to accommodate the shape of the proximal thoracic spine. Furthermore, the head position will most likely lie below the level of the chest, and adequate space beyond the head and below the face is important. This may be helped by a slight reverse Trendelenburg position. The Mayfield can also be used for attachment of the navigation reference arc.

The posterior aspect of the ribs at the level of the vertebra undergoing the PSO are exposed through the same incision to allow removal of approximately 3 cm of posterior rib on each side. Bilateral and partial costectomies allow good visualization of the lateral vertebral walls and aid correction. Limiting dissection to the extrapleural space is difficult and requires fastidious adherence to the rib when dissecting underneath. Frequently, a pleural perforation can occur. A chest radiograph may be performed in the recovery room postoperatively, and a chest drain may be inserted if a pneumothorax is evident radiographically. This resection (the removal of 3 cm of rib including the rib head) will allow avoidance of spinal cord mobilization during the osteotomy. It is best to remove each rib section en bloc as the free rib end (once cut laterally) can be mobilized to aid hemostasis as it is dissected medially, with the aid of a Penfield dissector from the costotransverse and costovertebral joints.

A modified transdiskal PSO (Schwab osteotomy grade 4) is our routine correctional procedure for the cervicothoracic and thoracic spine (▶ Fig. 23.6). The resection allows for a closed–open wedge osteotomy. The apex is not at the anterior aspect like a type 3 PSO but at the junction of the middle and anterior thirds of the superior endplate, aided if necessary by fluoroscopy or navigation. The result is that the fulcrum is more posterior and achieves a higher correction than at the anterior border, lowering the risk of cord kinking (less cord shortening) and increasing the probability of fusion (bone-to-bone contact). The distal cut is made below the pedicle, and the proximal cut is just above the inferior endplate of the cephalad vertebra. The size of the oblique cut surface of the osteotomized vertebra should approximate the opposing cephalad surface. The posterior annulus is incised on both sides of the cord with the use of a long scalpel and removed completely, and as much of the disk as possible is removed from posterior to anterior; the posterior half of the lateral annulus is also removed to increase global flexibility and avoid lateral nonunion. The curettes typically used for cage insertion (transforaminal lumbar interbody fusion [TLIF], etc.) are ideal as they can ensure a uniform endplate preparation. The osteotome is ideally directed in a transverse fashion toward the anterior midline so that it is less likely to slip mediolaterally, aiming toward the upper half of the vertebra, the level of the pedicle (▶ Fig. 23.7).

No temporary rod is required during the osteotomy (before the correction). Although the anterior wall is thin, the Mayfield frame and wedge apex's anterior limit of 1 cm provide adequate stability during the procedure. The posterior wall is removed with a 45° angulated pituitary forceps, inserted from laterally anterior to the dura. The forceps' jaws are opened outside the vertebra, and the upper jaw is inserted carefully between the anterior dura and the posterior wall. Then the bone is pushed anteriorly into the vertebra.

Simultaneous internal and external maneuvers achieve the final correction. An experienced operator (outside of the surgical field) who is familiar with the workings of the Mayfield frame is best placed so that he or she can steadily maintain the Mayfield frame as an assistant loosens the table attachments (▶ Fig. 23.8). Two precontoured cobalt chrome rods connected by a domino are applied across the PSO site. The head and neck are then extended to create closure of the osteotomy and telescoping of the rods. If the kyphosis is such that the proximal and distal rods do not meet before correction, then the rods are applied distally, and as the head is lifted, the rods are guided into the proximal screws (cantilever bending) (▶ Fig. 23.9). These combined maneuvers allow posterior closing of the

wedge site, ultimately leading to a smooth correction while avoiding spinal cord trauma at the osteotomy level. Once correction has been achieved, the Mayfield frame is fixed in place, but vigilance is required in case of vascular or neurological deterioration to reverse the correction before starting decortication and wound closure.

The Schwab type 4 PSO is particularly relevant in the proximal thoracic spine given the smaller thoracic vertebra and overlapping oblique spinous process. The cancellous bone quality in this region allows generous bone healing potential. Furthermore, the wedge closure does not require a large effort during the correction maneuvers. While the posterior wedge closes, there is a slight opening across the resected disk space, which allows for a larger angular correction with a smaller posterior shortening, while avoiding dural kinking.[10]

23.5.3 Vertebral Column Resection

Navigation, as mentioned previously, is a useful guide for deformity correction but particularly with VCR. The intraoperative scan can be done at the outset after the screws are inserted or after bone resection. Given the acute deformity angle present in most VCRs, screw insertion is aided by navigation. It can help achieve an

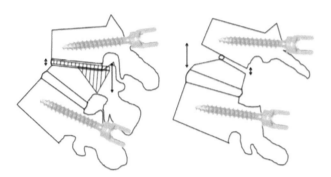

Fig. 23.6 Modified grade 4 osteotomy where the apex at the junction of the middle and anterior thirds of the superior endplate and resection includes the cephalad disk. This is particularly useful in short vertebrae such as the proximal thoracic spine or L5.

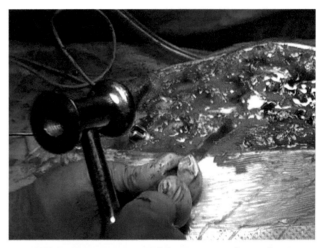

Fig. 23.7 Transverse orientation of the osteotome when performing pedicle subtraction osteotomies around the thoracic spine. Adequate posterolateral access is achieved by removal of posterior rib head (3 cm) thus avoiding manipulation of the spinal cord.

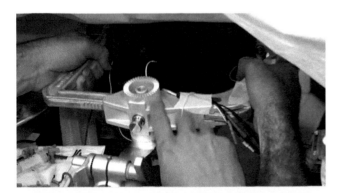

Fig. 23.8 External maneuver of the Mayfield frame incorporating the head to aid in closure of the cervicothoracic/proximal thoracic osteotomy, requiring the intervention of an experienced colleague who is familiar with the workings of the frame and the fragility of the spinal column during this procedure.

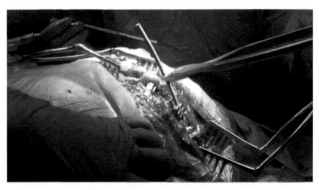

Fig. 23.9 Internal maneuver involving lowering of the cephalad rod into the caudal pedicle screws as the osteotomy closes.

adequate yet safe bone resection, particularly as navigation attachments can be mounted on the high-speed burr. After exposure (with rib resection in the thoracic spine) and pedicle screw insertion to the fixation levels, the pedicles are then removed from the vertebral body. Prior to removing the anterior body, a temporary, stabilizing rod is placed and attached to at least two or three pedicle screws both above and below the resection area. With a coronal deformity (kyphoscoliosis), the temporary rod is best applied to the concave side as most of the resection is performed at the convex side, and one should always remember that the spinal cord is resting on the concave apical pedicle. The burr is used to decancellate as far as the anterior cortex. Diskectomies are then performed with curettes and an anterior cage should be considered to prevent overshortening of the deformity and to act as a hinge to provide further kyphosis correction.

Finally, the posterior vertebral wall is removed as previously described. It is imperative that the ventral spinal cord is completely free of any bony prominences to avoid impingement during closure. For reduction, convex construct-to-construct compression is performed, using dominoes. The dominoes are placed at the apex of the resected area after breaking the temporary rod with the first assistant holding the two parts of the broken rod. It is imperative to compress slowly as subluxation and/or dural impingement can occur at any time.

Once closure is completed, a contralateral rod is inserted after removal of the broken temporary rod. Appropriate compression and distraction forces, in situ contouring, and other correction techniques may be performed while being mindful of any resultant effect on the resected area with respect to subluxation or dural impingement. One should avoid excessive spinal shortening in the thoracic spine to avoid spinal cord kinking, which can lead to neurological complications (▶ Fig. 23.10).

VCD is slightly different in that it does not completely remove the vertebral body, which is less destabilizing with less resected bone and without the need for anterior support. It involves removal of cancellous bone through both pedicles; the cortex of the anterior and lateral walls is made as thin as possible, and the posterior wall is removed so that it can collapse under

pressure during the reduction maneuver. This technique may be applied at multiple adjacent levels, and the remnants of the different vertebral bodies may serve as natural anterior support cages (▶ Fig. 23.11).

23.5.4 Congenital Kyphosis

Congenital kyphosis manifests in the growing child, and the patient can present at any point with this deformity. While it can occur in any part of the spinal column, the apex is often located between T10 and L1 (▶ Fig. 23.11). The anterior aspect of the spine has failed either in formation, in segmentation, or a mix of both. The degree of kyphosis increases during adolescence and decelerates once growing stops. Hemivertebrae, butterfly vertebrae, and wedge vertebrae occur as a result of the formation failure of the vertebral body.[20] Whereas management of these cases in children less than five is not described here, they may require only posterior fusion (uninstrumented epiphysiodesis on the convex side) if the kyphotic angle is lower than 55°.[6] However, treatment at a young age is much easier than after skeletal maturity where a 3CO is usually needed. In the adult setting, osteotomies at the apex are often necessary. In some cases, the deformity is so severe that one PSO is not enough to obtain an acceptable correction. Instead of performing VCRs with their associated risks, adjacent osteotomies may be a preferred option. These can be performed at the same setting. This technique enables bone-on-bone contact between the two PSO sites and between the proximal PSO and the level above after the closure, which significantly decreases the pseudarthrosis rate and avoids a complementary anterior approach for grafting; this technique permits use of the vertebral body between the two PSOs as a bony cage, decreasing the risk of spinal cord kinking and increasing fusion rate. The desired correction here is slightly kyphotic or neutral as opposed to lordotic, thus not ideal in the lumbar spine. It is preferably indicated in the thoracic and thoracolumbar junction and, moreover, it is more difficult at the lumbar spine because of the lordotic shape of these segments.

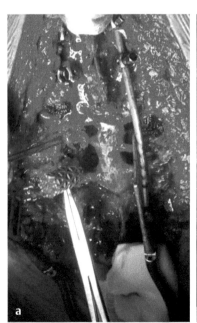 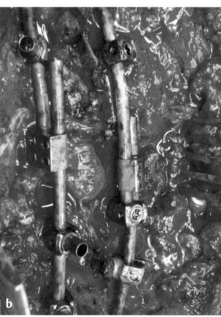

Fig. 23.10 Vertebral column resection of three vertebrae for major kyphosis. This caused a postoperative left limb monoplegia; the vertebral body replacement cage was small **(a)**, leading to spinal cord kinking **(b)**. This patient was reoperated on the same evening and the symptoms were relieved after distraction with a temporary rod and insertion of a larger cage.

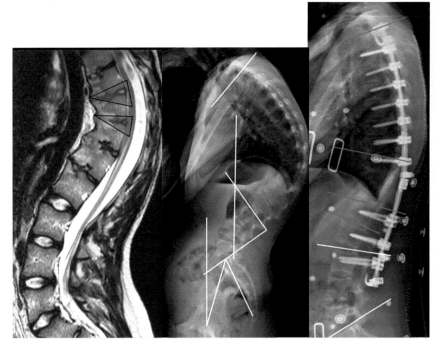

Fig. 23.11 Two adjacent pedicle subtraction osteotomies were performed at T11 and T12 for thoracic and thoracolumbar kyphosis. In this case, the disks were removed above the vertebrae. At T12, the distal third of the pedicle and the posterior arch were left attached. Preoperative parameters: PI = 48, TK = 97, LL = 83, L3-S1 = 81, T10-L1 = 72, PT = 18. Postoperative parameters: PI = 48, TK = 36, LL = 47, L3-S1 = 40, T10-L1 = 12, PT = 8. PI, Pelvic incidence; TK, thoracic kyphosis; LL, lumbar lordosis, PT, pelvic tilt.

23.5.5 Posttraumatic Kyphosis

Severe thoracolumbar deformities can be seen after a vertebral fracture, which predisposes to further contiguous fractures and worsening deformity. Particularly in fragile or elderly patients, the surgeon must take advantage of all segmental mobility possibilities to obtain a good correction with the least aggressive surgery. Any mobile level should be used to improve the correction even when a 3CO is indicated. Location of the correction, while typically at the apex of the deformity, may also in these cases be more caudal at the lumbar spine to avoid a second additional correction in the thoracolumbar spine (▶ Fig. 23.12). This may create a lumbopelvic mismatch in a patient with a small PI, and these parameters should warrant careful preoperative evaluation. An anterior reconstruction may also be required to fill the gap at the fracture site thus promoting correction and potential for osseous union.

23.6 Complications

Infection is more associated with long operating times, significant blood loss, and muscle dissection—all factors in surgery for deformity. Factors to address this include regular lavage with povidone-iodine solution, soaking the bone graft in the povidone solution, vancomycin powder application to the wound layers upon closure, glove change with any external interaction, and all the routine theater preventative standards for infection.

The prevalence of radiographic and implant-related complications is 31.7% when achieving Schwab's target values (pelvic tilt [PT] < 10%, PI-LL < 10%, SVA < 4 cm), and 52.6% of the patients with these complications require a reoperation for mechanical revision.[21] Full osseous union in some cases may take up to 3.5 years. The strength of the construct is reliant on its longevity until union is achieved, hence the use of satellite or accessory rods. Pseudarthrosis is thus common and can be foreseen by assessment with CT. Neurological complications experienced by our center include temporary quadriceps weakness (recovers within 3 months) and prolonged thigh numbness.

Techniques employed to reduce the risk factors for adjacent segment degeneration include the following:
- Preservation of at least one caudal and two cephalad spinous processes and the associated superspinous ligament.
- Tension-free (no involvement in the correction) rod segments at both ends.
- Mild kyphosis of the cephalad aspect of the rod.
- Topping off hooks at the cephalad transverse processes without grafting.
- Lumbar corset for 6 months with daily spinal extension exercises.

The documented learning curve of one of the authors demonstrated a progressive improvement over time in both the surgical strategy and the techniques used for the osteotomy, which resulted in a significant decrease of complications and a shorter hospital stay. With time, there was a tendency to select fewer levels in the instrumentation and a lesser number of TLIF procedures (probably related to the increase of grade 4 osteotomies), which made the surgical procedures less globally invasive. There were more L5 and S1 PSOs in the latter group, which are more complicated and riskier, and which may correlate with a better surgeon's confidence related to skill improvement.[22]

23.7 Rehabilitation

Rehabilitation in a brace is routinely required postoperatively. The patient may stand up the first time as early as day 2 with a thoracic lumbar sacral orthosis and with assistance from a physical therapist. This helps the stability of the fixation, reminds

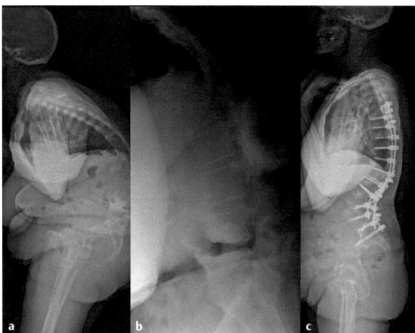

Fig. 23.12 Lateral spinal radiographs of an elderly female with a severe thoracolumbar and lumbar kyphosis. **(a)** Preoperative erect view. **(b)** Hyperextension radiograph (rotated) with evidence of significant opening of the L4-L5 disk space (compared to **a**). The intradiskal correction contributed to the overall correction. **(c)** Postoperative view demonstrating L3 pedicle subtraction osteotomy and L4–L5 Ponte osteotomy with L3-L4 and L4-L5 cages. Postoperative L1-S1 lordosis was 67° with pelvic incidence of 48°. This lumbar hypercorrection compensated for thoracolumbar kyphosis and allowed a good global alignment.

the patient to assume a more upright posture, and protects against PJK and muscular stretching. As PJK is most evident in the first 6 months, a brace helps lower this risk. A brace helps stretch out the anterior abdominal muscles. Contractures of the hip flexor muscles are usually present also. Extensive physiotherapy is necessary to aid thoracic extension and hip extension. Postural elements of both gait and standing are optimized. At first, walking is attempted without any support; if needed, a walker or a cane are proposed to help the patient adapt to the new posture. Early active spinal extension muscle reinforcement is used. The patient is requested to undergo 50 to 100 sustained head and trunk extension exercises in the prone position every day (divided into three stints).

Occupational needs change postoperatively also. Whereas previously, activities of daily living were adapted to the stiff flexed spine, the patient must learn to adapt to a stiff straight spine. This may affect eating and drinking, toileting, putting on shoes and socks, and so on.

23.8 Conclusion

AS spinal deformity cases require significant amounts of planning, multidisciplinary input, and expertise. Careful analysis of the imaging is necessary to identify the osteotomy level and whether multiple osteotomies are required. Planning for staged procedures allows some recovery with reassessment of sagittal balance. Intraoperative reducibility assessment is helpful after complete inferior and superior bilateral facetectomy so that lesser correctional procedures may be sufficient. A three-column osteotomy (PSO, VCR) is a more powerful technique than posterior-only osteotomy (Ponte) but has more bleeding and neurological injury potential, longer times, and a higher pseudarthrosis rate. Thus, with progression through a stepwise approach—from exposure, soft-tissue release, posterior elements resection, pedicle resection, cage insertion to vertebral body resection—increments of correction

may be achieved that are sufficient to cease bony resection and finish the procedure expediently. Postoperative rehabilitation should be closely guided by a multidisciplinary team so that patient satisfaction is achieved.

References

[1] Roussouly P, Nnadi C. Sagittal plane deformity: an overview of interpretation and management. Eur Spine J. 2010; 19(11):1824–1836

[2] Schwab F, Blondel B, Chay E, et al. The comprehensive anatomical spinal osteotomy classification. Neurosurgery. 2015; 76(1) Suppl 1:S33–S41, discussion S41

[3] Obeid I, Boissière L, Vital JM, Bourghli A. Osteotomy of the spine for multifocal deformities. Eur Spine J. 2015; 24(1) Suppl 1:S83–S92

[4] Smith-Petersen MN, Larson CB, Aufranc OE. Osteotomy of the spine for correction of flexion deformity in rheumatoid arthritis. J Bone Joint Surg. 1945; 27(1):1–11

[5] Adams JC. Technique, dangers and safeguards in osteotomy of the spine. J Bone Joint Surg Br. 1952; 34-B(2):226–232

[6] Winter RB, Moe JH, Lonstein JE. The surgical treatment of congenital kyphosis. A review of 94 patients age 5 years or older, with 2 years or more follow-up in 77 patients. Spine. 1985; 10(3):224–231

[7] Obeid I, Bourghli A, Boissière L, Vital JM, Barrey C. Complex osteotomies vertebral column resection and decancellation. Eur J Orthop Surg Traumatol. 2014; 24(1) Suppl 1:S49–S57

[8] Hu X, Thapa AJ, Cai Z, et al. Comparison of Smith-Petersen osteotomy, pedicular subtraction osteotomy, and poly-segmental wedge osteotomy in treating rigid thoracolumbar kyphotic deformity in ankylosing spondylitis a systematic review and meta-analysis. BMC Surg. 2016; 16(1):4

[9] Liu H, Yang C, Zheng Z, et al. Comparison of Smith-Petersen osteotomy and pedicle subtraction osteotomy for the correction of thoracolumbar kyphotic deformity in ankylosing spondylitis: a systematic review and meta-analysis. Spine. 2015; 40(8):570–579

[10] Obeid I, Diebo BG, Boissière L, et al. Single level proximal thoracic pedicle subtraction osteotomy for fixed hyperkyphotic deformity: surgical technique and patient series. Oper Neurosurg (Hagerstown). 2018; 14(5):515–523

[11] Chang KW, Tu MY, Huang HH, Chen HC, Chen YY, Lin CC. Posterior correction and fixation without anterior fusion for pseudoarthrosis with kyphotic deformity in ankylosing spondylitis. Spine. 2006; 31(13):E408–E413

[12] Qian BP, Qiu Y, Wang B, et al. Pedicle subtraction osteotomy through pseudarthrosis to correct thoracolumbar kyphotic deformity in advanced ankylosing spondylitis. Eur Spine J. 2012; 21(4):711–718

[13] Chang KW, Tu MY, Huang HH, Chen HC, Chen YY, Lin CC. Posterior correction and fixation without anterior fusion for pseudoarthrosis with kyphotic deformity in ankylosing spondylitis. Spine. 2006; 31:E408–E–413

[14] Kim KT, Lee SH, Suk KS, Lee JH, Im YJ. Spinal pseudarthrosis in advanced ankylosing spondylitis with sagittal plane deformity: clinical characteristics and outcome analysis. Spine. 2007; 32(15):1641–1647

[15] Kim KT, Lee SH, Son ES, Kwack YH, Chun YS, Lee JH. Surgical treatment of "chin-on-pubis" deformity in a patient with ankylosing spondylitis: a case report of consecutive cervical, thoracic, and lumbar corrective osteotomies. Spine. 2012; 37(16):E1017–E1021

[16] Zhang HQ, Huang J, Guo CF, Liu SH, Tang MX. Two-level pedicle subtraction osteotomy for severe thoracolumbar kyphotic deformity in ankylosing spondylitis. Eur Spine J. 2014; 23(1):234–241

[17] Obeid I, Boniello A, Boissiere L, et al. Cervical spine alignment following lumbar pedicle subtraction osteotomy for sagittal imbalance. Eur Spine J. 2015; 24(6):1191–1198

[18] Obeid I, Cawley DT. Sagittal balance concept applied to the cranio-vertebral junction. In: Tessitore E, ed. Surgery of the Cranio-Vertebral Junction; in press

[19] Barrey C, Perrin G, Michel F, Vital JM, Obeid I. Pedicle subtraction osteotomy in the lumbar spine: indications, technical aspects, results and complications. Eur J Orthop Surg Traumatol. 2014; 24(1) Suppl 1:S21–S30

[20] Tsou PM, Yau A, Hodgson AR. Embryogenesis and prenatal development of congenital vertebral anomalies and their classification. Clin Orthop Relat Res. 1980; 152:211–231

[21] Soroceanu A, Diebo BG, Burton D, et al. Radiographical and implant-related complications in adult spinal deformity surgery: incidence, patient risk factors, and impact on health-related quality of life. Spine. 2015; 40 (18):1414–1421

[22] Bourghli A, Cawley D, Novoa F, et al. 102 lumbar pedicle subtraction osteotomies: one surgeon's learning curve. Eur Spine J. 2018; 27(3):652–660

24 Surgical Failures Mechanisms and Their Treatment

Pierre Roussouly, Hyoungmin Kim, Amer Sebaaly, and Daniel Chopin

Abstract

Several studies have demonstrated a very high level of compli- cation in the surgical treatment of adult spinal deformities. Among them, mechanical failures comprise the bigger share with pseudarthrosis, proximal junctional kyphosis (PJK), loss of correction, and instrumentation breakage. Recently, numerous authors pointed out the role of the spinopelvic sagittal balance and the correlation between balance resto- ration and functional quality of life. Strong correlations between pelvic parameters, pelvic incidence (PI), pelvic tilt, and sacral slope, and the spine curvatures, mainly lumbar lordosis (LL), showed a direct relation between PI and LL (PI-LL). Improvement of techniques of osteotomies permitted very strong correction and lordosis restoration. But at the same time, the level of PJK increased dramatically. In this chapter, we describe the various mechanisms of failure based on the effect of a surgical fusion on the spinopelvic alignment. Mechanical compensations described in Chapter 11 may happen with local kyphosis induced by fusion such as adjacent hyperextension of the spine above and below, and/or pelvis retroversion. A primary good reduction may be lost by secondary disk degen- eration and collapse inside a fusion area, inducing a delayed kyphosis and loss of balance. Anterior stabilization by interbody cages is required. After these general considerations, the strategy of reduction has to be based on PI value, which is the only signature of the initial status. The Scoliosis Research Society classification considers PI-LL and sagittal vertical axis values to quantify the balance. It generally works well, but two conditions seem to limit this classification: patients with small PI (nonretroverted pelvis) and kyphosis–lordosis interaction based on lordosis length and repartition. In the case of low PI, there is a poor possibility of compensation by pelvic retro- version. The ideal restitution is type 1 or 2 in Roussouly's classi- fication. The main mistake is correction by an excessively long and curved lordosis (type 3), inducing an anteverted pelvis. Repartition of lordosis is another cause of error when posi- tioning surgical correction up to L4 (L3 pedicle subtraction osteotomy, for instance). Increasing the upper arc of lordosis instead of the lower arc (L4-S1) induces by angle reciprocity an increase of the lower arc of kyphosis and is probably one of the main causes of PJK.

Keywords: balance compensatory mechanism, contact force, lumbar lordosis, pelvic incidence, postoperative unbalance, proximal junctional kyphosis

24.1 Introduction

The recent information on sagittal balance has allowed a better understanding of spinopelvic organization. Pelvic and spinal parameters are now quite well-known to the spinal specialists; however, their role (or application) in surgical strategy for treating spinal disorders is still confusing and misunderstood, leading to a common source of serious mistakes. The

development of very efficient surgical techniques for correction of spinal alignment, such as posterior column osteotomy or three-column osteotomy (3CO), has allowed dramatic transfor- mation of spinal alignment; at the same time, the need for a better understanding of well-balanced spinal alignment has become more crucial.

Recently, various publications have highlighted poorer clinical outcomes of patients with spinal deformities when the correction was far from an ideal restoration of sagittal balance.[1, 2,3] Although the mechanism of an unbalanced spine is assessed and understood in a very schematic and simplistic way, such as pelvic retroversion and increasing sagittal vertical axis (SVA), numerous other mechanisms remain unexplained, or are still not found.[4]

As we have seen in other chapters, understanding of sagittal balance relies on the knowledge of the pelvic parameters pelvic incidence (PI), pelvic tilt (PT), and sacral slope (SS) (PI being a morphometric [or anatomic] parameter, whereas PT and SS are positional parameters), spinal parameters (lordosis and kyphosis), and global balance assessed by C7 or external auditory canal positioning. The strong correlation between PI and SS, as well as SS and spinal lordosis, has simplified our understanding; that is, within the ideal sagittal balance, an adaptable reciprocal value of PI-lumbar lordosis (LL) should be almost constant, so that surgical strategy focuses on restoration of this ideal angular value of LL determined by the individual PI.[5] However, things are not that simple, and this simple, clear strategy often results in surgical failures.[6,7]

As presented in Chapters 6 and 20, we may describe the specific types in different geometries of sagittal alignment in an asymptomatic population as well as its particular degeneration pattern. We could then hypothesize that a different patho- logical alignment should evolve from a different "normal" or "premorbid" alignment.[8,9] By recognizing these particular patterns of pathological alignment and then, within this context, by understanding how PI, their main driver (or a major determinant), is related with responses to other parts affecting whole spinal balance, we can determine the more proper, or ideal, restoration of spinal alignment.

Regardless of the cause of misalignment—natural degen- eration, trauma, iatrogenic, etc.—a local hyperkyphosis or hypo- lordosis is the main culprit of sagittal misalignment and they induce two means of compensation: (1) hyperextension (to decrease kyphosis or to increase lordosis) of the flexible spine above and below the kyphotic area, and (2) retroversion of the pelvis around the femoral heads (FHs). This last mechanism is dependent on PI: a very small range of adaptation with small PI and a higher range of adaptation in higher PI.

Recent identification of a new type of sagittal alignment, anteverted type 3 or, type 3 with anteverted pelvis, in an asymptomatic population allowed our understanding of the mechanisms of adaptive positioning of the pelvis in the case of hyperlordosis by inducing an increasing SS and decreasing PT (to values less than 0).[8] This very anteverted unbalanced situa- tion may occur in the case of hypercorrection of the lordosis.

In this chapter, we will analyze the occurrence of simple deleterious compensation in response to PI and, in more complicated cases, the association of several mechanisms inducing the most common sagittal balance-related complication after surgery, proximal junctional kyphosis (PJK).

24.2 Compensation to Spinal Imbalance

In Chapter 11, mechanisms of compensation for a loss of balance either by decreasing lordosis or by increasing kyphosis depend on spinal flexibility and muscular contraction. When the spine is flexible, the part of the spine above and below the deformity area compensates using hyperextension. When the spine is rigid, pelvic retroversion is engaged to compensate.

24.2.1 Compensation by Extension

Short Fusion for Local Degeneration

As this mechanism needs a flexible spine, this method of compensation is found typically in younger patients with local degeneration like one level diskopathy, with or without stenosis and/or previous disk herniation, without multiple levels of degeneration.

When local fusion is done with insufficient lordosis, extension of the flexible spine above and below the fusion area is the common rule. In types 3 and 4, lordosis is mainly located in the lower arc between the apex and S1 plateau. In other words, the extension with sufficient lordosis between L4 and S1 has to be maintained in the case of local fusion. The classical situation is the fusion between L4 and L5 or L4 and S1—for local degenerative L4-L5 spondylolisthesis—with insufficient lordosis. This induces an adjacent compensation by L3-L4 hyperextension (i. e., the first nonfused level). Various technical errors are involved in this problem. The rod bending must be done according to the curve restoration. A polyaxial system often fails to maintain an adequate degree of lordosis and only fixes the motion segment, frequently in an improper angle rather than correcting the deformity. In addition, especially in cases with posterior lumbar interbody fusion/transforaminal lumbar interbody fusion, using a nonlordotic cage or with a cage placed too posteriorly (near to the posterior longitudinal ligament), sufficient extension, or lordosis, is limited by the tension of the anterior longitudinal ligament, which interferes with posterior closing (▶ Fig. 24.1).

The first step of compensation by adjacent-level hyperextension is a forward opening at the junctional disk level, followed by posterior facet subluxation and, in addition, a true retrolisthesis. Of course, this situation is painful and may induce back and even radicular pain (▶ Fig. 24.2). One treatment option is to extend the fusion to the adjacent level and to stabilize the junctional disk. But, from a sagittal balance point of view, this is not enough because this leaves the previously fused distal levels in insufficient lordosis and restoring the lordosis angle is performed only by increasing the proximal lordosis (upper angle). If the apex of LL is above the level where it should exist naturally, it is known to be related to a higher risk of PJK occurrence.[6] In our opinion, it is necessary to restore the distal

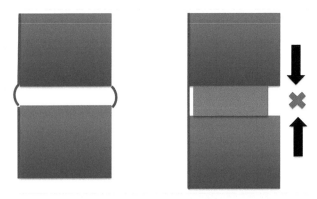

Fig. 24.1 When introduced by the posterior approach as in posterior lumbar interbody fusion, the tension of the anterior longitudinal ligament may impede lordosis restoration.

lordosis (lower angle) where the previous fusion was performed, and to extend the fusion on this physiologically restored alignment.

Fracture Treatment

Spine fractures occur in younger patients and frequently at the thoracolumbar (TL) level.[10] With increased local kyphosis, there is a compensatory increase of lordosis by extension in the lumbar area. If the surgical reduction does not address the traumatic kyphosis correctly, the compensatory lumbar extension exceeds the physiologic range of intervertebral motion and generates pain, usually arising from increased pressure on facet joints. The lumbar ability for extension may allow a local compensation for a slightly increased kyphosis. This is the case in types 3 and 4 spines where lumbar flexibility is better than in type 2. In type 2, a traumatic kyphosis in the TL junction area turns the spinal alignment into the pattern of type 1, with distal hyperlordosis, on a spine that is not adapted for such hyperextension. In type 1, a fracture commonly occurs in the TL area because of the characteristic TL kyphosis, and the compensatory lordosis of the distal lumbosacral area easily exceeds the segmental extension capacity as it has already greatly increased.

24.2.2 Compensation by Simple Retroversion

When the spine is rigid as after a long fusion, and when the sagittal balance reduction is insufficient, the main mechanism of compensation is by pelvic retroversion (increasing PT). This mechanism depends on both the individual value of PI and the ability of the hips for extension. The greater the PI, the greater the possibility of PT compensation. But when PT increases, the hips are more extended. When the PT needs to be increased more than the range of hip extension, femoral shaft tilting (with knee flexion) occurs, allowing the additional pelvic retroversion. There are two steps of PT compensation: (1) pure hip extension with vertical femurs, and (2) hip extension and femur tilting with knee flexion. Even if efficient in restoring overall balance, the retroversion mechanism is uneconomical. First, to maintain the retroverted pelvis, gluteal and hamstring muscle overuse is necessary, thus inducing posterior thigh pain from

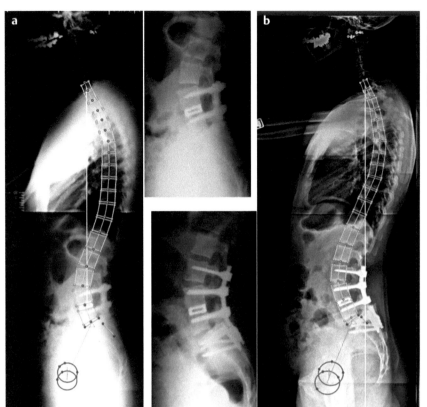

Fig. 24.2 (a) L4-L5 degenerative listhesis previously treated by posterior fusion with posterior lumbar interbody fusion L4-L5; the local lack of lordosis induces a compensation by hyperextension of the adjacent level L3-L4. (b) Extension of fusion to L3 maintaining the hyperextension restored enough but not harmonious lordosis.

muscle fatigue. In addition, when walking, at the time of the posterior step with the hip limited in extension, the pelvis has to follow the femoral forward tilt, inducing a global forward tilt of the trunk. Incidentally, even if the patient with a retroverted pelvis seems quite balanced in the standing position, when walking, the forward unbalance emerges dramatically (▶ Fig. 24.3). In some patients with a great ability of hip extension, pelvic retroversion may be quite well accepted without trouble walking. Of course, the mechanism of knee flexion and femoral tilting used in severe unbalance remains a very bad situation with limited walking. Frequently, there are no complaints of pain in such patients; they just feel tired and limited when walking. The Oswestry Disability Index questionnaire based on lumbar pain is completely inadequate to assess unbalance with a pelvic retroversion compensation.

Restoring a standard lordosis by osteotomies can be considered the better plan for decreasing PT. In severe unbalance, many authors have integrated the femoral shaft tilting in correction planning. Le Huec et al[11] have described the full balance integrated technique, which includes the angle of femoral tilting in the strategy of 3CO calculation. However, if PT reduction is included in the preoperative planning, when reducing PT, the femoral tilt angle is automatically reduced because it is a part of PT.

With a small PI, this compensatory mechanism by pelvic retroversion is poor. This is the reason why an equivalent quantity of kyphosis seems more unbalanced with a greater SVA (and C7 tilt) in small PI compared with higher PI. Nonetheless, with a small PI, less lordosis is required to correct sagittal imbalance with 3CO than in cases with higher PI. In simple terms, it is easier to restore good balance in severe sagittal imbalance with low PI than in the same case with high PI.

Many controversies appear in the literature regarding the best level for 3CO. van Royen et al[12] demonstrated geometrically that the more distal the osteotomy site, the more efficient it was (▶ Fig. 24.4). Because of an easier approach with fewer

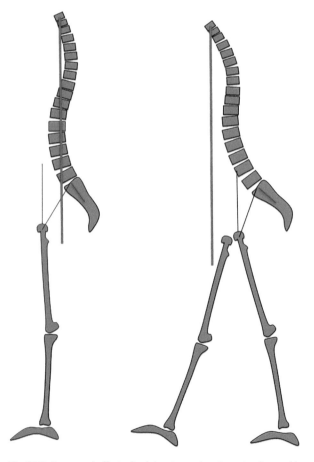

Fig. 24.3 Compared effect of pelvic retroversion: in a standing stable position, the balance seems correct, but when walking, the hip extension is overpassed in the posterior gait and induces an anterior pelvic tilt with forward trunk unbalance.

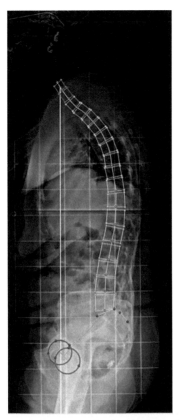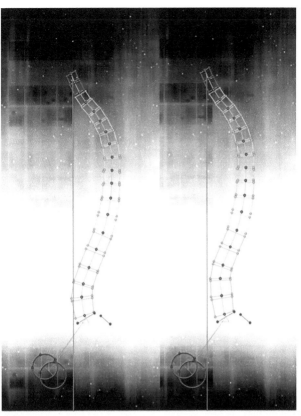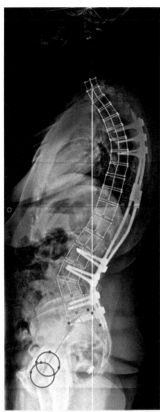

Fig. 24.4 Previous long stable fusion to S1 for scoliosis with insufficient lordosis compensated for by pelvic retroversion. Restoration of a better balance after L4-three-column osteotomy (3CO). Using KEOPS simulation, for a same value of pelvic tilt and a same angle of 3CO, the sagittal vertical axis is slightly higher with L3–3CO than on L4.

complications, Schwab defended the level L3 as the most appropriate for LL restoration.[13] If the overall LL angle is the only concern, regardless of the level of osteotomy placement and the location of the new apex of lordosis, this assertion can be right and, in this context, the surgical strategy will focus simply on the target lordosis angle. However, unfortunately, things are not so simple. We have seen in Chapter 6 that by lordosis segmentation, dividing the spinal lordosis into two arcs of circles, in higher angulated curves, the lower arc (between L4 and S1) concentrates the bigger part of the angle. Physiologically, if the lordosis is lost in this area, it is necessary to restore it by treating the same area; an L4–3CO is expected to restore alignment much closer to normal than L3. Recently, Obeid et al published a description for a 3CO at L5 with promising results.[14] Sebaaly et al showed, in a recent publication, that a higher level of a postosteotomy apex of lordosis was one of the most reliable negative factors in PJK occurrence[6,15] (▸ Fig. 24.5).

24.3 Secondary Loss of Balance by Disk Degeneration

One of the most common failures is the delayed loss of sagittal balance after spinal fusion, although initial postoperative spinal balance was good. The mechanism is a progressive loss of disk height by secondary disk degeneration within or adjacent to the fusion level. The latter situation is commonly found in cases of loss of lordosis in spite of an apparently good posterior fusion,

which is often compensated for by pelvic retroversion. In such cases, a narrowing of the highest disk is found on X-rays, inducing a shortening of the anterior column and the loss of lordosis. To avoid this consequence, the fusion technique should be changed with the use of interbody cage placement combined with posterior fusion and instrumentation. This anterior supporting cage has dual advantages: maintaining the disk height and increasing stability. We will not discuss here the different techniques of the surgical approach for anterior cage placement, such as anterior lumbar interbody fusion, oblique lumbar interbody fusion, and extreme lateral interbody fusion, as they have their own advantages and disadvantages. However, regardless of surgical approach, anterior stabilization with an interbody cage is necessary when planning spinal fusion for treatment of adult spinal deformity (▸ Fig. 24.6).

24.4 Fusion to L5 and the Resulting Consequence

Fusion to L5 is still one of the main controversies in adult spinal deformities treatment: fuse to only L5 or include the sacrum and pelvis in the fusion level? Of course, when there are degenerative changes in the L5-S1 segment (stenosis, instability, etc.), there is no doubt that fusion to the sacrum is the preferred option. Long-level spinal fusion, including the L5-S1 segment, has a bad reputation with higher risk of complications and of revision surgery.[16] This is the reason why many surgeons still prefer to stop fusion at L5 when there is no disk degeneration at the L5-S1 level. The main failure of this strategy is a delayed L5-S1 diskopathy. Depending on the individual value of PI, its pattern of degeneration, and influence on the spinal balance may be different. In type 2 alignment with a small PI and a flat lordosis, the increasing vertical pressure on the disk may destroy the disk without changing the global spinal balance, although this can be

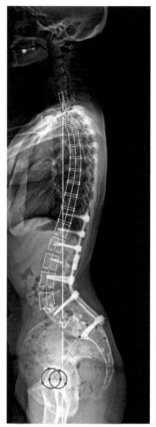
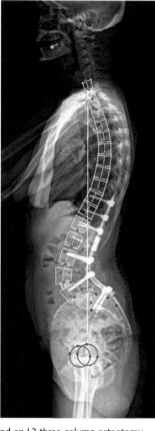

Fig. 24.5 After several surgeries and an L3-three-column osteotomy (3CO), in this L5 spondylolisthesis with a hyper–pelvic incidence (PI) (PI = 90°), even if the quantity of lordosis seems correct, the forward projection of the spine at level L4-L5-S1 did not permit a good balance. A 10° L5–3CO restored a better lordosis repartition and allowed relaxation of the thoracic spine with a more adequate kyphosis.

a disabling pain generator. However, if this distal diskopathy at L5-S1 involves a local kyphosis, severe global imbalance can easily happen as the compensation mechanism by pelvic retroversion is limited in this type, possibly associated with the small PI and small PT (▶ Fig. 24.7). On the other hand, and in spines with higher PI as in type 3 or 4 alignments, the decreased disk height at L5-S1 even with evident kyphosis can be easily compensated for by pelvic retroversion. Even though it is effective, as this mechanism is not economical, it may induce discomfort and fatigue related to increased muscular activity to maintain pelvic retroversion. It can also be disabling, especially when patients are walking, as a retroverted pelvis can limit hip extension.

In some patients who have lumbosacral pain without evidence of L5-S1 diskopathy following spinal fusion to L5 only, it is recommended to check whether there is a local hyperextension at the L5-S1 segment in compensation for insufficient lordosis of the fused segment. In such cases, increased pressure on the posterior elements, such as facet joint and impinged spinous process, can be a source of the pain. It is interesting that, occasionally, this kind of pain from increased pressure on posterior spinal elements can also be found in patients without spinal fusion surgery when they have distal hyperextension (lumbar hyperlordosis), especially in types 1 and 4 alignment.

24.5 Excessive Lordosis Resulting in Compensatory Anteverted Pelvis

Even though failures resulting from a residual kyphosis or an insufficient LL are well described in the literature, the effect of an excessive lordosis is not yet recognized. Laouissat et al[8] introduced a new type in the Roussouly classification: anteverted type 3 or type 3 with anteverted pelvis. The spinal lordosis looks like a type 3 lordosis with SS between 35° and 45° but is associated with small PI (<50°). This situation is found frequently in young people, but it is rarer in older people with degenerative changes. In fact, 16% of the young adult population had this type of spine as found in Laouissat et al,[8] whereas it is present in only 1.5% of the adult population with degenerative changes as found in Sebaaly et al.[9] The identification of this spinopelvic disorganization demonstrates that hyperlordosis can induce a pelvic anteversion bringing the

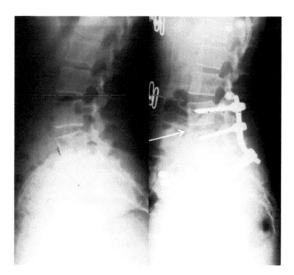
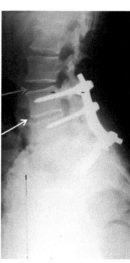

Fig. 24.6 Initial excessively extended fusion L3-S1 with good height of the disk L3-L4. Five years later, degenerative narrowing of the disk L3-L4 inside the fusion area induced compensation in hyperextension of the adjacent disk L2-L3.

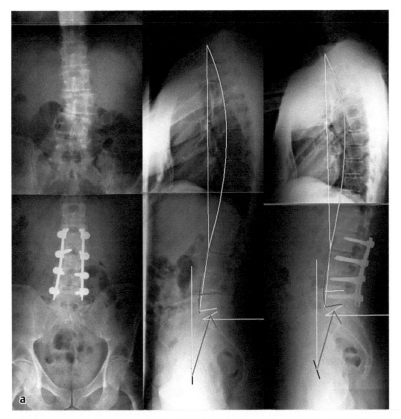
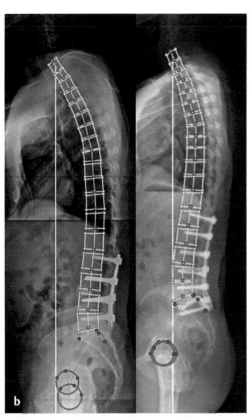

Fig. 24.7 **(a)** Degenerative scoliosis in a 54-year-old man treated by fusion L2-L5. **(b)** Six years later, the degenerative collapsing of the disk L5-S1 led to a forward loss of balance in this low-grade pelvic incidence (PI) back (PI = 45°). The extension of the fusion to S1, restoring the disk L5-S1 height, allowed a good balance.

sacral plateau just above the FHs, even sometimes in front of it. This is an inadequate position that brings the trunk center of mass in front of the FH, creating a kind of forward unbalance. Although their possible thoracic compensation with reduced kyphosis is difficult to identify on lateral X-rays, it may explain their common symptom of dorsal discomfort.

This kind of failure is rarely identified, mainly in patients with very small PI. Ferrero et al[17] have described patients with small PT and apparent good balance (small SVA) but with bad functional results. Analyzing the surgical treatment in patients with previous type 1 TL kyphosis, Scemama et al[18] have shown that patients obtain the worse result when their alignment changes to the anteverted type 3 after surgery, although within a small cohort. As in type 2 lordosis, the global angle of lordosis is small; an excessive lordosis does not appear. It is only the very small or negative PT that must signal an excess of lordosis as a cause of patient discomfort. We attempted surgical reduction by decreasing lordosis with excellent functional and radiological results. On X-rays, the decreasing lordosis restitutes an adequate LL in relation to PI and a better PT (▶ Fig. 24.8).

24.6 Combined Decompensation: Proximal Junctional Kyphosis

PJK was first described in adolescent idiopathic scoliosis[19] and Scheuermann's kyphosis.[20] The most commonly used definition for PJK is the one described by Glattes et al; PJK angle was determined by the angle between the lower endplate of the last instrumented vertebra and the upper endplate of the two supra-adjacent vertebrae. PJK was present when the angle was superior to 10° and at least 10° greater compared its preoperative value.[21] Many risk factors for PJK were described like increased age, obesity, osteoporosis, posterior elements disruption, proximal anchor types, female sex, etc.[22] Analysis of risk factors for PJK is beyond the scope and objectives of this chapter. However, two important aspects will be focused on the importance of an adequate degree of correction and the importance of achieving an individualized correction that corresponds to each patient's own type of sagittal alignment.

In a recent evaluation of a large database of adult deformity patients[23], adequate correction of the sagittal balance according to patient's age was evaluated. Patients with an adequate degree of correction resulted in low incidence of PJK, while both under- and overcorrection of the sagittal imbalance resulted in higher incidence of this complication. One important finding is that PJK in undercorrected patients was milder (< 20°) while PJK in overcorrected patients was more severe (≥ 20°) and frequently required surgical revision.

Restoring the sagittal apex of the lordosis and its effects on the incidence of PJK was also recently analyzed by the authors.[6] When postoperative sagittal apex of the lumbar curve was identical to the theoretical apex, PJK occurred in 13.5% of the cases, whereas it occurred in 41.4% of cases where the theoretical and actual apex were different (*p* = 0.01) with an odds ratio [OR] = 4.6. When compared to other predictive methods,

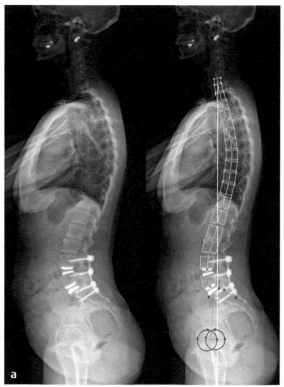
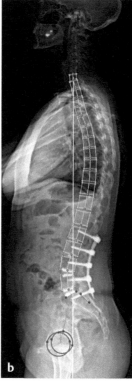

Fig. 24.8 **(a)** Pain for a woman of 50 years, with previous double disk arthroplasty, then fused L4-S1. Pelvic tilt (PT) was very small as a result of too much lordosis. The spinal shape resembled an anteverted type 3. **(b)** Extension of fusion to L2, reducing lumbar lordosis and restoring a better PT and balance.

restoring the sagittal apex of the lordosis was found to be the most important predictive factor. This could have several implications for degenerative spine surgery. The first implication is the choice of the level of a 3CO when treating adult deformity as discussed above. For instance, some authors found no difference in global balance correction or complication rate with level of pedicle subtraction osteotomy (comparing L3 and L4 osteotomy),[13] whereas others found better sagittal balance correction as well as PT correction with L4 osteotomy compared to L3 osteotomy.[23] We think that the osteotomy placed at L4 is better at restoring the apex of the lordosis at the theoretically desired level. The second implication is for the anterior correction techniques of adult scoliosis or anterior indirect decompression techniques. For instance, these techniques rely on anterior release of the diskoligamentous complex and to insert lordotic cages. Nonetheless, restoring the correct sagittal apex of the lordosis is important. Thus, proper choice and placement of lordotic cages (very lordotic cages in L5-S1 and L4-L5 disks) helps avoid inadequately elongated LL with higher apex and decreases mechanical complications in general and PJK in particular.

24.6.1 Possible Mechanisms of Proximal Junctional Kyphosis

Sebaaly et al demonstrated that the change of spinal alignment or orientation determined by a surgical deformity correction was a key factor in PJK production.[6] On another hand, we see in Chapter 9 that each vertebral unit is under the influence of a contact force, a combination of gravity and muscle counterbalance; this contact force is dependent on the spinal orientation. When a spinal surgery changes the spinal orientation, the adjacent contact forces are changed, and a new overstress may appear and induce the PJK.

24.6.2 What Kind of Change in Spinal Architecture May We Expect?

We divide PJK localization into low thoracic PJK (LT PJK) when proximal instrumentation finishes between T12 and T9 and upper thoracic PJK (UT PJK) when instrumentation finishes up to T4.

Low Thoracic Proximal Junctional Kyphosis

- Hypokyphosis compensation by insufficient lordosis correction was the first sagittal balance mechanism described as a cause of PJK. In high-grade PI (types 3 and 4), when the spinal lordosis restoration angle is insufficient, there may be a double compensation by pelvis retroversion (increasing PT) and flattening of the thoracic area when this compensation existed previously. Fracture of the first proximal instrumented vertebra is common, creating a local kyphosis. If we analyze the junctional contact force, there is a conjunction of several circumstances furthering flexion forces; the gravity line is displaced forward because of insufficient lordosis, compensation by increasing PT is apparently effective in a static position but during ambulation this compensation usually fails, and the distinct positive sagittal imbalance tends to unfold. Posterior muscle compensation at the level of the erector spinae is increased tremendously to compensate for both the gravity moment and maintaining the thoracic spine flattening. As we have seen in Chapter 6, the hypolordotic and hypokyphosis conjunction induces a vertical orientation of the spine by decreasing curvatures (▶ Fig. 24.9). This situation increases the pressure resulting from the contact force on vertebral bodies and disks. Evidently, in older female patients, osteoporotic bone is prone to be broken under this condition with significantly increased contact force. In this situation, restoration of an adequate lordosis is necessary, emphasizing the distal lower angle of lordosis at L4, even L5–3CO. As

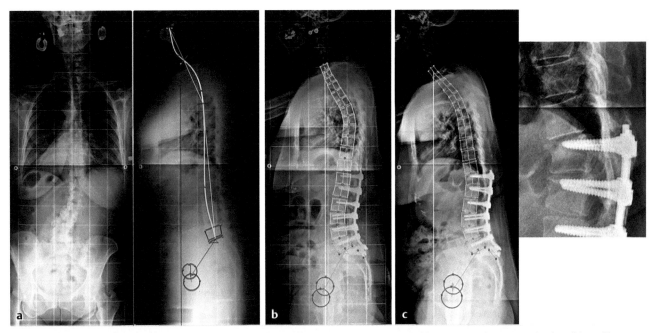

Fig. 24.9 (a) A woman of 60 years with degenerative lumbar scoliosis (pelvic incidence = 60°), false type 2 with retroverted pelvis. **(b)** Insufficient lordosis restitution, remaining retroverted pelvis with flat compensated thoracic hypokyphosis. **(c)** First instrumented vertebra (T12) fracture with proximal junctional kyphosis by junctional vertebral body hyperpressure.

we have seen, the lordosis restoration induces a physiological increase in thoracic kyphosis (TK); the extension of the fusion instrumentation to the UT spine has to restitute the kyphosis by sufficient bending of the rods, taking into account the flattening of the spine in the prone position on the operating table.

- Restoration of a "normal" TK: when lordosis is restored at the lumbar level, this is the most common situation. In Chapter 11, thoracic hypokyphosis compensation has been described as a way of maintaining balance when the LL is insufficient, the second mechanism being the pelvic retroversion. This thoracic flattening is a result of erector muscle activity and is an active compensation. This mechanism is mainly used in patients with high PI (previously types 3 or 4) where sagittal contour is more curved both in thoracic and lumbar areas than in types with low PI. When the surgery restores a more normal curved LL, the TK flattening is no longer necessary and, automatically, the flat thoracic area returns to its natural kyphosis. This spontaneous recovery of the TK effect after restoration of LL is concentrated at the junctional level of the uppermost instrumented vertebra, especially when the rods are not contoured properly, anticipating this change in curve orientation. The typical case is the false type 2, associating flat LL and flat TK with a retroverted pelvis (▶ Fig. 24.10). Although the amount of lordosis required for correction can be accurately predicted, the behavior of thoracic curve following fusion is very difficult to predict. With a medium length fusion (S1 to T12 or T10), there is great risk, as we have described above; but if we extend the fusion to the UT spine with insufficient rod bending of TK, there is a risk of proximal instrumentation loosening even in some cases of UT PJK. A practical strategy is, with a patient's consent, to choose the medium length fusion initially, then, if the spontaneous kyphosis adaptation overpasses a balanced situation with sometimes a junctional fracture, it is possible to extend the

fusion to the proximal thoracic vertebrae, maintaining the kyphosis. In some cases, there occurs a mild junctional fracture that allows kyphosis adaptation without compromising balance and without significant pain.

- Induction of an inadequate TK by restoration of an inadequate LL: in Chapter 6, lordosis and kyphosis repartition were described around the inflection point where lordosis transitions to kyphosis. With the geometry described by Berthonnaud et al,[24] each curve is characterized by angle, length, and curvature distribution. Based on the sacral plateau orientation, the spinal lordosis may be divided into two angles through a horizontal line drawn by the apex. The lower angle is geometrically equal to the SS, and the upper arc, from the apex to the inflection point, is geometrically equal to the lower arc of kyphosis as complementary angles. From this construct, we may deduce that
  - As the lower arc is equal to SS, to modify SS, it is necessary to concentrate the lordosis correction on the distal lumbar between L4 and S1 or on the disks L4-L5 and L5-S1.
  - An increasing upper angle of lordosis increases the corresponding lower angle of kyphosis creating an inadequate excessive lower kyphosis (or reduced lordosis). In other words, if a loss of lordosis is produced by distal degenerative disks collapsing (L4-L5 and L5-S1), and the surgical correction compensates by increasing the proximal lordosis at the level of the upper arc of lordosis, this induces an increasing angle of the corresponding lower angle of kyphosis. Two different lordoses do not have the same effect on the global spinal shape if, with the same angle, the distribution of lordosis is different. Numerous PJKs have been induced by this mechanism when correction is performed in adherence to the dogma that the angle of lordosis in correspondence with PI decides everything. We shall develop later the production of UT PJK by the same mechanism (▶ Fig. 24.11).

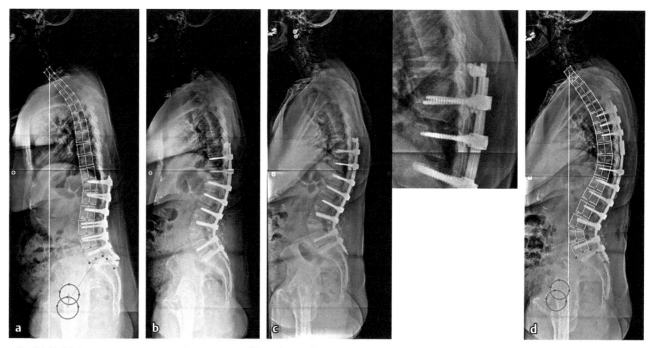

Fig. 24.10 **(a)** Same patient as in ▶ Fig. 24.9 at stage c. **(b)** L4-three-column osteotomy with extension fusion to T10. **(c)** Immediate postop proximal junctional kyphosis by restoration of "normal" thoracic kyphosis. **(d)** Extension of fusion to T6 following the new thoracic kyphotic status.

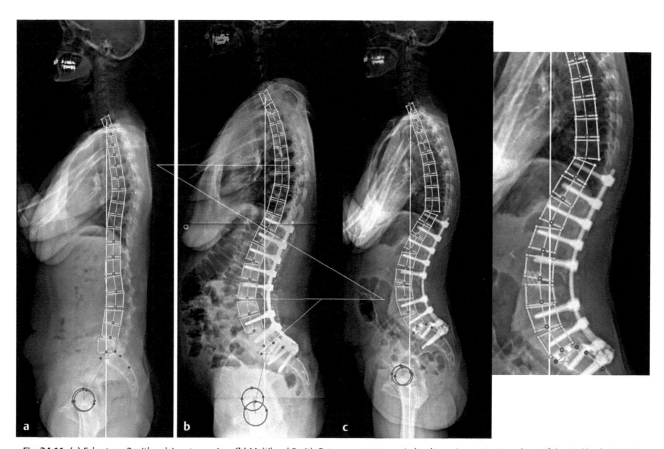

Fig. 24.11 **(a)** False type 2 with pelvic retroversion. **(b)** Multilevel Smith-Petersen osteotomy in lumbar spine, restoring a beautiful spinal lordosis (T10-S1). Apex at L2-L3 and the upper angle of lordosis is equal to 30° and increases the lower angle of kyphosis. **(c)** Proximal junctional kyphosis T8-T9 by induction of an abnormal kyphosis by excessive spinal lordosis restoration.

Upper Thoracic Proximal Junctional Kyphosis

UT PJK involves a high risk of neurologic compromise causing difficulty in choosing a proper surgical treatment option. Naturally, cervicothoracic kyphosis is required only to compensate for distal hypokyphosis or lordosis. But UT PJK is, in the great majority of cases, an iatrogenic production. It is always the result of a fusion instrumentation up to T4. These PJKs typically appear quickly in the first weeks following the instrumentation and probably initiate in the very first days. A localized kyphosis may lead to intervertebral dislocation at level T1-T2 or T2-T3 with cord compression and severe neurologic compromise.

UT PJK never appears above a kyphotic thoracic spine. As for LT PJK, thoracic evolution may be a "normal" kyphosis restoration after lordosis restoration or may be abnormal hyperkyphosis compensation.

As described previously, when correcting a false type 2, which is actually type 3 but associated with compensation by retroverted pelvis and flattened thoracic curvature, restoration of LL is accompanied by spontaneous restoration of TK. When the construct goes up to T4, in T3, if the rod bending does not address this reactive evolution of TK and only maintains a flattening thoracic spine, there will be a conflict between the flattened rods and the tendency of the thoracic spine to return to its natural kyphosis, which will increase stress at the uppermost instrumented vertebra. This increases the possibility of upper instrumentation pullout and/or screw loosening. Reinforcement of distal fixation is not a solution without the thoracic rod contour matching the natural TK in balance with restored LL. Those patients with stable overcorrection are very uncomfortable, with upper dorsal pain and complaints of a constant feeling of backward traction in their upper back. At the first stage of correction, this is a difficult situation to deal with, because the final thoracic positioning is not easy to predict and leads to rod bending in an improper contour. The situation is easier when the false retroverted type 2 is associated with a TK. This TK does not change after lordosis correction and balances the corrected spinal lordosis as in a true type 3 or 4.

The second issue of abnormal hyperkyphosis as a failure of the compensation mechanism just above the instrumentation is more disabling and difficult to treat. Combination of bad architecture and muscle insufficiency is probably the cause of UT spine collapse.

- In ▶ Fig. 24.12, a patient with an insufficient lordosis restoration after an old arthrodesis presents a progressive cervicothoracic kyphosis by muscular impossibility to counterbalance the anterior unbalance. Restoration of a better lordosis by L4–3CO allows a spontaneous cervicothoracic balance restoration with less muscle action to balance the system.
- Sometimes the patient develops a PJK above the uppermost instrumented vertebra of T4, with enough or even an excessive amount of lordosis restoration. The TK is too small for the LL and the proximal rods appear to be bent too straight.
  - First hypothesis: lordosis is excessive and the thoracic spine is too flat. The patient is positioned too posteriorly by the instrumentation. The head is projected forward and the balance gravity muscles are strongly displaced forward. PJK appears.

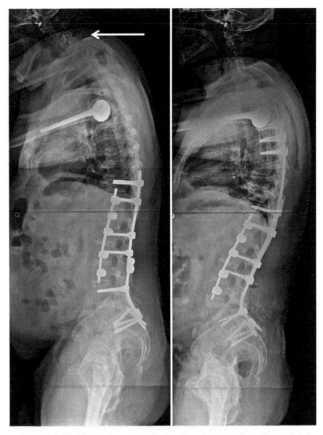

Fig. 24.12 (Left) Development of a functional cervicothoracic proximal junctional kyphosis (PJK) 5 years after a T10-S1 fusion. The progressive thoracic kyphosis dragged the PJK by muscle weakness. (Right) After restoration of the sagittal balance by L4-three-column osteotomy, the patient was able to rebalance the cervicothoracic spine spontaneously.

  - Second hypothesis: as described previously, angle of lordosis corresponds with PI, but lordosis distribution favors the upper angle and does not sufficiently reduce the lower angle of lordosis. The complementary lower angle of kyphosis is augmented following the upper angle of lordosis. If the instrumentation does not follow this new kyphotic inflection, the UT spine is projected posteriorly, and the same mechanism of cervicothoracic flexion occurs (▶ Fig. 24.13).
- In any case, an excessive lordosis correction is as bad as an insufficient correction. It is the same for the TK where too much correction with rods that are too straight does not allow a natural thoracic adaptation, inducing a junctional stress in flexion to compensate for the inadequate hypokyphosis (▶ Fig. 24.14).

24.7 Conclusion

It is no longer possible to consider the sagittal balance and alignment of the spine as an accessory element of treatment strategy. A majority of mechanical failures depend on this fundamental feature. Because of the sagittal pelvic shape variation

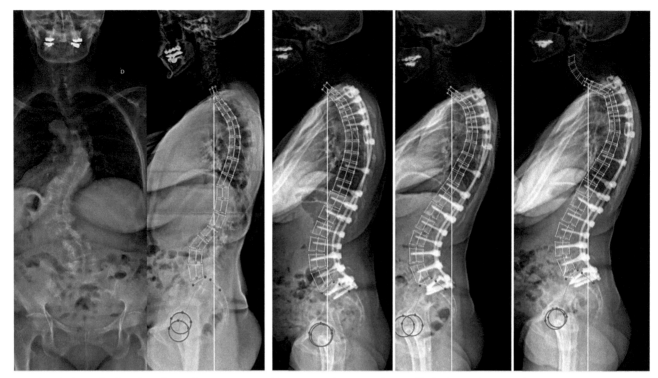

Fig. 24.13 Thoracolumbar idiopathic scoliosis in a 55-year-old woman, with an "anarchic" profile (pelvic incidence = 50°). An excessive lordosis restoration shown by the pelvic anteversion, leading the top of the thoracic spine in a backward position regarding the vertical head projection. Flexion of the proximal thoracic spine is the result of a forward positive balance force. The increasing PJK induced pelvis retroversion compensation, bringing backward the top of the instrumented spine. A vicious cycle was created: the posterior head-thoracic spine offset increased, increasing the need of PJK compensation.

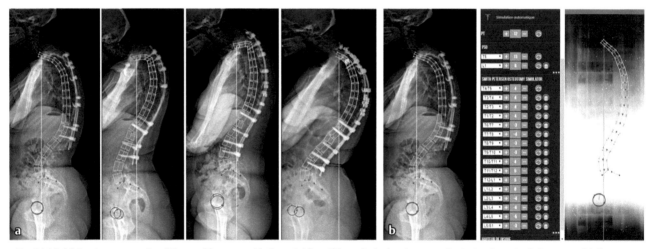

Fig. 24.14 **(a)** Previous surgery in a 25-year-old woman with thoracic idiopathic scoliosis showing several mistakes in sagittal alignment: (1) flattening of the thoracic kyphosis; (2) thoracolumbar kyphosis; (3) lumbar hyperlordosis (anteverted pelvis); (4) high thoracic proximal junctional kyphosis (PJK); and (5) bad strategy of revision with L1-three-column osteotomy (3CO) without restoring the thoracic kyphosis. This induced an insufficient global kyphosis increasing the upper angle of lordosis. The spine was globally tilted backward (negative sagittal vertical axis) inducing the PJK. At the last revision, thoracic Smith-Petersen osteotomy (SPO) allowed restoration of kyphosis but without PJK reduction. This hyperkyphosis was compensated for by a short distal hyperlordosis. **(b)** Reduction simulation with KEOPS software showed very complex sequences of osteotomies with association of T5 and L1–3CO and several levels of negative SPO in the previous thoracic fusion for restoring the thoracic kyphosis.

issuing from human phylogenies, one may identify distinct variable spinal shapes and variable degeneration changes. The very powerful technical means now used in spinal surgery have resulted in overcorrections and overcompensations. Even if the failure mechanism is well understood, it can be difficult to find an efficient and economical correction to such failures, and therapeutic escalation is the rule. Probably the best option would be to prevent rather than treat, and for that, a good understanding of sagittal alignment is needed based on two rules:

- The only signature of the previous situation is the PI.
- The sagittal correction must be predicted accordingly with PI values.

References

[1] Glassman SD, Bridwell K, Dimar JR, Horton W, Berven S, Schwab F. The impact of positive sagittal balance in adult spinal deformity. Spine. 2005; 30 (18):2024–2029

[2] Smith JS, Shaffrey CI, Glassman SD, et al. Clinical and radiographic parameters that distinguish between the best and worst outcomes of scoliosis surgery for adults. Eur Spine J. 2012; 22(2):402–410

[3] Bourghli A, Aunoble S, Reebye O, Le Huec JC. Correlation of clinical outcome and spinopelvic sagittal alignment after surgical treatment of low-grade isthmic spondylolisthesis. Eur Spine J. 2011; 20(Suppl 5):663–66–8

[4] Le Huec JC, Charosky S, Barrey C, Rigal J, Aunoble S. Sagittal imbalance cascade for simple degenerative spine and consequences: algorithm of decision for appropriate treatment. Eur Spine J. 2011; 20(Suppl 5):699–703

[5] Schwab F, Ungar B, Blondel B, et al. Scoliosis Research Society-Schwab adult spinal deformity classification: a validation study. Spine (Phila Pa 1976). 2012; 37(12):1077–10–82

[6] Sebaaly A, Riouallon G, Obeid I, et al. Proximal junctional kyphosis in adult scoliosis: comparison of four radiological predictor models. Eur Spine J. 2018; 27(3):613–621

[7] Yilgor C, Sogunmez N, Boissiere L, et al. Global alignment and proportion (GAP) score: development and validation of a new method of analyzing spinopelvic alignment to predict mechanical complications after adult spinal deformity surgery. J Bone Joint Surg Am. 2017; 99(19):1661–1672

[8] Laouissat F, Sebaaly A, Gehrchen M, Roussouly P. Classification of normal sagittal spine alignment: refounding the Roussouly classification. Eur Spine J. 2018; 27(8):2002–2011

[9] Sebaaly A, Grobost P, Mallam L, Roussouly P. Description of the sagittal alignment of the degenerative human spine. Eur Spine J. 2018; 27(2):489–496

[10] Sebaaly A, Rizkallah M, Bachour F, Atallah F, Moreau PE, Maalouf G. Percutaneous cement augmentation for osteoporotic vertebral fractures. EFORT Open Rev. 2017; 2(6):293–299

[11] Le Huec JC, Leijssen P, Duarte M, Aunoble S. Thoracolumbar imbalance analysis for osteotomy planification using a new method: FBI technique. Eur Spine J. 2011; 20(Suppl 5):669–6–80

[12] van Royen BJ, de Kleuver M, Slot GH. Polysegmental lumbar posterior wedge osteotomies for correction of kyphosis in ankylosing spondylitis. Eur Spine J. 1998; 7(2):104–110

[13] Lafage V, Schwab F, Vira S, et al. Does vertebral level of pedicle subtraction osteotomy correlate with degree of spinopelvic parameter correction? J Neurosurg Spine. 2011; 14(2):184–191

[14] Alzakri A, Boissière L, Cawley DT, et al. L5 pedicle subtraction osteotomy: indication, surgical technique and specificities. Eur Spine J. 2018; 27(3): 644–651

[15] Kharrat K, Sebaaly A, Assi A, Ghanem I, Rachkidi R. Is there a correlation between the apical vertebral rotation and the pelvic incidence in adolescent idiopathic scoliosis? Glob Spine J. 2016; 6(1)(S)(uppl)–s-0036–1583044–s-0036–1583044

[16] Kim YJ, Bridwell KH, Lenke LG, Cho K-J, Edwards CC, II, Rinella AS. Pseudarthrosis in adult spinal deformity following multisegmental instrumentation and arthrodesis. J Bone Joint Surg Am. 2006; 88(4):721–728

[17] Ferrero E, Vira S, Ames CP, et al. Analysis of an unexplored group of sagittal deformity patients: low pelvic tilt despite positive sagittal malalignment. Eur Spine J. 2016; 25(11):3568–3576

[18] Scemama C, Laouissat F, Abelin-Genevois K, Roussouly P. Surgical treatment of thoraco-lumbar kyphosis (TLK) associated with low pelvic incidence. Eur Spine J. 2017; 26(8):2146–2152

[19] Lee GA, Betz RR, Clements DH, III, Huss GK. Proximal kyphosis after posterior spinal fusion in patients with idiopathic scoliosis. Spine. 1999; 24(8):795–799

[20] Lowe TG, Kasten MD. An analysis of sagittal curves and balance after Cotrel-Dubousset instrumentation for kyphosis secondary to Scheuermann's disease. A review of 32 patients. Spine. 1994; 19(15):1680–1685

[21] Glattes RC, Bridwell KH, Lenke LG, Kim YJ, Rinella A, Edwards C, II. Proximal junctional kyphosis in adult spinal deformity following long instrumented posterior spinal fusion: incidence, outcomes, and risk factor analysis. Spine. 2005; 30(14):1643–1649

[22] Liu F-Y, Wang T, Yang S-D, Wang H, Yang D-L, Ding W-Y. Incidence and risk factors for proximal junctional kyphosis: a meta-analysis. Eur Spine J. 2016; 25(8):2376–2383

[23] Sebaaly A, Sylvestre C, El Quehtani Y, et al (2018) Incidence and Risk Factors for Proximal Junctional Kyphosis: Results of a Multicentric Study of Adult Scoliosis. Clin spine Surg 31:E178–E183. doi: 10.1097/BSD.0000000000000630

[24] Sebaaly A, Kharrat K, Kreichati G, Rizkallah M. Influence of the level of pedicle subtraction osteotomy on pelvic tilt change in adult spinal deformity. Glob Spine J. 2016

[25] Berthonnaud E, Dimnet J, Roussouly P, Labelle H. Analysis of the sagittal balance of the spine and pelvis using shape and orientation parameters. J Spinal Disord Tech. 2005; 18(1):40–4–7

Index